Health and the City

YORK MEDIEVAL PRESS

York Medieval Press is published by the University of York's Centre for Medieval Studies in association with Boydell & Brewer Limited. Our objective is the promotion of innovative scholarship and fresh criticism on medieval culture. We have a special commitment to interdisciplinary study, in line with the Centre's belief that the future of Medieval Studies lies in those areas in which its major constituent disciplines at once inform and challenge each other.

All enquiries of an editorial kind, including suggestions for monographs and essay collections, should be addressed to: The Academic Editor, York Medieval Press, University of York, Centre for Medieval Studies, The King's Manor, York, YO1 7EP (E-mail: gmg501@york.ac.uk).

Publications of York Medieval Press are listed at the back of this volume.

Health and the City

Disease, Environment and Government in Norwich, 1200–1575

Isla Fay

THE UNIVERSITY *of York*

YORK MEDIEVAL PRESS

First published 2015

A York Medieval Press publication
in association with The Boydell Press
an imprint of Boydell & Brewer Ltd
PO Box 9, Woodbridge, Suffolk IP12 3DF, UK
and of Boydell & Brewer Inc.
668 Mt Hope Avenue, Rochester, NY 14620–2731, USA
website: www.boydellandbrewer.com
and with the
Centre for Medieval Studies, University of York

ISBN 978-1-903153-60-4

A CIP catalogue record for this book is available
from the British Library

The author and publishers are grateful to
the trustees of the Marc Fitch Fund
for their grant towards the costs of publishing this book

FOR MY FAMILY
AND
FOR MIKE

CONTENTS

ILLUSTRATIONS

Maps

Figures

ACKNOWLEDGEMENTS

My sincere thanks are due to the following people, without whom the current publication would not have been realized. Firstly, I owe to Carole Rawcliffe my deepest gratitude for introducing me to the subject, for her excellent advice, her many readings of the manuscript and her stimulating comments on it, as well as her support over many years. Professor Rawcliffe has spearheaded the study of medicine, hospitals and environmental health for both the city of Norwich and the country as a whole, and I am fortunate to have her as my guide and mentor. The final text ought to be read in conjunction with her *Urban Bodies: Communal Health in Late Medieval English Towns and Cities* (Woodbridge, 2013). Also essential to the development of the manuscript was the tutoring and gentle shepherding of Sachiko Kusukawa, Trinity College, Cambridge, and of Nicholas Jardine, Department of History and Philosophy of Science (HPS), University of Cambridge, as was the generous encouragement of Lauren Kassell, Department of HPS, University of Cambridge, who pushed me to rethink the text. I am very grateful indeed to each of them. Jayne Bown, NAU Archaeology, and Ann Stirland were extremely generous in allowing me access to the unit's archive and the pre-publication reports on St Margaret's Fyebridge, and I owe them too my deepest thanks. For their comments, analysis and suggestions, my sincere thanks are also due to Andy Wood, formerly of the University of East Anglia (UEA), Sarah Rees Jones, Centre for Medieval Studies, University of York, Elizabeth Rutledge, UEA, Andrew Cunningham, Department of HPS, Silvia De Renzi, Open University, and an anonymous reviewer. Caroline Palmer, Peter Biller, Jocelyn Wogan-Browne at York Medieval Press and Boydell and Brewer were guardians of the text in its final stages. Peter taught me as a second-year undergraduate in a module on Medieval Medicine at the University of York. Memories of what I learned from him then inspired me here: I feel very fortunate to benefit (for a second time) from his guidance and inexhaustible knowledge.

The research was completed with funding from the Institute of Historical Research (six-month Scouloudi fellowship) and a small grant from the Norfolk and Norwich Archaeological Society; and awards from the Arts and Humanities Research Council (AHRC) and the University of East Anglia. The images were reproduced following a very generous grant from the Marc Fitch fund. My sincere gratitude is due to the trustees of the fund. Nicholas Jardine, Sachiko Kusukawa and Liba Taub, the investigators of the AHRC-funded project *Diagrams, Figures and the Transformation of Astronomy, 1450–1650*, allowed me time to finalize the manuscript in 2013, and I am very grateful to them.

For carefully reading parts, versions or all of the text and for making stimulating suggestions, as well as saving me from awful mistakes, my indebted and appreciative thanks also go to: Brian Ayers, School of History, UEA, and Butrint Foundation; Karin Ekholm, Department of HPS, Cambridge; Mary Fissell, Johns Hopkins University, Baltimore; Roberta Gilchrist, Reading University; Chris Knüsel, University of Exeter (who was also an inspirational tutor at the University of Bradford in Human Osteology and Palaeopathology in 2001–02); Helen Lacey, Mansfield College, University of Oxford; Elaine Leong, Max Planck Institute for the History of Science, Berlin; Peter Murray Jones, King's College, Cambridge; Gabriella Zuccolin, Open University; as well as colleagues and research students at the Department of HPS. For sharing ideas and sources, my thanks also to Elizabeth Shepherd Popescu, Cambridge Archaeological Unit; Francesca Boghi, NAU Archaeology; Giles Emery, Norvic Archaeology; Richard Hoggett, formerly of the Historic Environment Service, Norfolk County Council; and Caroline Erolin, University of Dundee. Audiences in Cambridge, Leeds, Lyon and Norwich also pointed me in the right direction at various times. I am also grateful to the search room staff at the NRO and Norfolk Museums and Archaeology Service for answering several queries and requests. Phillip Judge drafted several maps for me, which have been redrawn by Tamsin Preston. Mike Evans is due especial thanks for innumerable acts of heroism, and for his technical expertise in drafting further maps with no complaint, whilst Alasdair and Gerrie Fay showed equal stamina and forbearance and proved insightful readers of various drafts. Any errors are, of course, entirely my responsibility alone. For encouragement of a different kind my thanks to Maria and Rob and family; to Isla North; to Janka Rodziewicz and Sam Earl; to Tamara Hug and friends; and to the 'Dirty Harriers'.

Finally, for their loving support and understanding, my deepest gratitude go to Mike Evans, to my parents, Rod and Gerrie Fay, and to my brother, Alasdair. My book is dedicated to each of them.

ABBREVIATIONS

Atkin, Carter and Evans, EAA 26	M. Atkin, A. Carter and D. H. Evans, *Excavations in Norwich 1971–1978: Part II*, East Anglian Archaeology 26 (Norwich, 1985)
Atkin and Evans, EAA 100	M. Atkin and D. H. Evans, *Excavations in Norwich 1971–1978: Part III*, East Anglian Archaeology 100 (Norwich, 2002)
Ayers, EAA 37	B. Ayers, *Excavations at St. Martin-at-Palace Plain, Norwich, 1981*, East Anglian Archaeology 37 (Dereham, 1987)
Ayers, *NAFC*	B. Ayers, *Norwich: Archaeology of a Fine City* (Stroud, 2009)
BAR BS	British Archaeological Reports, British Series
BAR IS	British Archaeological Reports, International Series
BL	British Library
Blomefield, *Norfolk*	F. Blomefield, *An Essay Towards a Topographical History of the County of Norfolk*, 11 vols. (London, 1805–10)
Bown and Stirland, 'CAP'	J. Bown and A. Stirland, 'Criminals and Paupers: Excavations at the Site of the Church and Graveyard of St Margaret *in combusto*, Norwich, 1987' (unpublished site excavation report, Norfolk Archaeological Unit, Norfolk Museums Service)
CA	Chamberlains' Accounts
CBA	Council for British Archaeology
Cuningham [Kenningham], *A&P* 1558	*A Newe Almanacke and Prognostication … Made for the Meridian of Norwich and … Serving for All England*. (London: John Daye, 1557 for 1558)

Cuningham, *A&P* 1564	*A New Almanach and Prognostication … Faithfully Calculated for the Longitude of London and Pole Articke of the Same* (London: Rowland Hall, 1563 for 1564)
Cuningham, *A&P* 1566	*A New Almanach and Prognostication … Diligentlye Calculated for the Longytud of London and Pole Articke of the Same* (London: Richard Serll for William Jones, 1565 for 1566)
Cuningham, *CG*	William Cuningham, *The Cosmographical Glasse: Conteinyng the Pleasant Principles of Cosmographie, Geographie, Hydrographie or Navigation. Compiled by William Cuningham Doctor in Physicke* (London: John Day, 1559)
DCN	Dean and Chapter of Norwich
EAA	East Anglian Archaeology
EETS ES	Early English Text Society, Extra Series
EETS OS	Early English Text Society, Original Series
Emery, EAA 120	P. A. Emery, *Norwich Greyfriars: Pre-Conquest Town and Medieval Friary*, East Anglian Archaeology 120 (Dereham, 2007)
HER	Historic Environment Record
Hippocrates, *AWP*, ed. Lloyd	Hippocrates of Cos, *Airs, Waters, Places*, in *Hippocratic Writings*, ed. G. E. R. Lloyd (London, 1978), pp. 148–69 (revising *The Medical Works of Hippocrates*, ed. J. Chadwick and W. N. Mann (Oxford, 1950))
LJ, ed. Hudson	*Leet Jurisdiction in the City of Norwich during the XIIIth and XIVth Centuries*, ed. W. Hudson, Selden Society 5 (London, 1892)
LP	*Letters and Papers, Foreign and Domestic, Henry VIII*, ed. J. S. Brewer et al., 21 vols. (London, 1880–91)
Margeson, EAA 58	S. Margeson, *Norwich Households: The Medieval and Post-Medieval Finds from Norwich Survey Excavations, 1971–1978*, East Anglian Archaeology 58 (Norwich, 1993)
MC	Minor Collections
MN, ed. Rawcliffe and Wilson	*Medieval Norwich*, ed. C. Rawcliffe and R. Wilson (London, 2004)
NA	*Norfolk Archaeology*

NCR	Norwich City Records
NRO	Norfolk Record Office, Norwich
NRS	Norfolk Record Society
NS1550, ed. Rawcliffe and Wilson	*Norwich Since 1550*, ed. C. Rawcliffe and R. Wilson (London, 2004)
Pelling, *CL*	M. Pelling, *The Common Lot: Sickness, Medical Occupations and the Urban Poor in Early Modern England* (London, 1998)
Pelling and Webster, 'MP'	M. Pelling and C. Webster, 'Medical Practitioners', in *Health, Medicine and Mortality in the Sixteenth Century*, ed. C. Webster (Cambridge, 1979), pp. 165–235
PMR	*Calendar of Plea and Memoranda Rolls Preserved Among the Archives of the Corporation of the City of London*, ed. A. H. Thomas and P. E. Jones, 6 vols. (Cambridge, 1926–61)
Rawcliffe, *MFTS*	C. Rawcliffe, *Medicine for the Soul: The Life, Death and Resurrection of an English Medieval Hospital: St Giles's, Norwich, c. 1249–1550* (Stroud, 1999)
RCN	*The Records of the City of Norwich*, ed. W. Hudson and J. C. Tingey, 2 vols. (Norwich, 1906–10)
Shepherd Popescu, EAA 132	E. Shepherd Popescu, *Norwich Castle: Excavations and Historical Survey 1987–98*, East Anglian Archaeology 132, 2 vols. (Dereham, 2009)
Soden, EAA 133	I. Soden, *Life and Death on a Norwich Backstreet, AD 900–1600: Excavations in St Faith's Lane*, East Anglian Archaeology 133 (Northampton, 2010)
SR	*Statutes of the Realm, from Original Records and Authentic Manuscripts (1101–1713)*, ed. A. Luders, T. E. Tomlins, J. France, W. E. Taunton, J. Raithby, 11 vols. (London, 1810–28)
Stirland, EAA 129	A. Stirland, with contributions by B. Ayers and J. Bown, *Criminals and Paupers: The Graveyard of St Margaret Fyebriggate in combusto, Norwich*, East Anglian Archaeology 129 (Dereham, 2009)
UH	*Urban History*

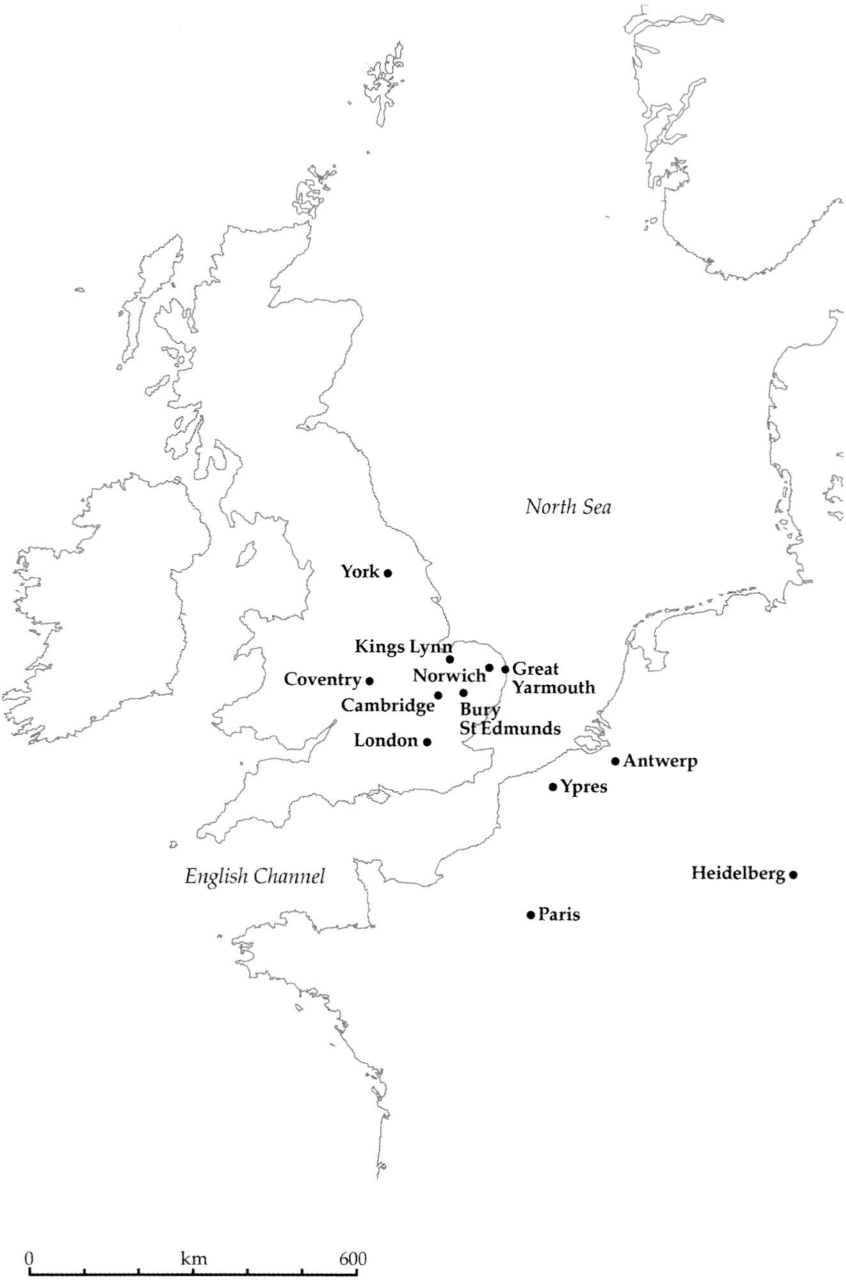

Map 1: Norwich and other towns and cities mentioned in the text.

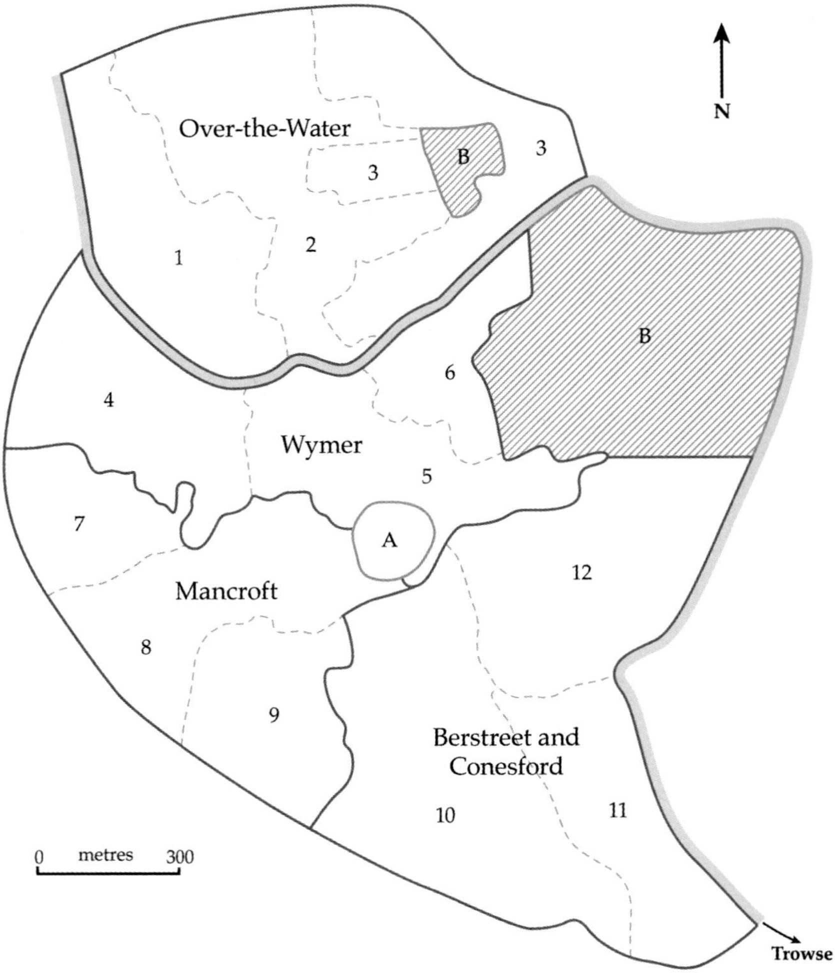

1. Coslany
2. Colegate
3. Fyebridge
4. West Wymer
5. Mid Wymer
6. East Wymer
7. St Giles
8. St Peter Mancroft
9. St Stephen
10. Berstreet
11. South Conesford
12. North Conesford

A Castle
B Cathedral liberty

Map 2: The wards of Norwich.

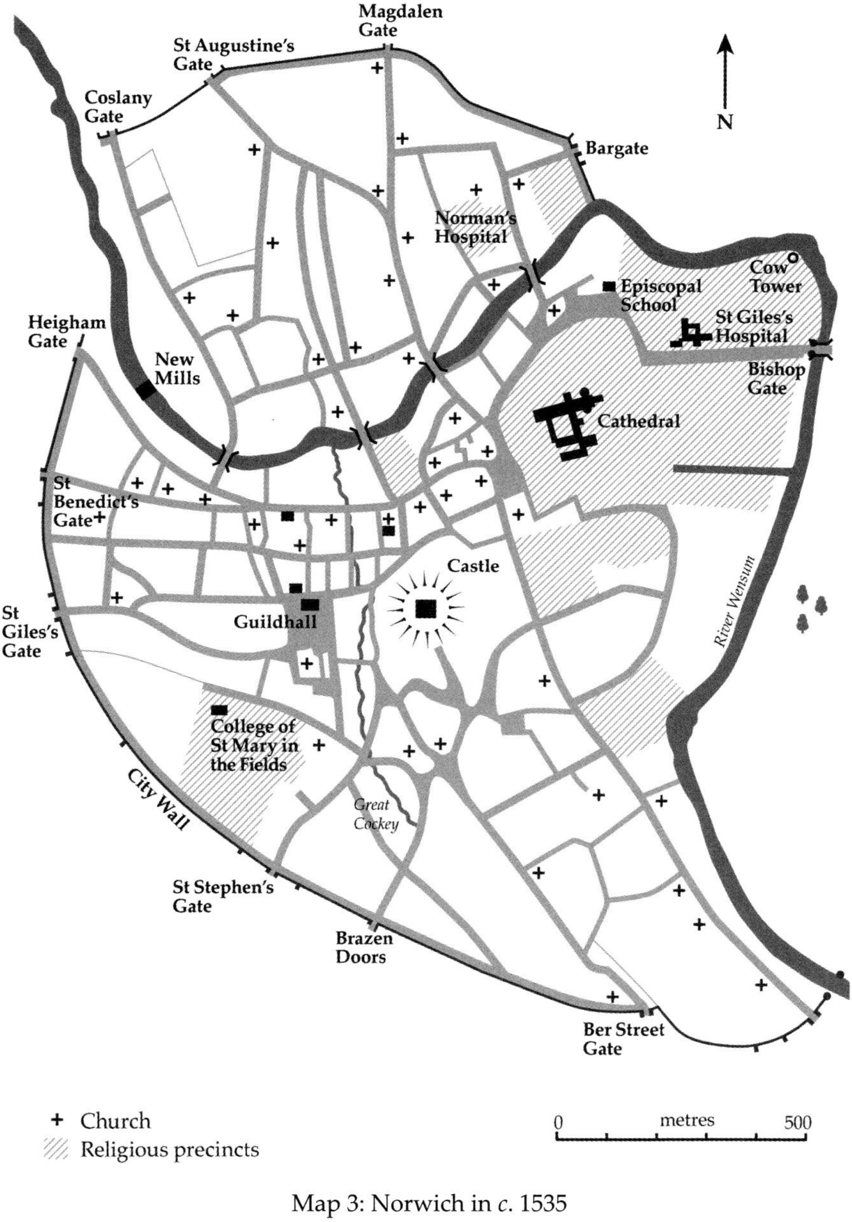

Map 3: Norwich in *c.* 1535

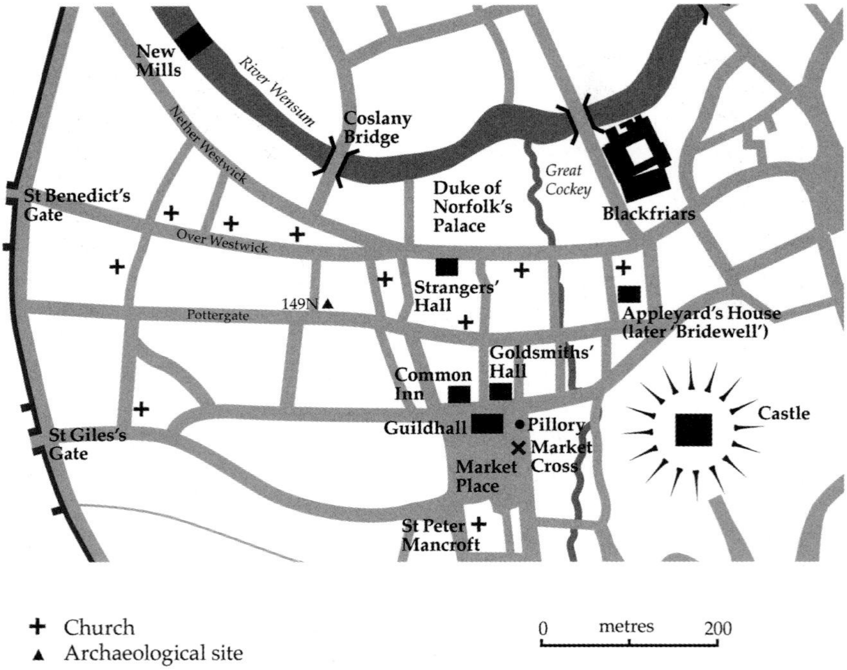

Map 4: Central Norwich in *c.* 1535

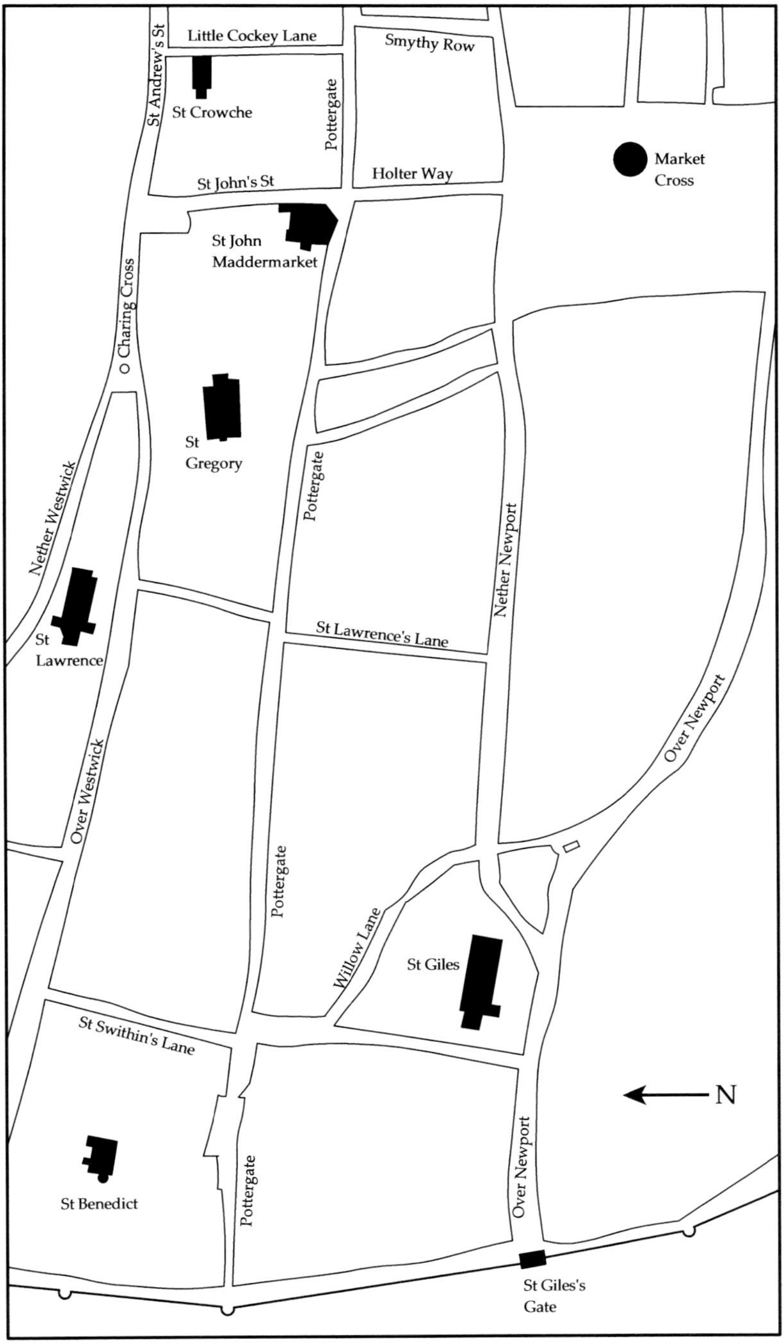

Map 5: The actual topography of the streets and churches shown in figure 8.
Based on Campbell, 'Norwich', map 2.

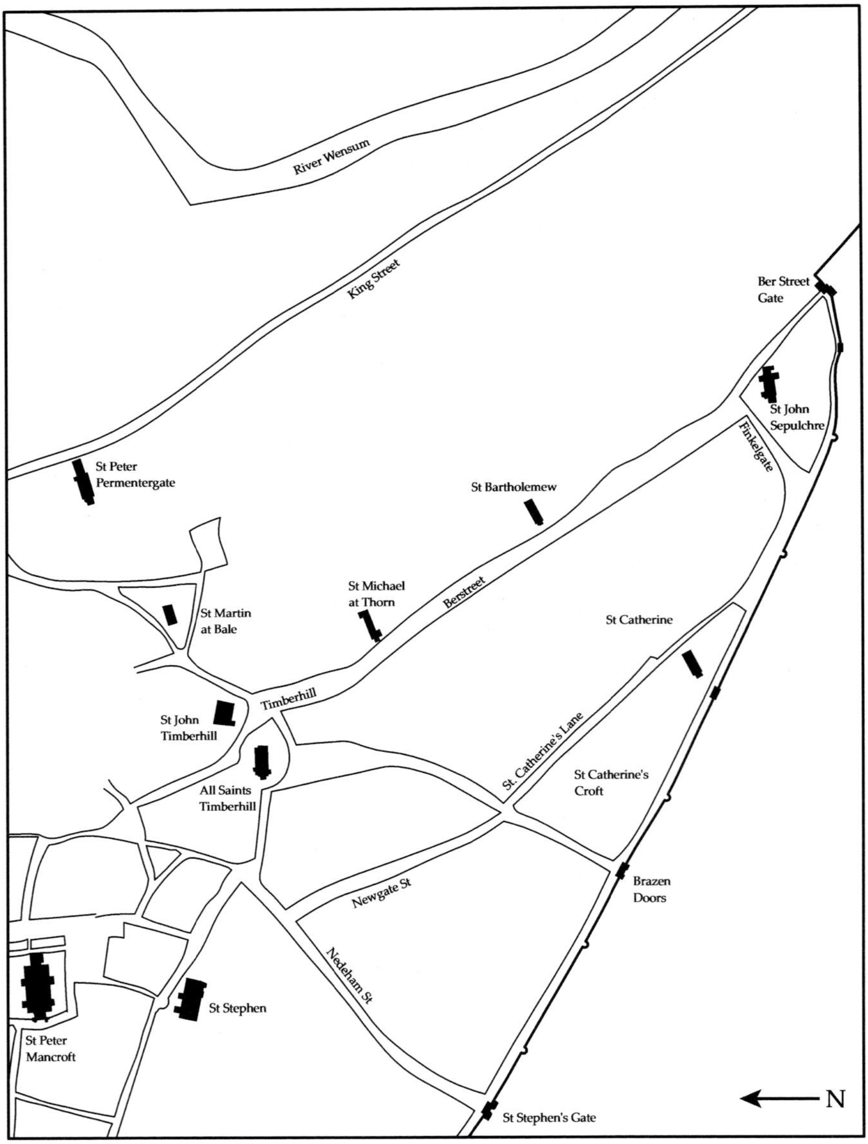

Map 6: The actual topography of the streets and churches shown in figure 10. Based on Campbell, 'Norwich', map 2.

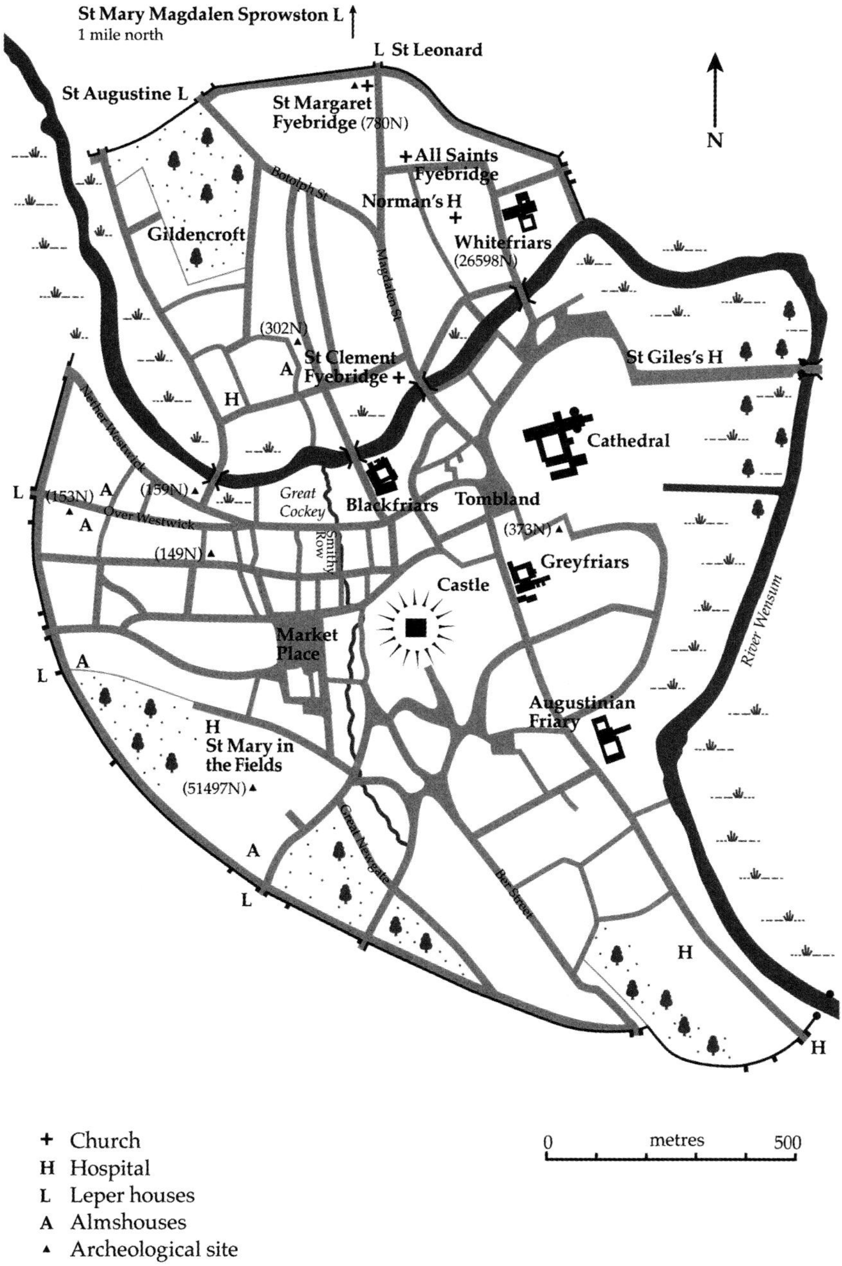

Map 7: Places mentioned in chapters 3–6.

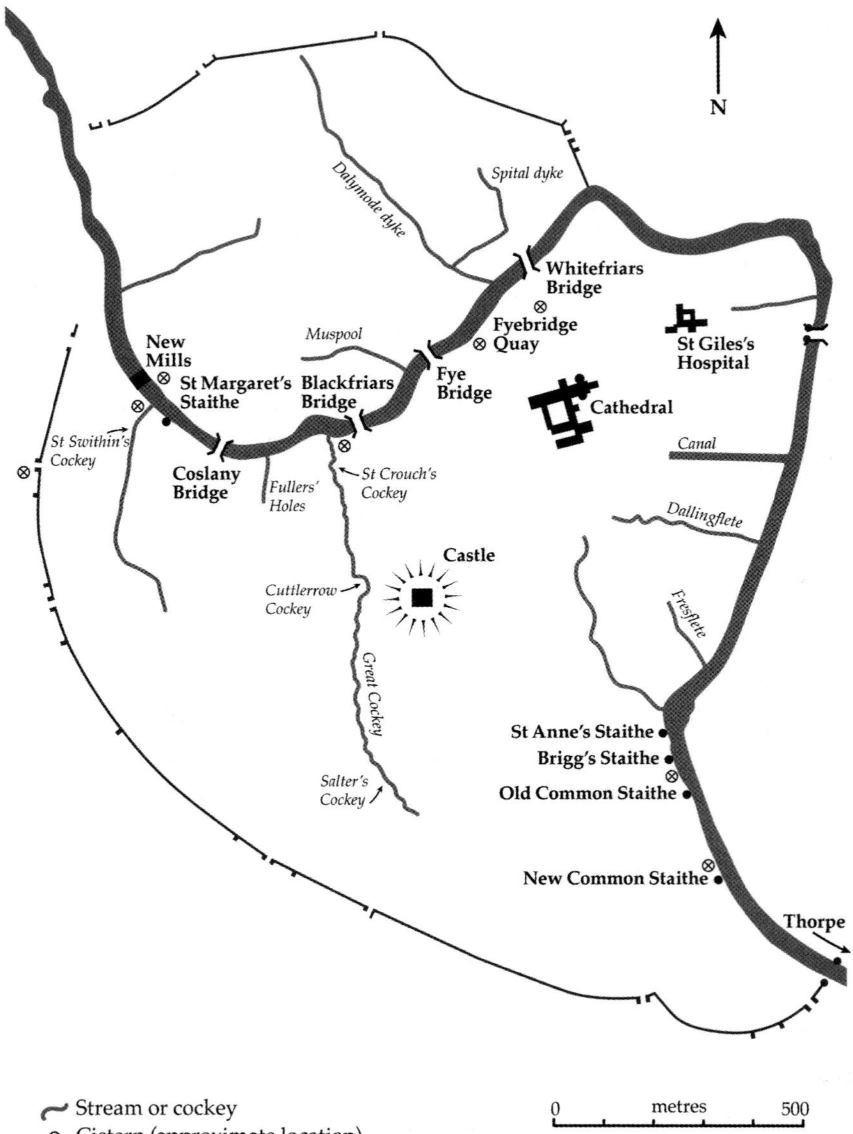

Map 8: Norwich's watercourses.

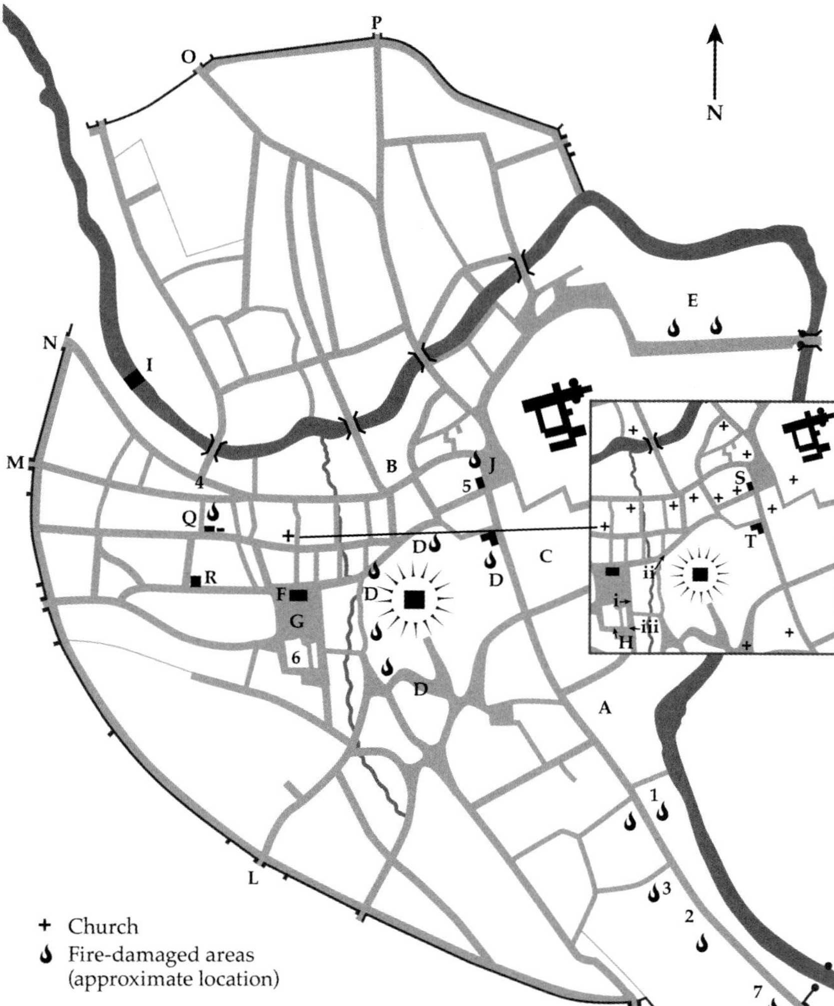

1.	St Clement Conesford	G	Market		
2.	St Edward	H	Market: Cobblerrow		
3.	St Etheldreda	I	New Mills	i	Cockey Lane
4.	St Lawrence	J	Tombland	ii	Cuttlerrow
5.	St Mary the Less	K	Ber Street Gate	iii	Sporrerrow
6.	St Peter Mancroft	L	St Stephen's Gate		
7.	St Peter Southgate	M	St Benedict's Gate		
		N	Heigham Gate		
A	Augustinian friars	O	St Augustine's Gate		
B	Blackfriars/Common Hall	P	Magdalen Gate		
C	Greyfriars	Q	Excavated fire-damaged plots, Pottergate		
D	Castle Fee	R	Rede's tenements		
E	St Giles's Hospital	S	St Mary's tenements		
F	Guildhall	T	Suffragan's tenements		

0 metres 500

Map 9: Dilapidation and renovation in mid-sixteenth-century Norwich.

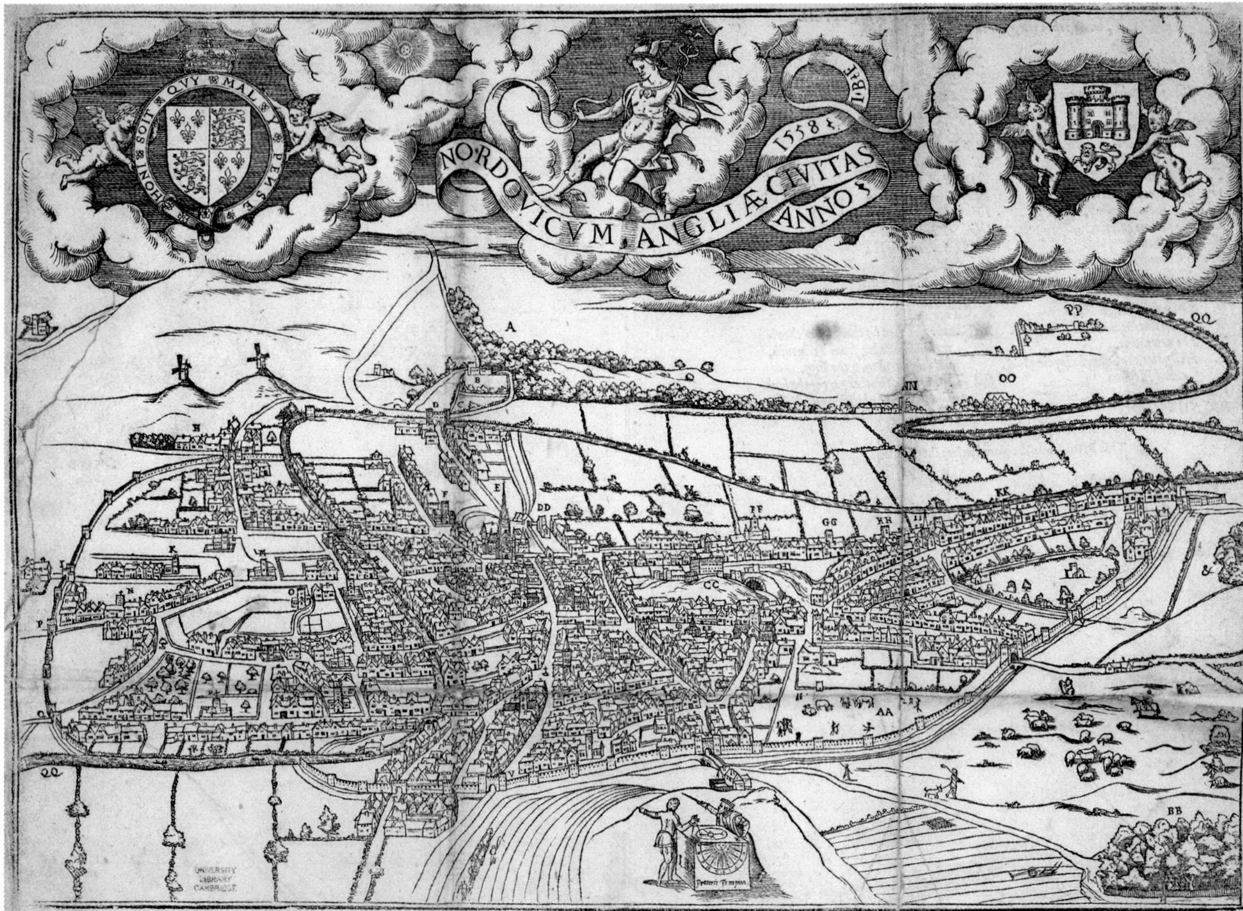

Figure 1: Prospect of Norwich from William Cuningham's *The Cosmographical Glasse* (1559).

INTRODUCTION

A 'HEALTHFULL AND PLEASANT' CITY

In 1559, the physician and cosmographer William Cuningham published a long and beautifully produced textbook under the title *The Cosmographical Glasse*. One of the most arresting features of the text was a printed illustration of what was, in the physician's opinion, an exceptionally 'healthfull and pleasant' city (fig. 1).[1] The city was Norwich in the county of Norfolk, then England's largest and wealthiest provincial centre, and the place in which Cuningham was born. In the woodcut, Norwich appears as a paradigm of urban hygiene: it is well situated in the landscape; blessed with enviable natural resources; beautifully adorned with fine and imposing buildings all in the very best state of repair; and free from any obvious sources of pollution, disorder or corruption. Though clearly an idealized representation, Cuningham's vision had at least some basis in reality. The municipal authorities of Norwich had recently implemented various schemes to help improve sanitary standards in public areas by cleansing waterways, repaving the streets, refurbishing buildings and employing labourers to remove waste materials from public spaces.[2] Local residents might, however, have raised a sceptical eyebrow when confronted with Cuningham's exemplary image of cleanliness and order. No one who had lived there

[1] William Cuningham, *The Cosmographical Glasse: Conteinyng the Pleasant Principles of Cosmographie, Geographie, Hydrographie or Navigation. Compiled by William Cuningham Doctor in Physicke* (London: John Day, 1559), p. 174 (*hereafter*, Cuningham, *CG*).

[2] See, for example, Norwich, Norfolk Record Office (NRO), Norwich City Records (NCR) 16d/2 Assembly Proceedings 1491–1553, fol. 211r (1549), which records the implementation of a system for carting accumulations of 'filtie and vile matter' out of the streets (a revision of earlier measures). For the election of a permanent committee which oversaw sanitary provisions from 1552, see 'The Norwich River and Street Accounts, 1557–61 and 1570–80', ed. I. Fay, in *Health and Hygiene in Early Modern Norwich*, ed. E. Phillips and I. Fay, NRS 77 (Norwich, 2013), pp. 105–200 (pp. 109–10), and see below, chapter 5.

during the preceding twenty-year period could ignore the fact that Norwich had suffered grievously from a series of damaging disasters: fire, plague, floods, food shortages and economic recession had all hit in quick succession, and the infrastructure suffered as a result.[3] At one point manure was piling up in the streets,[4] whilst many buildings and structures were left in ruins following arson and artillery attacks during Kett's rebellion (a regional uprising in 1549 inspired by damaging economic and social circumstances).[5] Residents viewed these conditions as a direct threat to health. Perhaps the ultimate irony was that, even as Cuningham's woodcut was being prepared for the press, a virulent, protracted, influenza-like virus was raging through the city, decimating the population.[6] However, no hint of such misfortunes can be detected in the plan. Indeed, Cuningham – a practised draughtsman and surveyor as well as a medical professional – greatly misrepresented aspects of the actual topography to achieve his end. What, exactly, motivated him? And what light does his endeavour shine on urban hygienic culture in an age before germ theory?

Of the various scholarly interests that inspired Cuningham to produce his image in this particular form, accurate cartography (as we might judge it) was of relatively minor importance. More significant to Cuningham was the extent to which the image captured the essential qualities of the place:[7] its 'pleasantness' and 'healthfulness'. Consequently, his approach was influenced as much by a recent revival of Hippocratic environmental theory within medical literature[8] (a system

[3] For fire, floods, and food shortages see below, chapters 2, 5 and 6; for plague in Norwich in 1544–45 and 1554–55, see P. Slack, *The Impact of Plague in Tudor and Stuart England* (Oxford, 1985), p. 61; on the mid-century slump in one of the city's important exports, see K. J. Allison, 'The Norfolk Worsted Industry in the Sixteenth and Seventeenth Centuries [Part] 1', *Bulletin of Economic Research* 12 (1960), 73–83 (pp. 79–82), and R. Wilson, 'The Textile Industry', in *NS1550*, ed. Rawcliffe and Wilson, pp. 219–41 (p. 221).

[4] See below, p. 156.

[5] A. Wood, *The 1549 Rebellions and the Making of Early Modern England* (Cambridge, 2007), pp. 13–14.

[6] Slack, *Impact of Plague*, p. 71.

[7] Cuningham's agenda was therefore closely allied to that of the draughtsman of the most famous of all sets of city plans, the *Nuremberg Chronicle*: see the analysis in A. McLean, *The Cosmographia of Sebastian Münster: Describing the World in the Reformation* (Aldershot, 2007), p. 116.

[8] Silvia De Renzi's forthcoming monograph on the early modern Roman physicians explores this revival and its importance in both medicine and politics in the Christian world's premier city. For context, see also M. Jenner, 'Environment,

of ideas to which Cuningham paid homage in the accompanying text of *The Cosmographical Glasse*), as to contemporary developments in geography and map-making. In the Hippocratic tradition, the main topographical features credited to Norwich by the physician – an ample, clean water supply, an easterly situation and lush vegetation – were considered to be intrinsically health-promoting. Cuningham's version of an ideal city was, therefore, a playful, visual summary of ancient doctrine, executed using the principles of perspective drawing. Secondarily, his plan served a political agenda. In the decades prior to the publication of Cuningham's book, England's home-grown 'civic humanists'[9] had agonized over the poor physical condition of the country's towns and had condemned their relative insalubriousness compared to continental models. The physician's plan was a counterblast against such pessimism.[10] Derivative versions of it were published across Europe which helped to spread the message about the healthy credentials of this English city.[11] We will return in later portions of this book to consider Cuningham's plan and the wider political and intellectual climate in greater detail. For the time being, his portrait of Norwich serves as a window onto the main subject of this book: the vibrant, native culture of urban hygiene and healing *in*

Health and Population', in *The Healing Arts: Health, Disease and Society in Europe 1500–1800*, ed. P. Elmer (Manchester, 2004), pp. 284–314 (p. 286); N. G. Siraisi, *History, Medicine and the Traditions of Renaissance Learning* (Ann Arbor, 2007), *passim*; A. Wear, 'Place, Health, and Disease: *The Airs, Waters, Places* Tradition in Early Modern England and North America', *Journal of Medieval and Early Modern Studies* 38 (2008), 443–65; S. Cavallo and T. Storey, *Healthy Living in Late Renaissance Italy* (Oxford, 2013).

[9] That is, individuals who wrote analytically about the structure and reform of society, government and the economy with reference to ideal models.

[10] Symbolic of the demand for accessible literature on this theme was the publication eight years earlier of the first vernacular translation of More's iconic *Utopia*: Thomas More, *A Fruteful and Pleasaunt Worke of the Beste State of a Publyque Weale and of the newe Yle called Utopia*, trans. Raphe Robynson (London: Abraham Vele, 1551). Amongst other themes, More's serioludic text (which purported to describe an ideal civic 'commonwealth') commented upon the social and governmental structures of contemporary London: S. Rees Jones, 'Thomas More's *Utopia* and Medieval London', in *Pragmatic Utopias: Ideals and Communities, 1200–1630*, ed. R. Horrox and S. Rees Jones (Cambridge 2001), pp. 117–35.

[11] Examples were produced in Cologne, Venice, Frankfurt, Nuremberg and Amsterdam, as well as London, until the early eighteenth century: see R. Frostick, *The Printed Plans of Norwich 1558–1840: A Carto-Bibliography* (Norwich, 2002), pp. 1–20, 23–5.

which Cuningham was tutored, but of which the kinds of academic interests he displayed constituted only a part.

Cuningham's familiarity with the Hippocratic tradition arose out of his reading as a medical student at the University of Cambridge. The format of his particular brand of 'environmental health' – which incorporated astrology as well as medicine, topography and cosmography – was contingent upon the systems of knowledge generation and dissemination of the late 1550s and 1560s.[12] In earlier periods, other young people growing up in Norwich and its surrounding market towns and villages who did not benefit from such an advanced education would nevertheless have understood Cuningham's fascination with the fundamental link between location and health. Here, as in other urban centres, a distinctive philosophy existed concerning the importance of the city's landscape and of its population in creating and maintaining corporate and individual well-being: a philosophy rooted in the evaluation of places on the basis of their relative orderliness and purity.[13] According to received medical theory (familiar in broad terms at least to Norwich residents for at least two hundred years before *The Cosmographical Glasse* was written), the internal processes of the human body were influenced by a place's air and water quality, or by changes in the prevailing weather, or by atmospheric conditions. By extension, different types of urban space – a street, a house, a garden or an empty plot – were invested with particular significances for corporate health, in line with their prevailing characteristics. Individuals were expected to take steps to care for and maintain the quality of such spaces just as they were expected to preserve their own livelihood or keep

[12] The European educational and intellectual culture in which Cuningham was trained and attempted to operate can be understood by examining the more fully documented life of his older contemporary Girolamo Cardano: see N. G. Siraisi, *The Clock and the Mirror: Girolamo Cardano and Renaissance Medicine* (Princeton, 1997), and A. Grafton, *Cardano's Cosmos: The Worlds and Works of a Renaissance Astrologer* (Cambridge MA, 1999). Additionally, the continental literature which fuelled Cuningham's fascination with instruments, navigation and cartography is introduced in *The Worlds of Oronce Fine: Mathematics, Instruments and Print in Renaissance France*, ed. A. Marr (Donington, 2009). For the kind of tradition in which he was probably initially tutored, see references to the work of J. Greatrex below, p. 54, n. 78.

[13] On the nationwide context, see C. Rawcliffe, *Urban Bodies: Communal Health in Late Medieval English Towns and Cities* (Woodbridge, 2013).

their bodies in the best possible condition.[14] The emphasis placed by medico-moral culture on personal responsibility seemed particularly compelling to urban men and women because it complemented wider concepts of neighbourliness and duty which, when infringed, resulted in heated disagreements at street level.[15] Norms, aspirations and condemnations were built upon such conflicts; ideals of corporate hygiene were generated when attitudes to the social hierarchy and to decorum collided with the realities of urban living.

This book assesses the two cultures in tandem: the native, civic ideology represented by documents and objects produced in Norwich, and the theoretical tradition maintained in the region's intellectual centres. It examines how each tradition was seeded, how they grew together and how they nourished one another. In this light, English urban hygiene culture appears not as a pale imitation of better-known schemes devised by Italian city-states in the fifteenth and sixteenth centuries,[16] nor as the direct product of the circulation of printed advice literature on the subjects of epidemic disease or daily regimen,[17] but rather as a collection of responses to the quotidian concerns of city dwellers reacting to physical imperatives, such as waste, dilapidation and disease.[18] Like the 'alternative tours' sold to sightseers in many European cities today, our route through pre-modern Norwich takes us

[14] On the personal obligation to maintain livelihood and bodily state, see William Marshall, *The Forme and Maner of Subvention or Helpyng for Pore People* (London: Thomas Godfray, 1535), sig. B3r and *passim*.

[15] See, for example, a series of complaints made by Norwich men and women to the authorities in February 1551. One property owner, Nicholas Manne, offended neighbours because he heaped 'manure' in the highway, blocking traffic and damaging a drainage gutter. As if to add fuel to the fire, it was also noted that he failed to resurface the street following the removal of the obstruction, a situation which (as urban governors were apt to point out) was liable to cause even more unsanitary conditions: NRO, NCR 5c/3 Leets before the City Sheriffs (1551) [ward not legible].

[16] On Italian urban Health Boards, see C. M. Cipolla, *Public Health and the Medical Profession in the Renaissance* (Cambridge, 1976), and see J. Henderson, 'Coping with Epidemics in Renaissance Italy: Plague and the Great Pox', in *The Fifteenth Century XII: Society in an Age of Plague*, ed. L. Clark and C. Rawcliffe (Woodbridge, 2013), pp. 175–93.

[17] On which, see Part I of this book.

[18] In this I follow a path indicated by Margaret Pelling's 'Medicine and the Environment in Shakespeare's England', in Pelling, *CL*, pp. 19–37, which – in a historiographical climate then dominated by analyses framed in terms of semiotics and rhetoric – put material concerns back into the writing of British pre-modern medical history.

to some hidden and insalubrious spaces: we will witness the burial of deformed and diseased paupers; seek out the location of muck-heaps and burnt-out tenements; reflect on the state of cesspits, drains and gutters; glimpse, through open shutters, the efforts of men and women to minister to their families and friends by preparing remedies, by observing urine samples or by offering devout prayers; hear anxious exclamations about infected air, insanitary neighbours and diseased beggars; and ponder the motives of civic officers working to improve conditions in the streets, rows of houses and local watercourses. We will find strongly articulated and medically informed sentiments concerning cleanliness and wholesomeness (broadly conceived) in each arena. This book is, therefore, a history of a city's health culture viewed through its landscape. It is inspired by a mode of medical history writing 'grounded in the particularity of place',[19] and gives a twist to the medieval cosmological view of human physiology (in which pathological processes were influenced by events in the natural world) by arguing that individuals used concepts of health to categorize and order their experiences and surroundings.

Themes and arguments: a map of the text

From what goes before, it will be clear that *Health and the City* is a materialist account of health culture. Texts, images, human skeletal remains, objects and landscapes form the substrate of my enquiry; I treat each as a form of *artefact*, that is, as an item which through handling, shaping, use and treatment bears witness to types of behaviour, social practices and attitudes. This kind of evidence base demands a strongly interdisciplinary outlook: I draw upon existing scholarship in medical history, urban archaeology, literary analysis and landscape studies to address themes such as attitudes to the body, the built environment, disease, disability and sanitary technology. But here we must pause to make an acknowledgement. There are risks involved in writing such a book. Aside from the perennial hazards any investigator must face when collating evidence from a range of sub-disciplines (namely, that he or she disappoints specialists in all fields), it is fair to note that materialist accounts of pre-modern hygiene have not always been well

[19] M. Jenner, 'Underground, Overground: Pollution and Place in Urban History: Review Essay, *Journal of Urban History* 24 (1997), 97–110 (pp. 104–5).

received by medical historians.[20] Bones, sewers and books necessarily provide very different vantage points from which to view the medical culture of the past. Nonetheless, the subject demands that we strive to develop a large methodological toolkit. Pre-modern hygiene culture was not limited to the philological pursuits, nor to doctor–patient interactions. The underlying attitudes, beliefs and ideas are also evident in the creation of objects, structures, ceremonies and technologies. For a richer, more comprehensive view of the medical history of medieval and early modern England, we must attempt to interpret the impulses which prompted these acts of creation of all sorts – of enacted events, and of scribed, engraved, manufactured and constructed items. My aim is to suggest what such a method can achieve.

Like this book, my enquiries began with Cuningham's plan, although they led me both backwards and forwards from that point in time. Tracing the roots of the enviro-medical culture celebrated in the image took me to the first relevant surviving archival records from Norwich, that is, to the documents generated by the local law courts during the late thirteenth century, and (still earlier) to the largely undocumented responses to disease attested in the osteoarchaeological record. After its publication, Cuningham's map directly inspired fresh treatments of the theme of topography and health in the works of a new generation of topographical writers: I followed these too as they extend into the later sixteenth century.[21] As a result, the old periodization that characterizes the history of science and medicine which takes as a starting point the elitist, Latinate, academic literature of the sixteenth and seventeenth centuries is circumvented in the pages that follow. Instead, this book argues for the existence of a shared and generative culture of urban environmental health which bridged social and intellectual constituencies.

The text itself is divided into three thematic sections. Part I considers how ideas about cleanliness, climate and location were incorporated into local and regional medical writing about preventative health care up to and beyond the publication of Cuningham's plan of Norwich. The component elements of pre-modern hygiene – the significance of

[20] See Appendix I.

[21] Developments in Norwich health culture from the late sixteenth century onwards are addressed in Pelling, *CL*, and M. Pelling, 'Health and Sanitation to 1750', in *NS1550*, ed. Rawcliffe and Wilson, pp. 117–37.

putrefying substances in causing disease; the impact of cosmic fluctuations and seasonal changes upon the body; and the necessity of carefully managing the so-called 'non-naturals'[22] of air, food, exercise, sleep, excretion and thoughts or feelings – comprised a reservoir of common medical knowledge in which the physical world was given central importance. How was this knowledge developed and sustained in urban communities such as Norwich? Several agents played a part in the process: graduates like Cuningham, academics, licensed physicians, members of Norwich cathedral priory and of the regional nobility and gentry all transported concepts into the city from elevated scholarly and social circles. But the traffic in ideas did not move in only one direction. The governing mercantile elite also propagated and shaped notions of civic hygiene, and – alongside various kinds of healers (surgeons, apothecaries, nurses, domestic ministrators of 'cures', and carers) – helped transact exchanges between the proponents of extrinsic and indigenous forms of knowledge. The picture of health culture that emerges throughout chapters 1 and 2 is, therefore, necessarily *urban* in its nature. The institutions, people and circumstances that facilitated, created and disseminated its concepts were dependent upon aspects of civic life (the market economy, a basically stable government and a large population).

The exchange of ideas benefited from reading and recording in many different mediums. Personal notes and letters, manuscript compilations of medicinal recipes, and the minutes of civic or guild meetings each indicate crucial events which stimulated the diffusion of concepts. Equally important but less accessible to the researcher were forms of communication such as (of course) the conversations taking place between a healer and a patient, or a carer and the cared for, but also the instructions given by tutors to pupils, or the directives issued in the city's administrative hub to labourers working on cleansing and rebuilding projects. The opening chapters of this book help to pinpoint the media in which the pre-modern provincial culture of hygiene developed, and the various loci in which ideas about health and the environment were voiced.

With this knowledge, we can see how Cuningham could reasonably expect viewers of his plan of Norwich – a visual commentary on the interrelationship between 'health and place' – to decode his allusions.

22 That is, factors or processes that the human body was bound to encounter or perform in its daily life.

Chapter 2 provides a dissection of the form and message of the plan. The ways in which that physician chose to represent (and, in places, misrepresent) the actual topography were directly informed by his familiarity with the city (he knew its most and least salubrious parts), and by an appreciation of the themes and 'packaging' that would most strongly appeal to the kind of civic-minded gentleman reader at whom his work was marketed.

Part II moves us along a different path. The physical remnants of Norwich's enviro-medical culture give us an opportunity to penetrate further the mentality of individuals who leave little or no mark on the documentary record. In chapter 3, the human body itself is given centre stage. The appearance and physical characteristics of the people of Norwich varied across its different districts, with some impoverished areas containing a much larger proportion of diseased, impaired and deformed individuals than other, more affluent enclaves. The treatment of the body after death provides our points of access to this phenomenon; the grave is a platform upon which ideas about the body, hierarchy and landscape coalesce. Osteoarchaeological evidence demonstrates that one of the most marginal and poverty-ridden areas of Norwich contained, over an extended period of time, concentrations of individuals suffering from a range of manifest or disfiguring diseases and serious physical impairments. The corpses of certain of these people received substandard funerary provisions. Here are individuals who lacked or forfeited economic and social capital, and whose deaths failed to attract the community's interest; their situation gives us an insight into a nexus of ideas concerning personal behaviour, worth and disease.

Chapter 4 inverts the lens to capture a different view, one which accords much more closely with the image produced by Cuningham. The inhabitants of Norwich constructed their own mental maps of the city's component parts, in which beneficial zones or places (such as health-promoting gardens) were especially valued. A diverse range of sources from the civic archives and Norwich's archaeological record help us to reconstruct those concepts of local salubriousness, including legal records of property holdings, the remains of domestic objects, and the documentary accounts of theatrical performances. The chapter draws out the close associations between space, air, health, exercise, therapeutics and food in local health culture.

The theme of the conflict between ideals and reality which dominated the discussion of Cuningham's plan resurfaces again as the subject of Part III of this book, but this time our source material constitutes the manuscript records of the civic government. Here we focus on the attempts of the residents of Norwich and its governing elite to improve standards of health, healing services and civic cleanliness. In chapter 5, the emphasis is on the difficult question of what to do with the vast quantities of animal and human waste, industrial effluent and rubbish generated by the population. The chapter takes the long view of attempts to marshal and corral these materials. In so doing, it explores themes of personal and corporate responsibility, and considers the language in which condemnations of unhygienic behaviour were constructed. The final parts of the book (the second part of chapter 5 and chapter 6) narrow the focus to the years just following the publication of the reformed version of the ancient Hippocratic text *Airs, Waters, Places.* To Sir Geoffrey Elton, the venerable historian of Tudor England, certain legislative programmes carried out by the central government at this time in the name of the 'commonwealth' were overspill from what he characterized as a 'splendid porridge of reformist yearning', that is, a mixed product of Protestantism, Christian humanism and social and political reformism consolidated into articulate written critiques of the status quo.[23] I suggest that – rather than producing stock solutions to apparently universal difficulties in a stereotypical language of reform – Norwich's civic elite attempted to formulate tailored schemes to counter observed problems in the city on the basis of hygienic theory. Their proposals were on occasion both idiosyncratic and self-serving but nonetheless constituted what in modern political parlance might be labelled 'a joined up policy'. This included attempts not only to preserve the quality of water and air, but also to identify individuals in need of healing assistance; to moderate the consumption of food amongst the wealthy; to sanitize and refurbish dilapidated properties; to reform hospitals; to punish the so-called indolent (who, it was asserted, brought disease upon themselves); to oversee the quality of medical and surgical services; and to petition parliament for powers to improve the state of the city fabric. In so doing, the ruling elite aggregated to its administrators and governors a degree of accountability for standards of health which complemented older, medieval notions of individual liability. Throughout this book, the subjects of decay, abnormality and corruption are placed in apposition

[23] G. R. Elton, *Reform and Renewal: Thomas Cromwell and the Common Weal* (Cambridge, 1973), pp. 1, 7.

to symbols of authority, orthodoxy, ownership and rank:[24] the friction created by these competing influences informed people's attitudes to the city environment as a deciding factor in promoting (or compromising) health.

Norwich: introducing a city and its people

"But why Norwich?"

Norwich today is a city of moderate size, home to approximately 200,000 people. This 'Fine City' (as it is known) gives the impression of being as salubrious and pleasant as its counterpart in Cuningham's plan. Situated centrally within the county of Norfolk, it is still surrounded by extensively farmed arable land, although the city's economy is dominated by retail, tourism and service industries. A university town, Norwich remains proud of its heritage. Indeed, several medieval structures survive within its core, and the outline of the pre-modern street pattern can be traced amid the thoroughfares. Few people nowadays – regardless of how predisposed to celebrate the city's merits they may be – would nominate Norwich for the title of being England's 'second city'. Yet immediately prior to the Industrial Revolution, its residents could reasonably stake such a claim.[25] Norwich in 1559 perhaps corresponded in its manufacturing capacity, cultural capital and wealth to modern Glasgow, Birmingham or Manchester.

For a start, Norwich was physically large. The area bounded by the city walls incorporated a piece of land equal in extent to that of contemporary London, although it probably contained about a quarter

24 The same themes surfaced in the ancient and medieval concept of the 'body politic'. On this, see P. Maddern, 'Order and Disorder', in *MN*, ed. Rawcliffe and Wilson, pp. 189–212 (pp. 205–10), and J. G. Harris, *Foreign Bodies and the Body Politic: Discourses of Social Pathology in Early Modern England* (Cambridge, 1998).

25 A. Dyer, *Decline and Growth in English Towns, 1400–1640* (Cambridge, 1995), pp. 56, 58, 62 (on the overall trend of population expansion in Norwich between 1377 and 1524/25, see p. 64). Prior to the sixteenth century, it always compared well (ranking in position five or six) in terms of its relative size and wealth compared to other English towns: A. Dyer, 'Appendix: Ranking Lists of English Medieval Towns', in *The Cambridge Urban History of Britain: Volume I, 600–1540*, ed. D. M. Palliser (Cambridge, 2000), pp. 747–70 (pp. 752, 754–5, 758, 761).

of the capital's population.[26] It also enjoyed a relatively stable government,[27] and benefited greatly from good trading connections to major continental towns as well as from a profitable hinterland (map 1).[28] Its essentially varied, widely based and adaptable market – which specialized in the production and sale of textiles, luxury goods, and services – was robust enough to weather periods of the local political instability and economic recession that caused crippling damage to other large towns and cities.[29] With prosperity and rising aspirations, however, came divisive social inequalities. By 1520, Norwich boasted some of England's wealthiest citizens in its ranks, but its resources were overwhelmingly concentrated in the hands of the social elite.[30]

These circumstances give us three compelling reasons to use Norwich as the case in our study. Firstly, the city developed something of an outward-looking culture, no doubt because significant intellectual, governmental and trading centres could be accessed with relative and equal ease from the city.[31] Secondly, and relatedly, Norwich developed

[26] J. Campbell, 'Norwich', in *The Atlas of Historic Towns: Volume II*, ed. M. Lobel (London, 1975), p. 11. By 1333, the resident population totalled about 25,000 people, although (as was the case across the county) this number shrank rapidly during the second half of the fourteenth century following repeated outbreaks of epidemic disease. For more on this subject, see Appendix II below.

[27] As an exception, see the account of outbreaks of factional fighting in government in 1433 and the 1440s in B. R. McRee, 'Religious Gilds and Civic Order: The Case of Norwich in the Late Middle Ages', *Speculum* 67 (1992), 69–97 (pp. 83–97).

[28] E. Rutledge, 'Economic Life', in *MN*, ed. Rawcliffe and Wilson, pp. 157–88 (pp. 158–81, 183–5); P. Dunn, 'Trade', in *MN*, ed. Rawcliffe and Wilson, pp. 213–34; *East Anglia and its North Sea World in the Middle Ages*, ed. D. Bates and R. Liddiard (Woodbridge, 2013); Atkin and Evans, EAA 100, pp. 245–6. On artefacts (and culinary traditions) imported from the Low Countries: Atkin, Carter and Evans, EAA 26, pp. 80, 84; Margeson, EAA 58, pp. 143, 166, 236.

[29] However, for a loss of diversity in the economy in the early fourteenth century, see Rutledge, 'Economic Life', p. 188, and for the city's mixed economic fortunes in the late fifteenth century, see 'Income Tax Assessments of Norwich, 1472 and 1489', ed. M. Jurkowski, in *Poverty and Wealth: Sheep, Taxation and Charity in Late Medieval Norfolk*, ed. M. Bailey, M. Jurkowski and C. Rawcliffe, NRS 71 (Norwich, 2007), pp. 99–156 (esp. pp. 117–19).

[30] J. F. Pound, 'The Social and Trade Structure of Norwich 1525–1575', *Past and Present* 34 (1966), 49–69 (pp. 49–54); J. Pound, 'Government to 1660', in *NS1550*, ed. Rawcliffe and Wilson, pp. 35–61 (p. 38).

[31] The premier family dynasties in the ruling oligarchy fostered powerful political connections reaching to Westminster. For example, the city's network of sixteenth-century mercantile families and their connections to the most powerful men in central government (including Thomas Cromwell) and with continental

a particularly strongly articulated policy with regard to the sanitization and improvement of the city's fabric. The civic government had the crucial income, administrative machinery and workforce at its disposal to enable it to set ambitious goals in this respect, and it was assisted by wealthy philanthropists seeking to augment their local standing through investment in glamorous projects. Finally (but importantly), Norwich benefits from an unusually rich base of archival and archaeological evidence, and a wide body of existing historiography, which enables us to mine down deeply into our subject.[32] In what remains of this introduction, the governmental, social and physical constitutions of the city – the constant backdrop of the rest of our enquiry – are brought into sharper focus.

The body politic: status and respectability

From a relatively early date, the governing class in Norwich exercised a good deal of executive authority. The city was granted a royal charter[33] in 1404 which recognized Norwich as a legal and jurisdictional entity separate from the county of Norfolk as a whole.[34] This permitted the citizens[35] to elect a mayor and two sheriffs,[36] thus replacing the four bailiffs who had dominated the urban government hitherto.[37] The

merchants can be traced in *History of Parliament: The House of Commons 1509–1558*, ed. S. T. Bindoff, 3 vols. (London, 1982).

[32] See Appendix III.

[33] Excerpted in *RCN*, I, 31–6. The value of this charter for the new corporation cannot be overestimated. It sanctioned the citizens' collective authority at a time when they were struggling to preserve their jurisdiction over significant tracts of land from the powerful Norwich Benedictine priory. On the wider context, see N. Tanner, 'The Cathedral and the City', in *Norwich Cathedral: Church, City, Diocese, 1096–1996*, ed. Atherton et al., pp. 255–80 (pp. 255–69); *RCN*, I, 320–4.

[34] R. Frost, 'The Urban Elite', in *MN*, ed. Rawcliffe and Wilson, pp. 235–53 (pp. 236–7).

[35] That is, enfranchised residents who were members of the freedom of Norwich. The distinction of belonging to the freedom brought with it not only status and electoral privileges but also specific financial obligations and was limited to a minority of Norwich inhabitants: Frost, 'The Urban Elite', p. 236.

[36] The sheriffs were elected from within the city government and had three main duties: they presided over personal lawsuits heard at the guildhall, they were the returning officers for parliamentary elections, and they were responsible for paying the city's Fee Farm (an annual land rent) to the Crown: T. Hawes, *An Index to Norwich City Officers, 1453–1835*, NRS 52 (Norwich, 1989), p. xi.

[37] On the structure of Norwich government prior to 1404, see B. McRee, 'Peacemaking and its Limits in Late Medieval Norwich', *English Historical Review* 109 (1994), 831–66 (pp. 835–8).

main administrative hub of the corporation, the guildhall, was completed not long afterwards in a prime location at the heart of the city.[38] For organizational purposes, Norwich was divided into four major wards or districts (see map 2), in which the corporation's policies were implemented by twenty-four senior officials ('aldermen'), who were themselves nominated from the ranks of the most powerful and influential families across the city.[39] Together, this group also formed an inner council that acted in an advisory capacity to the mayor.

After the 1404 charter was sealed, the governing elite set about carefully reordering its archive of procedural, financial and legal records.[40] This was an important resource: the restructured organization was beset by frequent outbreaks of factional infighting, and the archives served as an unambiguous guide not only to procedure and to landholdings but also as a protocol for good governance. Whilst drafting the corporation's cornerstone documentation, some clerks appropriated from political rhetoric the language of a healthy, effectively functioning and well-coordinated human body.[41] Here was a powerful linguistic tool which helped to add dignity and legitimacy to its innovations. Following mediations between rival factions in 1415, for example, the corporation reformulated its procedure for civic elections in a document that was suffused with the vocabulary of bodily

[38] The guildhall was finished in 1407–12 and remains the largest building of its type to survive in provincial England: Ayers, *NAFC*, pp. 117–18 and plate 22 therein.

[39] Hawes, *Index to Norwich City Officers*, p. xiv.

[40] On the archive, see M. C. McClendon, *The Quiet Reformation: Magistrates and the Emergence of Protestantism in Tudor Norwich* (Stanford, 1999), p. 16; P. Dunn, 'After the Black Death: Society and Economy in late Fourteenth-Century Norwich' (unpublished PhD thesis, University of East Anglia, 2003), pp. 9–20; *Records of Early English Drama: Norwich 1540–1642*, ed. D. Galloway (London, 1984), pp. xlv-lxxiv. For developments in archive keeping in other important English cities, see S. H. Rigby, 'Urban "Oligarchy" in Late Medieval England', in *Towns and Townspeople in the Fifteenth Century*, ed. J. A. F. Thomson (Gloucester, 1988), pp. 62–86 (pp. 62–3); S. Rees Jones, 'York's Civic Administration, 1354–1464', in *The Government of Medieval York: Essays in Commemoration of the 1396 Royal Charter*, ed. S. Rees Jones, Borthwick Studies in History 3 (York, 1997), pp. 108–40 (p. 110). For London, see, for example: John Carpenter, *Liber albus: The White Book of the City of London*, ed. H. T. Riley (London, 1861), esp. p. 3.

[41] In comparison – and on the necessity for all component parts to act together in both the physical body and in the figurative 'body politic' – see John Fortescue, *De laudibus legum Anglie*, trans. S. B. Chrimes (Cambridge, 1949), pp. 31–3 (1468–71); and S. B. Chrimes, *English Constitutional Ideas in the Fifteenth Century* (Cambridge, 1936), p. 175 (1483).

unity. The citizens reportedly gathered on the feast of St Valentine (14 February) to negotiate many long-standing disputes by which 'the cite hath be[en] divided, dissoyled and in poynt to ben distroyed'. Now, 'standynge ful onyd [oned]', they promised to: 'make pees, unite and acord, [both] poore and ryche to ben oon in herte, love, and charite, [and] nevermore fro this tyme forth to ben dissevered'.[42] Conversely, outbreaks of discord or political dissension were sometimes construed as pathologies in the body politic. In 1424, following further upheavals, an indenture was drawn up between the mayor, sheriffs and aldermen which ruled that 'non of the [twenty-four] aldermen ... xal speken sclaundrous wordes of non felawe of his alderman ne wyl [he] harm ne *disese* [distress] ne hevynesse [vexation] bern'.[43] The value placed on unity and order did not, however, extend to notions of equality: the most senior civic officials formed an oligarchy dedicated to preserving and advertising their power and material wealth to the exclusion of others.[44]

Slightly more representative in nature was the election of sixty 'common' councillors, that is, officials returned by the wider populace or 'commonalty'.[45] These men were a link between householders in the wards and the government machinery. The election process itself was something of a logistical feat. Over a period of four consecutive days 'alle the enfraunchised men housholders' from across Norwich were required to attend the guildhall. From this number were chosen

[42] *RCN*, I, 94.

[43] *RCN*, I, 111 (my emphasis).

[44] Election ceremonies for senior officials were an opportunity to physically demarcate, and thus reinforce, the proper order of precedence in the urban hierarchy. Distinctions of status within the civic body were confirmed by variations in the participants' costume and in the strict control of access to reserved spaces within the guildhall. During the proceedings, the mayor and twenty-four 'clothed in suyt after her [their] estat asketh' sat in a separate chamber while the election, determined by the 'voys of the poeple', took place in the hall: *RCN*, I, 95 (voice) and 102 (clothing). On these and other civic ceremonies in Norwich, see Frost, 'The Urban Elite', p. 238, and Maddern, 'Order and Disorder', pp. 208–9; cf. M. James, 'Ritual, Drama and Social Body in the Late Medieval English Town', *Past and Present* 98 (1983), 3–29 (p. 4), and see Rigby, 'Urban "Oligarchy"', p. 67, which argues that 'if the medieval town was a stage, then the message of much of its drama was that of social unity within a hierarchy'.

[45] Hawes, *Index to Norwich City Officers*, p. xiv. Unlike the aldermen, the common councillors were chosen from amongst the residents of the wards that they represented. Also in contrast to the aldermen, they were not appointed for life, and there was a high annual turnover of personnel in the ranks.

'suffisaunt men' for each ward whose role was to provide good and trustworthy counsel for the 'profit of the cite'.[46] The drawn-out observance helped to demonstrate what it meant to be an honourable denizen; an enfranchised male householder was a figure of authority within the community. In this way, the electorate had the opportunity to identify and to note responsible (and accountable) people in their districts.

Such a concept of personal respectability necessarily excluded – at least in theory – a significant proportion of the population that did not meet the criteria of maleness,[47] political privilege and residence. On one side of the balance-scale stood master craftsmen and merchants, and, on the other, a collection of individuals including journeymen (day-labourers), ungovernable women, outsiders, the young, the sick and the vagrant.[48] As in other cities, these groups of people were considered alarming precisely because they existed outside the normal systems of social control that were rooted in the structures of household and property ownership.[49] Apprehensions of this nature were explicitly addressed in the *Customal* of Norwich (a record of local customary laws) which was written in about 1308.[50] Under the heading 'concerning labouring servants who are evildoers through boldness of their poverty', the *Customal* condemned one batch of potential transients, namely, hirelings, 'because their masters are not answerable for them for they are not of their mainpast [i.e., a member of a household]' and have

[46] *RCN*, I, 99.

[47] Very few Norwich women obtained the freedom: Frost, 'The Urban Elite', p. 395, n. 13.

[48] F. Rexroth, *Deviance and Power in Late Medieval London*, trans. P. E. Selwyn (Cambridge, 2007).

[49] On the wider theme, see S. Rees Jones, 'Household, Work and the Problem of Mobile Labour: The Regulation of Labour in Medieval English Towns', in *The Problem of Labour in Fourteenth-Century England*, ed. J. Bothwell, P. J. P. Goldberg and W. M. Ormrod (York, 2000), pp. 133–53 (pp. 143–4); S. Rees Jones, 'The Household and English Urban Government in the Later Middle Ages', in *The Household in Late Medieval Cities: Italy and North-Western Europe Compared*, ed. M. Carlier and T. Soens (Leuven, 2001), pp. 71–88 (pp. 78–81); P. J. P. Goldberg, 'Migration, Youth and Gender in Later Medieval England', in *Youth in the Middle Ages*, ed. P. J. P Goldberg and F. Riddy (York, 2004), pp. 85–99; and see P. Griffiths, 'Masterless Young People in Norwich, 1560–1645', in *The Experience of Authority in Early Modern England*, ed. P. Griffiths, A. Fox and S. Hindle (Basingstoke, 1996), pp. 146–86. For an example of an ill-ruled house in Norwich in 1465, see Maddern, 'Order and Disorder', pp. 189–90.

[50] On the text, see *RCN*, I, cxx.

'nothing by which they can be attached'.[51] Other people whose presence or behaviour also seemed to threaten the established order – immigrants, the young and rootless, infectious 'lepers', or illegal traders – were likewise treated with occasional animus, and the citizens were periodically encouraged to inform on their movements.[52] Towards the end of our period, those suffering from the (often conjoined) afflictions of poverty and disease became particularly susceptible to the censure of civic leaders and their better-off neighbours.[53] Anxieties about both circumstances were allied to a wider discourse concerning deterioration and personal behaviour in civic consciousness.[54] A lexicon of condemnation duly developed: infectious or supposedly indolent and self-indulgent people seemingly threatened not only the social hierarchy, but also the precepts of self-management and moderation that lay at the heart of medieval and Tudor socio-medical theory. In this context, the manifest disfigurements and deformities of the sick poor – seemingly tokens of an inner physical corruption – acquired their own symbolism. Sixteenth-century medical texts portrayed conditions which caused the skin of the head to 'stynke thorowe the vaporynge of evyll and corrupte humours' or to run with 'matter bothe ugely to loke on and evyll smellynge to the nose' as both repellent and dangerous to

51 That is, they had no goods that could be seized during the enforcement of any judicial order: *RCN*, I, 189. On an influx of people during the early fourteenth century who, living by day labour and unable to purchase property, may have been the source of concerns of this type: see E. Rutledge, 'Landlords and Tenants: Housing and the Rented Property Market in Early Fourteenth-Century Norwich', *Urban History* 22 (1995), 7–24 (p. 12).

52 Historians have argued that anxieties like these – about transience, difficult interpersonal relationships and economic instability – were commonly expressed in terms of assaults upon the (urban) body: P. J. P. Goldberg, 'Pigs and Prostitutes: Streetwalking in Comparative Perspective', in *Young Medieval Women*, ed. K. J. Lewis, N. J. Menuge and K. M. Phillips (Stroud, 1999), pp. 172–93; P. J. P. Goldberg, 'Coventry's "Lollard" Programme of 1492 and the Making of *Utopia*', in *Pragmatic Utopias*, ed. Horrox and Rees Jones, pp. 97–116; M. S. R. Jenner, 'The Great Dog Massacre', in *Fear in Early Modern Society*, ed. W. G. Naphy and P. Roberts (Manchester, 1997), pp. 44–61.

53 On the lifestyle of the poor as a cause of plague, see A. Wear, *Knowledge and Practice in English Medicine, 1550–1680* (Cambridge, 2000), p. 283. More generally, on an increasing predilection amongst readers of plague literature after *c.* 1530 for an emphasis upon punishment, see G. R. Keiser, 'Two Medieval Plague Treatises and Their Afterlife in Early Modern England', *Journal of the History of Medicine and Allied Sciences* 58 (2003), 292–324 (p. 322).

54 Explored in P. Griffiths, 'Inhabitants', in *NS1550*, ed. Rawcliffe and Wilson, pp. 63–88.

any healthy people in the vicinity.[55] For this reason (that is, for covering up such sores), as well as for reasons of controlling sexual behaviour, the ordinances of Norwich's civic hospital produced at about this time insisted upon the provision of proper clothing for the sick poor.[56]

Beautifying by building: cityscape and city cleaning

In Norwich, as elsewhere, both the authority of the elite and social distinctions between persons were marked out through material means: members of the mercantile oligarchy sunk the profits accruing from their trade and manufacturing businesses into spectacular domestic and communal building projects.[57] By the mid-thirteenth century as many as sixty parish churches had been built in the city, although the number declined (along with the population) to forty-six by the eve of the Dissolution of the Monasteries.[58] As well as supplying spiritual services, these buildings were the mausoleums of wealthy citizens, and almost all of the many remaining examples show evidence of rebuilding or re-fenestration during the fifteenth century which was sponsored by the parishioners.[59] A very substantial donation by a single wealthy resident facilitated the completion of the most expensive and prestigious structures to grace Norwich's landscape: the city was completely enclosed by mural defences in about 1344 (map 3).[60] The symbolic value placed locally upon the city walls and other substantial buildings, and the ideals of power, protection and wealth to which they seemed to give concrete form, continued to reverberate down the centuries. In 1527, the mayor and other senior civic officials

[55] The quotations are from Andrew Boorde, *The Breviary of Healthe* (London: William Powell, 1552), fol. 11r (on leprous *allopecia*) and Marshall, *The Forme and Maner of Subvention*, sig. E4v. For similar concerns, see also Robert Copland, *The Hye Way to the Spyttell Hous* (London: Robert Copland, 1536), sig. A3v, and Ulrich von Hutten, *De morbo Gallico*, trans. Thomas Paynell (London: Thomas Berthelet, 1533), fol. 2r–v. On the wider context, see M. Pelling, 'Appearance and Reality: Barber-Surgeons, the Body and Disease', in *London 1500–1700: The Making of the Metropolis*, ed. A. L. Beier and R. Finlay (London, 1986), pp. 82–112 (pp. 89–91).

[56] E. M. Phillips, 'Charitable Institutions in Norfolk and Suffolk, *c.* 1350–1600' (unpublished PhD thesis, University of East Anglia, 2001), pp. 248–52.

[57] Ayers, *NAFC*, pp. 110–37.

[58] N. Tanner, 'Religious Practice', in *MN*, ed. Rawcliffe and Wilson, pp. 137–55 (p. 141).

[59] J. Finch, 'The Churches', in *MN*, ed. Rawcliffe and Wilson, pp. 49–72 (p. 60).

[60] Ayers, *NAFC*, pp. 89–94.

reflected upon how the walls and other architecture greatly impressed visitors in former times, claiming:

> the citie of Norwiche is and hath ben an auncient citie fortified with diches, envyround with walles, gates, toures, tourettes, beautified with goodly mansions and enhabited with substantiall merchauntes and craftysmen, whyche citie (as is beforesaid adorned) is the strength and comfort of all the countries adjoynaunt, and of all them that course and recourse to and from the same.[61]

Subsequent projects included the development of public wharfs or staithes (1379); the construction of a common inn (1397); the rebuilding of a defensive structure called the Cow Tower (1398–99); and the erection of water-driven corn mills known as the 'New Mills' (1410, effective in 1430). Although spearheaded by individuals, these schemes were frequently underwritten using funds generated by public taxes, and they were intended to benefit the commonalty of Norwich as a whole.

The economic and administrative nerve centre of Norwich was located at the marketplace, established in its present location by the late thirteenth century (map 4). The area also gradually came to be dominated by monuments to civic wealth, power and piety, many of which can still be seen today. The piazza contained a market cross, a centre for exchange,[62] and a pillory where public punishments were enacted. On the northern boundary stood (and still stands) the corporation's former guildhall, and the goldsmiths' hall, then home to one of the city's richest and most important trade guilds.[63] On the opposite side of the market, to the south, is situated the church of St Peter Mancroft, itself transformed by a series of magnificent rebuilding programmes during the fifteenth century. This edifice has recently been dubbed the 'merchants' cathedral' by one historian, owing to its imposing

[61] NRO, NCR 10f Draft for the Minutes of an Assembly held 12 August 19 Henry VIII (1527), no folio number. This rhetorical flourish was used to justify the levying of a rate, paid by property owners, towards the repair of the city walls which were actually in an appalling state of disrepair: see below, p. 22.

[62] Ayers, *NAFC*, p. 118. The cross and the guildhall were erected during the attempts by the corporation of Norwich to exert its control over the production and sale of manufactured goods, as well as other forms of commercial exchange.

[63] C. Garibaldi, 'The Guildhall of the Norwich Company of Goldsmiths', in *East Anglian Silver 1550–1750*, ed. C. Hartop (Cambridge, 2004), pp. 31–5 (with thanks to Brian Ayers).

architecture and its central importance in civic life.[64] The church was the spiritual home of the company of St George, a fraternity whose members dominated the ranks of civic government.[65] Those attending assemblies at the guildhall or services at St Peter's might have glanced across the Great Cockey (a large and fast-flowing natural stream which skirted the market) to the middle distance where the Norman castle and the college of St Mary in the Fields were situated: these two establishments further endorsed the corporation's authority (map 3).[66] By the late fifteenth and early sixteenth century, many of Norwich's most affluent and influential citizens owned property in the streets in this central area.[67]

The project to beautify Norwich had serious consequences for later generations of civic officials and local rate-payers. The combined costs of maintaining the city's public buildings, water and road infrastructure, its rental properties and the marketplace were significant: by the mid-sixteenth century, charges relating to refurbishments constituted between about one-fifth to about one-half of the administration's annual outgoings at any one time.[68] Nevertheless, the ruling elite

[64] R. Gilchrist, *Norwich Cathedral Close: The Evolution of the English Cathedral Landscape* (Woodbridge, 2005), p. 94.

[65] The company became a more or less formal adjunct of the municipal corporation in 1452: Tanner, 'Religious Practice', p. 149.

[66] For the good relations between the college of St Mary and the corporation – which used the college's premises for various activities – see C. Harper-Bill and C. Rawcliffe, 'The Religious Houses', in *MN*, ed. Rawcliffe and Wilson, pp. 73–119 (pp. 117–18). On the castle, see Shepherd Popescu, EAA 132, I, 464–5.

[67] L. G. Bollingbrook, 'St John Maddermarket, Norwich: Its Streets, Lanes and Ancient Houses and their Old-Time Associations', *NA* 20 (1921), 215–39. See also Ayers, *NAFC*, especially p. 114 and figure 59 for the 'Bridewell' (next to St Andrew's church). This house – constructed by the father of William Appleyard, first mayor of Norwich, in *c.* 1370 – unambiguously projected the affluence and social influence of its owners through the splendid, flint-fronted aspect of its north range. Similarly, on 'Stranger's Hall', the main residence of successive Norwich mayors, and on other merchants' houses, see C. King, 'The Interpretation of Urban Buildings: Power, Memory and Appropriation in Norwich Merchants' Houses, *c.* 1400–1660', *World Archaeology* 41 (2009), 471–88; and see map 4 in the present volume.

[68] Calculated from the Norwich series of chamberlains' accounts for 1531 to 1567, held at NCR 18a, and see Pound, 'Government to 1660', pp. 56–8, esp. p. 58. See also R. Tittler, *The Reformation and the Towns in England: Politics and Political Culture, c. 1540–1640* (Oxford, 1998), p. 108. Several minor campaigns, which were intermittently repeated or expanded, addressed the road and water infrastructure, the quality of the domestic building stock, the provision

continued to take on further commitments. Ranking high amongst its achievements following the Dissolution of the Monasteries was the constructive public use to which it put the dilapidated Blackfriars' site (which it acquired in 1540) and the former hospital of St Giles, thereafter known as the 'Great Hospital' (1546, map 3).[69] Both complexes were expensively refurbished. The conversion of the former Blackfriars' into a Common Hall alone accounted for about forty per cent of the city government's outgoings in 1542/43 and 1544/45.[70] When the works were complete, the corporation let out portions of the friars' garden and orchard as well as recently built domestic buildings in the precincts. These generated a substantial annual income, part of which was intended to be reinvested in civic schemes.[71] The Great Hospital's supervisory committee similarly modified and improved the hospital building for its new secular use as accommodation for the respectable – or potentially respectable – poor. Like the subsequent, more draconian, Bridewell, and in accordance with legislation mooted in parliament, the hospital endeavoured to rehabilitate inmates for an active working life. To this end it took the additional and seemingly

of suitable facilities and drainage in the marketplace, and the improvement of key civic amenities. These cost in the region of £30 to £60 each, and might be implemented over a two or three year period. During larger projects (specifically relating to the refurbishment of the walls and civic buildings), the bills could run into hundreds at a time. To take the 1540s as an example, a single repaving campaign totalled over £32; £26 was spent on refurbishing houses and rental properties in the corporation's possession; and £60 on improving rental properties, shops and drainage in the market, the Common Inn and Guildhall. At the same time, routine expenditure on the river and drainage systems cost between about £6 to £11 per annum: NCR 18a/7 CA 1541–49, fols. 15v, 18r–v, 19r, 24v, 54r–v, 59r, 64r, 66v, 105v, 107v, 110r–111r, 112v, 113r, 160r–v, 162r, 163r–v, 166v, 170r, 201r, 205v, 207v, 234r–v, 245v, 266v, 276v, 291v, 294r, 325r, 331v. To put this in context, the chamberlains' total expenditure for the decade, including rents, fees and wages, as well as work at the Common Hall, hospital and other properties, was over £3090.

69 For the wider theme (including the city's purchase of over £142 worth of property from the Court of Augmentations), see R. Tittler, 'Reformation, Resources and Authority in English Towns: An Overview', in *The Reformation in English Towns 1500–1640*, ed. P. Collinson and J. Craig (Basingstoke, 1998), pp. 190–201 (p. 287, n. 40).

70 In excess of £450 was spent on this project alone: NCR 18a/7 CA 1541–49, fols. 25v, 26r, 28r–29r, 31r–32r, 34v, 35v, 92r, 140v, 186r–v, 213r. The hall was subsequently used for civic and guild functions.

71 For the intended use of the orchard's revenue for maintaining a common granary in times of famine, see NRO, NCR 17b Mayor's Book (Book of Oaths), p. 152.

unprecedented step of employing a salaried surgeon at the corporation's expense.[72] During the renovations, quantities of timber, tile, wood and paving stone were stripped from these sites as well as from other religious precincts.[73] The resources, if not sold, were reused by the city corporation for repairs at the market and elsewhere, or were placed in the carefully audited 'common store' for future use.[74]

The commonalty's water mills (which alone cost the city over £116 to refurbish in 1562/63),[75] as well as the city's bridges, quays and staithes, the Common Inn and common close, the guildhall and cloth hall, and the walls, gates and towers all required expensive repair works. A survey undertaken in *c.* 1550, for example, reported that stretches of the walls were in a state of 'gret decaye', despite the positive rhetoric of the ruling elite. The document makes depressing reading: portions of wall had collapsed between the Black Tower and Ber Street gate; the southern 'tower with the iron door' was likely to be destroyed at any moment by flooding; four towers in the croft next to the college of St Mary in the Fields were in a parlous state, and one was on the point of falling down; St Augustine's gate had been hit by a cart and its portcullis required immediate attention; the roof of St Benedict's gate

72 On the Great Hospital's evolving remit and its employment of a civic surgeon, see Rawcliffe, *MFTS*, pp. 216–18, 226–8, and see references to John Porter below. For the rebuilding of the Great Hospital and its tenements (rental properties), see for example 'Account Rolls of The Great Hospital, Norwich, 1549–50 and 1570–71', ed. E. Phillips, in *Health and Hygiene*, ed. Phillips and Fay, pp. 1–99 (pp. 13–14); NRO, NCR 24a Great Hospital Account Rolls 1560–69, fol. 9r–v (1566/67); and *Norwich Landgable Assessment 1568–70*, ed. M. Rodgers and M. Wallace, NRS 63 (Norwich 1999), p. 90 for 'the tenements and shoppes late builded belongyng to the hospitall' in central Norwich. For the Bridewell, which was functioning by 1570, see Griffiths, 'Inhabitants', pp. 67–70.

73 For the dismantling and sale of parts of the Great Hospital's chancel, see NCR 16d/2 Assembly Proceedings 1491–1553, fol. 230r (modern foliation) and for the stripping of lead from the Blackfriars', see NCR 18a/6 CA 1537–47, fol. 179v. For the extraction and reuse of material from the Greyfriars: E. Rutledge, 'Documentary Evidence', in Emery, EAA 120, pp. 86–92 (pp. 86–9).

74 Resources from the common store were used during the renovation of the market stalls, corporation tenements and public watercourses, see, e.g. NCR 18a/8 CA 1551–67, fol. 124r–v (the materials used comprised nine chalder – or 288 bushels – of lime, 200 bricks, 4200 roofing tiles and 193 feet of wooden board).

75 Pound, 'Government to 1660', p. 57. The city's total expenditure on all aspects of its finances in that year was a little over £367: NCR 18a/8 CA 1551–67, fol. 262r.

had already fallen in, whilst those at Magdalen gate and St Giles's gate were perilously close to doing so (map 3).[76]

In addition to the decay caused to property by the passage of time, Norwich faced an additional threat to its fabric: the city's clay, wood and thatch building stock proved acutely vulnerable to outbreaks of fire. The toll taken by fire on the city landscape is a theme to which we will return periodically in this book, so it is worth briefly outlining the main events here. In particular, whole neighbourhoods had been destroyed in three major outbreaks: two that erupted in 1507 (in which perhaps as many as seven hundred or more houses were destroyed) and another during Kett's rebellion in 1549.[77] The mayor and aldermen made periodic attempts to stop the residents from building with highly inflammable materials,[78] balancing the risk of further catastrophic outbreaks with the need to stimulate rebuilding at an affordable cost.[79] Pockets of fire-damage remained when Cuningham was conducting his surveying expeditions around Norwich during the late 1550s. Property owners apparently proved reluctant or unable to incur the expense of repair. In these circumstances, the civic authorities laid the blame for declining economic conditions and for deteriorating hygienic standards on such apparent negligence.[80]

It was not until the close of the period studied here that the corporation took definitive steps to combat the problem of fire. In 1583,

[76] NCR 10f, Portion of a Wall Note *c.* 1550, no folio number.

[77] The figure of 718 houses, which is frequently cited in the secondary literature, derives from the assertion by the Norfolk antiquarian Francis Blomefield, although on the basis of exactly what evidence is not clear; he also suggested (using a different source) a total closer to 360: Blomefield, *Norfolk*, III, 182–3. See also Atkin, Carter and Evans, EAA 26, pp. 77–8, which estimates that the larger of Blomefield's figures equates to about forty per cent of the city's housing stock. The second of the 1507 outbreaks was elegized by John Skelton, 'Lamentatio urbis Norvicen', *The Poetical Works of John Skelton*, ed. A. Dyce, 2 vols. (London, 1843), I, 174.

[78] In early May 1509, the civic assembly issued a regulation that new housing should be covered with 'thacktyle [tiles]' rather than 'thakke [thatch]', to arrest the spread of any further conflagration. Offenders against this order risked a considerable 20*s.* fine: *RCN*, II, 107. The measure was intermittently revoked and reinforced: *RCN*, II, 120 (1532), 137–40 (1570); NCR 16a/5 Mayor's Court Book 1540–49, p. 545 (1549).

[79] Notably, the city corporation itself chose to re-roof its rental-tenements in thatch during the 1530s in order to free up funds to recondition other features of its properties: NCR 18a/5 CA 1531–7, fol. 31v.

[80] On this, see chapter 5 below.

the mayor and aldermen made an agreement with two London-based plumbers to provide high pressure water on demand to the centre of the city. The contract secured a supply of ten tonnes every day to an outlet at the west end of the guildhall, which could be used 'in tyme of casualtes for the safegarde of howses and buyldynges'. The plumbers were given permission to place the pump and the pipe in any location that best facilitated the scheme, as well as to dig up streets, lanes or other corporation-owned grounds as necessary. The system (impressive by any reckoning) was driven by a mill and floodgate situated in an inlet to the river Wensum close to Coslany bridge. The water was pushed through lead pipes to the parish church of St Lawrence, where the necessary pressure to convey the water over the 270 additional metres to the city centre was generated by forcing the water up the side of the church steeple.[81] Additionally, the plumbers agreed to supply smaller pipes to convey water to the households of select citizens able to pay for the privilege, and to deliver river water 'on tap' twice in every twenty-four hours.[82]

The citizens recognized that a well-governed and properly equipped city should also be a hygienic one. This was more than a matter of communal pride: Norwich's townsmen and women believed that, without proper regulation, the city's environment could damage them physically. The waste products that accumulated in the nooks and crannies of urban spaces (such as stagnant water, muck, blood and offal) seemed to pose particular health risks. For this reason, and on the basis of a sound grasp of contemporary disease theory, the parties involved in piping water to the guildhall in 1583 envisaged an additional benefit for the population from the planned works: the ample amounts of water supplied could be used to sluice down the 'gutters,

[81] NRO, NCR 22a/4 Agreement Concerning the Supply of Water and Cleaning of the Cockeys (1583).

[82] *RCN*, II, 392–4. On urban conduits, the motives compelling their construction, and their subsequent maintenance, see R. J. Magnusson, *Water Technology in the Middle Ages: Cities, Monasteries and Waterworks after the Roman Empire* (London, 2001), esp. pp. viii–ix, 22–30, 127–32 (and see pp. 55–115 on technological configurations); Rawcliffe, *Urban Bodies*, pp. 176–86, 211–13, 222–8; and (on the extent to which 'access to water was mediated by the micropolitics and material culture of neighbourhood'), see M. Jenner, 'From Conduit Community to Commercial Network? Water in London, 1500–1725', in *Londonopolis: Essays in the Cultural and Social History of Early Modern London*, ed. P. Griffiths (Manchester, 2000), pp. 250–72 (quote at p. 251).

channelles and cockeys [watercourses]' in the marketplace which would 'by the runeng of fresshe water in the channelles thear, ... bee claryfyed clensed and purged from stynche and yll savors whereuppon corrupcion and infeccion oft tymes ensueth'.[83] Though no mechanized solution had previously existed to cleanse gutters, the city's governors had waged regular campaigns to improve conditions in the drainage system and streets, and to clean up areas that were part of, or adjoined, the corporation's property, using the comparatively modest machinery of hand tools and muscle power (both human and animal), from at least the time of the pandemic known as the Black Death.[84] Additionally, civic officers put pressure upon property owners to clean the streets in front of their buildings, and to exercise due diligence in keeping the water supply as clear and pure as possible (and they instituted supervisory controls to ensure compliance).[85] The city's successes in these spheres led residents and visitors to assert that Norwich was an unusually salubrious place to live;[86] its periodic failures drew sharp derision from commentators who had become accustomed to the idea that magistrates had an obligation to oversee and protect the community's health. We will return to the nature of the corporation's schemes to sanitize Norwich in detail towards the end of this book. Now it is time to ask, on what particular ideas of health and hygiene did townsmen and women draw? What compelled their fear of stagnation and corruption? And how did these concerns fit within a wider body of ideas about the body and its place in the environment?

[83] NCR 22a/4 Agreement Concerning the Supply of Water and Cleaning of the Cockeys (1583). For comparison, see M. Dorey, 'Controlling Corruption: Regulating Meat Consumption as a Preventative to Plague in Seventeenth-Century London', *UH* 36 (2009), 24–41 (pp. 31–5).

[84] On this, see below, chapter 5.

[85] In 1467, for example, following a series of national and regional epidemics, the city government temporarily appointed supervisors in each district to ensure that the streets remained free from corruption. Residents who purchased commodities from suppliers living in the rural hinterland – especially hay, fuel, heather, hair or straw – were prevented from storing their purchases in the streets, because they might putrefy or wash into the drainage system: *RCN*, II, 98.

[86] On the image of Norwich in the sixteenth, seventeenth and eighteenth centuries, see C. Rawcliffe, 'Introduction', in *MN*, ed. Rawcliffe and Wilson, pp. xix–xxvi.

Part I

Health and Place in Texts and Images

MRS PANTS: But what about the privies?
BLACKADDER: Uhm, well, what we are talking about in privy terms, is the very latest in front-wall, fresh air orifices combined with a wide capacity gutter installation below.
MRS PANTS: You mean you crap out of the window?
BLACKADDER: Yes.
MRS PANTS: Well, in that case, we'll definitely take it. I can't stand those dirty indoor things.[1]

Thus the scriptwriters of the successful television comedy 'Blackadder II' (1986) satirized a prevailing belief that life in medieval England was unremittingly squalid, and the populace slovenly. Mrs Pants's retort (it's what you expect that matters) is reminiscent of an anthropological dictum: attitudes to dirt and disease are relative, circumstantial and socially constructed. Because of this, it is considered anachronistic to transpose biomedical notions of antibacterial sanitation on to the evidential record. Now historians are asking: by what standards did men and women of the period evaluate cleanliness, and what steps did they take to foster it? Part I of this book establishes the concepts of the body and of the natural world that were available to men and women living in medieval and early modern Norwich; the next few pages point to some particular landmarks which may help the reader to navigate what follows.

The fundamentals of hygienic theory in this period drew upon certain principles of health care that were already considerably over

[1] R. Curtis, B. Elton, J. Lloyd and R. Atkinson, *Blackadder: The Whole Damn Dynasty* (London, 1998), p. 186.

1,000 years old.[2] These originated in the Greek-speaking world, and are known from the works attributed to Hippocrates of Cos, b. 460 BC (actually, a collection of textbooks, lectures and polemics written by various authors between 430 BC and 330 BC), and 'his' intellectual heir, Galen of Pergamum, b. AD 129, a philosopher-physician. One of the most important texts arising out of this tradition was the Hippocratic treatise 'On the Nature of Man', which bequeathed the following precept: 'some diseases are produced by the manner of life that is followed; others by the life-giving air we breathe'.[3] The author went on to explain exactly how these circumstances could be distinguished. If a significant proportion of the inhabitants of a region or town fell ill with the same disease the cause was clearly something common to all, the most likely culprit being a 'morbid secretion' contained in the atmosphere. If, on the other hand, a number of different ailments afflicted a single population, then something individual to each case would be to blame, most likely a person's regimen.[4]

This scheme was not the only one available to men and women who sought to explain and alleviate their pathological experiences, nor did it survive unchallenged.[5] Even so, two of its concepts were

[2] For a concise overview of the textual tradition, see: H. Mikkeli, *Hygiene in the Early Modern Medical Tradition* (Helsinki, 1999), pp. 1–96. For these principles in civic and academic medicine during the late thirteenth and early fourteenth centuries (as represented in the works of Arnau de Villanova, especially), see M. R. McVaugh, *Medicine Before the Plague: Practitioners and their Patients in the Crown of Aragon, 1285–1345* (Cambridge, 1993), chapter 5, esp. pp. 144–53; and see J. Henderson, 'The Black Death in Florence: Medical and Communal Responses', in *Death in Towns: Urban Responses to the Dying and the Dead, 100–1600*, ed. S. Bassett (Leicester, 1992), pp. 136–50 (pp. 136–41).

[3] Hippocrates of Cos, *De natura hominis*, as translated in 'The Nature of Man', in *Hippocratic Writings*, ed. G. E. R. Lloyd (London, 1983), pp. 260–71 (p. 266), cf. e.g. Hippocrates of Cos, *De natura hominis* (Rome: Georg Herolt, *c.* 1481), p. [16]: 'morbi alii a victus genere: alii a spiritu quem trahentes vivimus proveniunt'.

[4] From the fifth century, the same ideas were adopted and adapted firstly by Latin and then by Muslim scholars, and were thence transmitted to medieval northern Europe.

[5] On, for example, care of the sick as a religious concern in local health culture, see C. Hill, *Women and Religion in Late Medieval Norwich* (Woodbridge, 2010), pp. 133–6, 141–3, 161–6. More broadly, on magical healing, see K. Thomas, *Religion and the Decline of Magic: Studies in Popular Beliefs in Sixteenth- and Seventeenth-Century England* (London, 1991), pp. 209–51. For schemes at the end of our period that sometimes rivalled and sometimes complemented Galenic and Hippocratic models, see L. Kassell, *Medicine and Magic in Elizabethan London: Simon Forman: Astrologer, Alchemist and Physician* (Oxford, 2005), and on the

appropriated unreservedly into English medical writing. The first emphasized the crucial importance of a person's immediate surroundings to well-being. The second supposed that an individual's habits and behaviour (and in particular an avoidance of, or abandonment to, idleness and self-indulgence) played crucial roles in preventing, and causing, disease. These twin notions were complemented by a third which also sprung ultimately from Greek roots, and which flourished in texts produced in Arabic towards the end of the first millennium AD. Disease seemingly not only originated within the body and its immediate environs (for example, from the putrid air emanating from some decaying material) but also in reaction to more distant causes: namely, the particular conjunctions of heavenly bodies. Indeed, the regular revolutions of the planets through the celestial spheres apparently influenced all aspects of the world below, not only human health but also the health of animals, the growth and condition of plants, meteorological events and the fortunes of cities. Because of this, patients and healers were required to turn scrutiny not only inwards (to gauge the state of the human body) but also outwards, to chart, measure and observe events in the natural world.

Before moving on to establish how the interrelation between the micro- and the macro- cosmoses were understood in the health culture of cities like Norwich, it is worth pausing briefly to situate ourselves more precisely amongst the wider developments taking place in English medical literature at this time. The concentration of epidemic outbreaks in the second part of the fourteenth century[6] led to an explosion in the production of reference works relating to the subjects of health, healing and the human body. To judge from the surviving Middle English manuscript compendia, medical recipe collections constituted the most popular type of information, although works on herbs, uroscopy, bloodletting and charms were also well represented.[7] One historian has suggested that, in this context, value was attached

perceived providential aspects of disease, see H. Newton, *The Sick Child in Early Modern England, 1580–1720* (Oxford, 2012), pp. 202–8. On chemical medicine, see A. G. Debus, 'The Paracelsian Compromise in Elizabethan England', *Ambix* 8 (1960), 71–97.

6 Rawcliffe, *Urban Bodies*, tabulates instances in England in an appendix: 'National and Urban Epidemics, 1257–1530', pp. 360–74.

7 L. E. Voigts, 'Multitudes of Middle English Medical Manuscripts, or the Englishing of Science and Medicine', in *Manuscript Sources of Medieval Medicine*, ed. M. R. Schleissner (New York, 1995), pp. 183–95 (p. 192); G. R. Keiser, *A Manual*

'to the very idea of information' as a means of 'expanding control over ... natural and social environments'.[8] From the later fifteenth century, readers with the requisite purchasing power could supplement collections of manuscript material with printed texts such as manuals of advice (or 'governances') on how to minimize the likelihood of contracting pestilential diseases, or with encyclopaedic treatments of the body and its component parts.[9] During a third phase of development, from the middle third of the sixteenth century onwards, an interest in the regimen and in the environment is discernible in new formats, that is to say, in printed vernacular medical textbooks (for a socially circumscribed readership),[10] and almanacs (for readers across different socio-economic boundaries).[11] This development complemented and was stimulated by the publication of Greek and Latin editions of parts of the Galenic and Hippocratic corpus by European printing houses.[12] Whilst the absolute number of textbooks in circulation was limited, the evidence from Norwich indicates that the aspects of information they

of the Writings in Middle English 1050–1500: Vol. 10, Works of Science and Information (New Haven, 1998), p. 3595.

8 P. Murray Jones, 'Information and Science', in *Fifteenth-Century Attitudes: Perceptions of Society in Late Medieval England*, ed. R. Horrox (Cambridge, 1994), pp. 97–111 (p. 100).

9 On epidemic literature, see, below, p. 37–8. On one influential encyclopaedia, see below, p. 34, n. 5.

10 The vernacular texts are explored in Wear, *Knowledge and Practice*, chapter 4 (esp. pp. 158, 165), and in P. Slack, 'Mirrors of Health and Treasurers of Poor Men: The Uses of the Vernacular Medical Literature of Tudor England', in *Health, Medicine and Mortality in the Sixteenth Century*, ed. C. Webster (Cambridge, 1979), pp. 237–73 (p. 243, table 1, and pp. 238–40, 246–7). On questions of literacy, book ownership and readerships for both English and Latin medical literature, see P. Murray Jones, 'Medical Literacies and Medical Culture in Early Modern England', in *Medical Writing in Early Modern English*, ed. I. Taavitsainen and P. Pahta (Cambridge, 2011), pp. 30–43 (p. 38); P. Murray Jones, 'Reading Medicine in Tudor Cambridge', in *The History of Medical Education in Britain*, ed. V. Nutton and R. Porter (Amsterdam GA, 1995), pp. 153–81; P. Murray Jones, 'Book Ownership and the Lay Culture of Medicine in Tudor Cambridge', in *The Task of Healing: Medicine, Religion and Gender in England and the Netherlands, 1450–1800*, ed. H. Marland and M. Pelling (Rotterdam, 1996), pp. 49–68 (p. 49).

11 L. Kassell, 'Almanacs and Prognostications', in *The Oxford History of Popular Print Culture, Volume One: Cheap Print in Britain and Ireland to 1660*, ed. J. Raymond (Oxford, 2011), pp. 431–42 (pp. 438–40); Murray Jones, 'Medical Literacies', p. 32.

12 Of significance for the discussion below is one particular text from the ancient corpus: Hippocrates, *De aere aquis et locis*, here cited in English translation (Hippocrates, *AWP*, ed. Lloyd).

contained (derived from medieval textual and cultural roots) enjoyed much wider currency.

The first chapter of this book, which is perhaps especially useful for readers unfamiliar with pre-modern medical theories, taps into a reservoir of common knowledge in Norwich and the region about the body's vulnerability to conditions and events in the wider environment. It serves to supply the 'what to expect' part of Mrs Pants's dictum and in so doing moves between a range of sources not often analysed together. These include letters, poems, notes and manuscript compilations, financial accounts, recipe books, printed pamphlets, almanacs and a legal deposition. As we will see, the people who collected, shared or dispensed knowledge in this wide range of formats came from diverse backgrounds. William Cuningham, who we have already met in the introduction to this book, reappears from time to time in what immediately follows. He is joined by members of the local gentry (represented by the Paston family, Nicholas Bacon and Thomas Butts); literary East Anglian Benedictines, namely John Lydgate and William Bokenham; certain of Norwich's civic officers, that is, its chamberlains and one mayor, Nicholas Norgate; a parish churchwarden, Robert Reynes; Valentyne Bourne (a compiler of an exceptionally lengthy medical commonplace book); as well as university-trained physicians, including Andrew Boorde and John Caius. Chapter 2 narrows the focus to dissect only one text, Cuningham's *Cosmographical Glasse*, and shows how the author drew on this body of shared ideas and beliefs when producing his plan of Norwich (fig. 1).

1

Air and Smell: Hygiene and Networks of Authority in an Urban Context

> The world so wyde, the ayre so remevable,
> The sely man so lytell of stature,
> The greve [grave] and the ground of clothyng so mutable,
> The fyre so hote and subtyle of nature;
> Watyr never in oon: What creature
> Made of these [four], whyche be so flyttyng,
> May stable be, here in hyr lyvyng?[1]
>
> 'The Pageant of Knowledge', fifteenth century

In the pre-modern natural philosophical scheme all animate and inanimate things located in the elemental spheres of the world were conceived as composites of the 'pure and unadulterated' qualities of heat, coldness, dryness and moisture.[2] It followed that each of the four humours (the bodily fluids present in man which were named in the English tradition as blood, phlegm, choler and melancholy) were mixtures of the absolute elements, and were sensitive to environmental and cosmological changes.[3] Theoretically, an optimally functioning body required appropriate levels of each of the different humours.

1 John Lydgate (attrib.), 'The Pageant of Knowledge', in *The Minor Poems of John Lydgate*, ed. H. N. MacCracken, 2 vols., EETS OS 192 (London, 1911), II, 730. The poet drew on principles derived from Hippocrates and Galen as laid out in Avicenna's *Canon* (see especially book I, part II, thesis II, chapters 1–14).

2 Galen, *De temperamentis* I.viii, cf. 'Mixtures', in *Galen: Selected Works*, trans. P. N. Singer (Oxford, 1997), p. 223. The physiological scheme described in this paragraph and below was systematized by Thomas Elyot in *The Castel of Helthe* (London: Thomas Berthelet, 1539), fols. 1r–12r.

3 S. K. Heninger, *The Cosmographical Glass: Renaissance Diagrams of the Universe* (San Marino, 1977), pp. 108–10, 147–9; Wear, *Knowledge and Practice*, pp. 37–9.

However, the ideal seemed impossible to achieve in practice. The overall bodily ratio of warmth and cold, moisture and dryness supposedly varied naturally through the seasons and in accordance with a person's age, sex and physical surroundings.[4] Minor variations were considered normal, but if the disproportion was great, or if the humours putrefied because of some external factor acting upon them, then disease (it was believed) would invariably result.[5]

A person might rebalance or strengthen their constitution by ingesting a substance in which the missing qualities predominated, be it in the form of a food, a plant product, a compound drug (customized to suit the individual patient) or a vapour.[6] The restorative power of food, for example, was recognized in the private correspondence of Norfolk's most famous gentry family, the Pastons, who (amongst other properties and estates) had a town house in Coslany in the west of Norwich. In late September 1443, Margaret Paston dictated this earnest message in a postscript to a letter to her husband, who had recently suffered a 'grete dysese':

[4] Newton, *The Sick Child*, especially chapter 1, 'Humid Humours: Children's Bodies and Diseases'; Galen, *De sanitate tuenda* I.ii, cf. *A Translation of Galen's Hygiene (De sanitate tuenda)*, trans. R. M. Green (Springfield, 1951), pp. 6–8 (on age and constitution).

[5] On the nature of each humour and their susceptibilities, see Bartholomaeus Anglicus, *De proprietatibus rerum*, trans. John Trevisa (London: Thomas Berthelet, 1535), fols. 27v–32r (book 4, chapters 6–11). On the reception of this systematic and highly successful encyclopaedia, written *c.* 1240, see H. Meyer, *Die Enzyklopädie des Bartholomäus Anglicus: Untersuchungen zur Überlieferungs- und Rezeptionsgeschichte von 'De Proprietatibus Rerum'* (Munich, 2000), pp. 261–80 (esp. pp. 266–71 on marks in manuscripts left by readers with medical interests), and see pp. 379–81 on English translations of the text. An edition of a fourteenth-century Latin manuscript version and late fourteenth-century French translation are now in production, with two volumes already in print: Bartholomaeus Anglicus, *De proprietatibus rerum: Volume I: Introduction générale, Prohemium, et Libri I–IV*, ed. B. Van den Abeele, H. Meyer, M. W. Twomey, B. Roling, R. J. Long, De Diversis Artibus 78, n.s. 41 (Turnhout, 2007); Bartholomaeus Anglicus, *De proprietatibus rerum: Volume VI: Liber XVII*, ed. I. Ventura, De Diversis Artibus 79, n.s. 42 (Turnhout, 2007). Trevisa's highly engaging and clear English translation was produced in *c.* 1398–99. For a modern edition, see *On the Properties of Things: John Trevisa's Translation of Bartholomaeus Anglicus De Proprietatibus Rerum*, ed. M. C. Seymour, 3 vols. (Oxford, 1975–88); and (on the 1535 edition and the (English) *editio princeps* by Wynkyn de Worde) see Meyer, *Die Enzyklopädie des Bartholomäus Anglicus*, pp. 403–4, 407.

[6] On food, for example, see K. Albala, *Eating Right in the Renaissance* (Berkeley, 2002), especially pp. 174–7.

> My modyr ... prayith yow, and I pray yow also, that ye be wel dyetyd of mete [food] and dryngke, for that is the grettest helpe that ye may have now to your helthe ward [i.e. for the guardianship of your health].[7]

In addition to augmenting or modifying his or her diet, a patient could undertake a range of activities to dispel a morbid plethora, release an internal blockage or counteract an unhealthy movement of humoral fluids within the body. These measures might include taking a bath, exercising or having one's blood let by a phlebotomist. As Galen put it: 'the attempt is to remedy an excess by the introduction of what is missing in order to bring about a state which may be described as well-balanced or median'.[8] Of course, it was better not to become ill in the first place. For a healthy individual the appropriate regimen was not corrective but preventative, prescribing foods, drinks, activities and surroundings that matched and maintained a person's natural composition or life stage.[9]

The non-naturals: the primacy of air

All bodies by necessity apparently performed functions and encountered things and experiences on an everyday basis which, if not carefully moderated, might harm them.[10] These factors – the so-called 'non-naturals' – fell under six broad headings, and were categorized as: contact with the ambient air; motion (or exercise) and rest; sleep and waking; substances consumed as food; substances evacuated or retained as nutriment; and 'things befalling the soul'. Of these factors, the first – air – was arguably the most important because it surrounded the body all the time, was drawn inside it by the process of respiration and was essential for life.[11] One vernacular poet, musing about

[7] *Paston Letters and Papers of the Fifteenth Century*, ed. N. Davis, 3 vols., EETS SS 20–2 (Oxford, 2004–05), I, 219.

[8] Galen, *De temperamentis* I.iii, cf. Galen, 'Mixtures', in *Selected Works*, trans. Singer, p. 206.

[9] On the appropriate times for applying either opposite or similar therapies, see Galen, *De sanitate tuenda* I.vii, cf. *Galen's Hygiene*, trans. Green, p. 23.

[10] K. van 't Land, 'Internal Yet Extrinsic: Conceptions of Bodily Space and their Relation to Causality in Late Medieval University Medicine', in *Medicine and Space: Body, Surroundings and Borders in Antiquity and the Middle Ages*, ed. P. A. Baker, H. Nijdam and K. van 't Land (Leiden, 2012), pp. 85–116.

[11] 'Ayre, among al thynges not natural, is chiefly to be observed, forasmoch as it doth both inclose us, and also enter into our bodyes, specially the most noble

the qualities of each of the four elements, described the underlying physiological process in this fashion:

> Ayre of kynde geveth inspiracion
> To mannys hert, thyng most temperatyf,
> And kyndly hete geveth respiracion,
> Of subtyll, rare, and a gret medegatyf,
> To tempre the spyrytes by vertew vegetatyf …[12]

A good supply of pure, clean air was thus essential to the functioning of one of the body's most important component parts: the heart. Conversely, bad air or vapours were considered to be especially injurious to the body. Whilst sweet smells might restore a person's senses, the *sensible virtue* (that is, the power rooted in the brain which governed the faculties of vision, hearing, olfaction, tasting and touch) risked being 'corupte[d] and greved by stynkynge smelles'.[13] The last non-natural – 'things befalling the soul' – loosely signified various aspects of thought or feeling, including the experiences of joy, hope, dread, sorrow, anger and love, all of which supposedly had a physiological basis.[14] Again, feelings could be manipulated according to one's surroundings or carefully planned sensory stimuli. The thirteenth-century *Regimen sanitatis Salerni* by Joannes de Mediolano, printed in a popular English translation in 1528, confirmed the interrelationship between the non-naturals when noting: 'nothinge maketh a man more jocunde and lesse hevye

member, which is the hart': Elyot, *Castel of Helthe*, fol. 12r.

12 The element of air, of its nature, causes breath to be drawn in to the heart, which is a thing most tempering; whilst the innate heat [of the body] gives rise to respiration. Air is fine, light, and a great palliative, balancing the spirits by the vegetative [or animating/life-giving] virtue: see 'The Pageant of Knowledge', in Lydgate, *Minor Poems*, II, 731. The poem, which survives in several manuscripts copies and fragments, and in print as part of Geoffrey Chaucer, *The Love and Complayntes bytwene Mars and Venus* (Westminster: Julian Notary, ?1500), sig. [B7r], is generally attributed to Lydgate though its exact provenance is not known. It may have originated in London, and parts of it may have been publicly performed: John Lydgate, *Mummings and Entertainments*, ed. C. Sponsler (Kalamazoo, 2010), pp. 125–6. For the divisions of the soul into a hierarchy of vegetable, sensitive and rational parts and the various powers allocated to each, see T. Dixon, *From Passions to Emotions: The Creation of a Secular Psychological Category* (Cambridge, 2003), pp. 29–61.

13 Bartholomaeus Anglicus, *De proprietatibus rerum*, trans. Trevisa, fol. 13v (book 3, chapter 12), see also 18r–v (book 3, chapter 19) on smell.

14 On sorrow and joy, see Elyot, *Castel of Helthe*, fols. 66r–70r.

[or oppressed] than to walke in clere aier'.[15] As befitted his status as an academically trained physician, our map-maker, William Cuningham, was expert in regulating such factors according to the needs of a patient. This is apparent in letter from Cuningham to the surgeon John Halle who consulted the physician over a case of *chamaeleontiasis cum icteritia nigra* (that is, of the *morbus gallicus* or pox with black jaundice) as part of a wider bid to gain Cuningham's endorsements for his (Halle's) own cures.[16] In addition to therapeutic bleeding, custom-made drugs and dietary modifications, Cuningham recommended a strict regimen. He suggested that the air surrounding the patient should be altered so that it was 'temparatt declyning to moystnes', that he should have neither too much or too little sleep, should exercise with lead weights and should be 'provokyd to urine[ate]'. With 'theis ways observyd', he reassured, 'all obstructyons shall be openyd, all dystemperaunce banyshed the venom extingwyshed and nature restoryd to her wontyd and pristynatt estatt'.[17]

Medical writers recognized, however, that in an urban context it was not always possible to avoid substances or situations that were risky for the body, particularly corrupt air or bad smells. Galen himself itemized the most dangerous things that a citizen was likely to encounter. These included decomposing animal or vegetable matter, manure, the kinds of stifling air found near particular rivers, marshes or topographical features, and closed-up, unventilated houses.[18] His list was rehearsed and invested with fresh importance by physicians and other commentators who witnessed the devastation wrought by the epidemic diseases of the fifteenth and sixteenth centuries.[19] For

15 Joannes de Mediolano, *Regimen sanitatis Salerni*, trans. Thomas Paynell (London: Thomas Berthelet, 1528), sig. I3v.

16 On the identity of *chamaeleontiasis*, and Cuningham as an authority therein, see Thomas Gale, 'An Excellent Treatise of Wounds made with Gonneshot', in *Certaine Workes of Chirurgerie* (London: Rowland Hall, 1563), fol. 9v.

17 Oxford, Bodleian Library, MS Bodley 178, fols. 34v–6v. On the astrological and meteorological causes of *chamaeliontiasis*, see Cuningham, *A&P* 1564, 'Prognostication', sig. A4v.

18 Galen, *De sanitate tuenda* I.xi, cf. *Galen's Hygiene*, trans. Green, pp. 35–6. Galen's words were made newly available to academics in a translation by Thomas Linacre published in Paris in 1517.

19 See, for example, a tract on escaping the English sweating sickness (1485) by the London-based physician Thomas Forestier: London, British Library, Add. MS. 27582, fol. 71v. Amongst other things, Forestier suggested avoiding 'stynken caryn [carrion] cast in the water nye to the cytees or townes, as the boles

example, a poem known to literary historians as the 'Doctrine for Pestilence' began with a general injunction that anyone 'who will been holle and kepe hym from sekenesse/ and resiste the strok of pestilence', should 'flee wikkyd heires [airs]' and 'eschew the presence/ Off infect placys', taking care always to 'smelle swote thynges and ... walk in cleene heir'.[20] This memorable advice was penned by John Lydgate (d. ?1451), an alumnus of Oxford University, and a Benedictine monk at the abbey of Bury St Edmunds, Suffolk (map 1), best known today as the author of the *Troy Book* and the *Fall of Princes*.[21]

Up to a point, urban men and women could rely on civic authorities to regulate day-to-day environmental hazards like those itemized by Galen.[22] The dumping of refuse, dung and other matter in the streets

[bowels] of bestes and of fysshes ... also of the castyng of stynkyng waters and many other foule thinges in the stretes [by which] the ayre is corrupte[d]'. See also Bengt Knutsson (attrib.), *Here Begynneth a Litill Boke Necessarye and Behovefull Agenst the Pestilence* (London: William de Machlinia, *c.* 1485), fols. [3v–4r], which similarly counselled that people ought to: 'eschewe every cause of putrifatcion and stinking ... [and] every foule stinche ... [namely] of stabyl, stinkyng feldes, wayes or stretes, and ... stinkyng dede careyn and moste of [all] stynking waters where in many places water is kepte 2 dayes or 2 nightes; or ellys [where] ther be gutters of water casten under therthe whiche causeth grete stinke and corrupcion ... Like wise in that place wher the wurtes [worts] and coles [cabbages] putrefied it maketh a noyfull [harmful] savour' (on this treatise, itself adapted from a very similar text attributed to Joanne Jacobi (d. 1384), see J. P. Pickett, 'A Translation of the "Canutus" Plague Treatise', in *Popular and Practical Science of Medieval England*, ed. L. M. Matheson (East Lansing, 1994), pp. 263–82; Keiser, 'Medieval Plague Treatises', pp. 318–22).

20 Lydgate, *Minor Poems*, II, 702.

21 Lydgate repeated the same counsel in his popular *Medecyne for the Stomacke* or *Dietary*, which circulated as an appendix to a treatise by John of Burgundy on regimen. According to one expert, this text 'ranks first amongst Lydgate's writings in the number of surviving [manuscript] copies, and third among all Middle English verse texts': L. R. Mooney, 'Diet and Bloodletting: A Monthly Regimen', in *Popular and Practical Science*, ed. Matheson, pp. 245–61 (p. 245). It was also printed twice in our period: John Lydgate and John of Burgundy, *In this Tretyse that is Cleped Governayle of Helthe* (Westminster: William Caxton, 1490) and *Here Begynneth a Lytell Treatyse Called the Governall of Helthe with the Medycyne of the Stomacke* (London: Wynkyn de Worde, *c.* 1506).

22 For example, *The Coventry Leet Book 1420–1555*, ed. M. Dormer Harris, 4 vols., EETS OS 134–5, 138, 146 (London, 1907–13), I, 23 (street cleaning and dung removal), 43 (disposal of offal and blood), 58–9 (paving, removal of privies emptying into watercourse), 91 (preserving cleanliness of the river), 113 (proper use of corporate muck-heaps), 170 (river cleansing), 192 (vegetable refuse), 199 (paving), 208 (river cleaning, entrails), 254 (cleaning of town ditch, urine disposal). For the capital, see *Calendar of Letter-Books of the City of*

and watercourses was controlled in many urban centres.[23] Ideally, however, people should not rely on corporate measures, but take their own sanitary precautions at home; in this way, they could secure their health before stepping out of the door.

Sanitation begins at home: cleansing buildings

The Paston letters testify to the perceived importance of warmth, hygiene and clean air within a household. One of John Paston II's first complaints to his mother, Margaret, when he arrived in new lodgings in London in the summer of 1479, was to note that neither his chamber nor his belongings were as clean as he supposed they ought to be.[24] He confessed the discovery greatly troubled him, no doubt because plague was cutting through the city, and he feared for his health. As a plague treatise published in London shortly afterwards reassured its readers, infected air would be kept out of a house if it was dirt-free, fumigated with herbs and had a clear burning wood fire flaming away inside it.[25]

Writing in the early 1540s, the physician Andrew Boorde (d. 1549) echoed these concerns when he argued that a person's health would benefit greatly from decent accommodation. Since he catered (or so he claimed) for a market of 'simple and unlearned' citizens, Boorde's advice could readily be scaled down into a basic philosophy for

London, 1275–1498, Books A-L, ed. R. R. Sharpe, 11 vols. (London, 1899–1912), A, 183 (street cleaning, *c.* 1275–81), 212 (clearing watercourse, 1286–87); D, 192, 201 (oath of scavengers and sergeants of the channel, fifteenth century), 312 (survey of pavements, 1312); F, 125 (streets, 1345); H, 108 (waterways, 1378); E. L. Sabine, 'City Cleaning in Medieval London', *Speculum* 12 (1937), 19–43; *PMR* (1364–81), II, 140–1 (filth at Tower Hill, 1372); *Memorials of London and London Life, 1276–1419*, ed. H. T. Riley (London, 1868), pp. 435–6 (street cleaning, 1379). For Norwich, see Part III below.

23 See Rawcliffe, *Urban Bodies*, pp. 134–52, 197–210; D. Jørgensen, '"All Good Rule of the Citee": Sanitation and Civic Government in England, 1400–1600', *Journal of Urban History* 36 (2010), 300–15. For the European context, see J. Henderson, 'Public Health, Pollution and the Problem of Waste Disposal in Early Modern Tuscany', in *Economic and Biological Interactions in Pre-industrial Europe from the Thirteenth to the Eighteenth Centuries*, ed. S. Cavaciocchi (Florence, 2010), pp. 373–82.

24 *Paston Letters and Papers*, ed. Davis, I, 515.

25 Knutsson, *A Litill Boke … Agenst the Pestilence*, fol. [4r].

everyday domestic management.[26] He elaborated on the point in a section of his *Dyetary of Helth*, a text that he dedicated to his erstwhile employer, the premier magnate of England, Thomas Howard, 3rd duke of Norfolk.[27] (Thomas's son, Henry, earl of Surrey, was himself considering what site to choose in Norwich for a new residence at the time.)[28] Boorde argued that a house should provide a good view. He went on to explain that if the eye was not content with what it saw, the brain would also suffer, for if:

> the mynde can not be contended, the herte can be not pleased; yf the herte and mynde be not pleased, nature doth abhorre. And yf nature do abhorre, mortyfyeacyon of the vytall, and anymall and spyrytuall powers [the life-giving forces of the body] do consequently folowe.[29]

But the most important consideration in Boorde's opinion, was, of course, that the air surrounding the house 'can not be to[o] clene and pure'. Houses which stood next to 'stynkynge and putryfyed standyng waters ... stynkynge dyches, gutters ... canelles [water channels] ... [and] corrupt dunghylles' were liable to infect the blood and engender poisonous humours in the human body, putrefying the brain and corrupting the heart with fatal consequences.[30] For this reason, Boorde noted, a housebuilder should ideally give thought to providing access to 'a fayre gardain repleted with herbes of aromatyck and redolent savours', and to properly maintaining the external parts of a property such as stables, privies and ponds.[31] Such dire warnings certainly impressed very wealthy housebuilders. The statesman Sir Nicholas

[26] In reality, only a tiny minority had the financial means to erect the kind of 'mansion' house he describes. For context, see Leon Battista Alberti, *De re aedificatoria* I.iii–iv; IV.ii; V.xiv; V.xvii, cf. *On the Art of Building in Ten Books*, trans. J. Rykwert, N. Leach and R. Tavernor (Cambridge MA, 1988).

[27] Boorde, whilst lodging with Sir Robert Drury, had been called upon to provide medical treatment for the duke in 1530: F. J. Furnivall, 'Forewords', in Andrew Boorde, *The Fyrst Boke of the Introduction of Knowledge*, ed. F. J. Furnivall, EETS ES 10 (London, 1870), pp. 48–9.

[28] E. A. Kent, 'The Houses of the Dukes of Norfolk in Norwich', *NA* 24 (1932), 73–87.

[29] Andrew Boorde, *Dyetary of Helth* (London: Robert Wyer, 1542), sig. B3v. Boorde's advice on building and maintaining a healthy house was subsequently extracted into a short black letter pamphlet: Andrew Boorde, *The Boke for to Learne a Man to be Wyse in Buyldyng of his Howse for the Helth of Body* (London: Robert Wyer, 1550).

[30] Boorde, *Dyetary of Helth*, sig. B4r–v.

[31] Ibid., sig. C2v.

Bacon (d. 1579), a man of considerable influence and property in Norfolk and Suffolk, conveyed concern to his kinsman, the royal minister William Cecil, when he noted that the latter had situated a privy too near to the main lodgings at his new palatial dwelling at Theobalds: a rash decision given the risk of offensive smells. Bacon opined that, in this case, it would have been 'bettr to have offendyd yor yey outward than yor nose inward'.[32]

The records of Norwich's government from the mid-sixteenth century show that civic officers were similarly anxious to sanitize the corporation's buildings. In the accounting year 1537/38, the city's principal financial officer, the chamberlain, recorded a payment for frankincense 'to heire the counsell chamber' at the guildhall.[33] Frankincense was considered a particularly effective domestic fumigant in times of pestilence or sweating sickness.[34] However, in this instance the resin was apparently purchased for a different purpose: to freshen the area following construction works.[35] Boorde later urged would-be architects to take similar precautions. He suggested that recently erected houses should always have 'a fyre kept contynually for a space to drye up the contagyous moysters of the walles, and the savour of the lyme and sande'. This done, he reassured, the building could be

[32] *Calendar of the State Papers Relating to Scotland and Mary, Queen of Scots, 1547–1603: Vol. I. A.D. 1547–1563*, ed. J. Bain (Edinburgh, 1898), p. 425 (17 June 1560), also cited in R. Tittler, *Nicholas Bacon: The Making of a Tudor Statesman* (Ohio, 1976), p. 66. For context, see also H. Smith, 'Concept and Compromise: Sir Nicholas Bacon and the Building of Stiffkey Hall', in *East Anglia's History: Studies in Honour of Norman Scarfe*, ed. C. Harper-Bill, C. Rawcliffe and R. Wilson (Woodbridge, 2002), pp. 159–88.

[33] NCR 18a/6 CA 1537–47, fol. 13r. A condensed English version of the longer of two Latin manuscripts of John of Burgundy's plague treatises – the most widely circulating authority on the disease in fifteenth-century England – suggested the burning of juniper or, if this could not be found, frankincense, 'if the ayre [in a house] be corrupte'. Under the title *The Myrour or Glasse of Helthe*, this recommendation reached a wide readership, twenty-one imprints of the text being made between *c.* 1530 and 1580: Keiser, 'Medieval Plague Treatises', pp. 294, 307. John Caius also recommended frankincense – burnt with myrrh and dry rose leaves – for a fumigant against the sweating sickness: John Caius, *A Boke or Counseill Against the Disease Commonly Called the Sweate or Sweatyng Sicknesse* (London: Richard Grafton, 1552), fol. 24r. The supplies would have been available to residents of Norwich in the nearby 'spicery', the apothecaries' row in the market, on the location of which, see John Kirkpatrick, *The Streets and Lanes of the City of Norwich*, ed. W. Hudson (Norwich, 1889) p. 32.

[34] Boorde, *Dyetary of Helth*, sig. L3v.

[35] NCR 18a/5 CA 1531–37, fols. 28r, 56v, 63r, 83v.

put to use 'without takynge any inconvenyence of syckenes'.[36] Civic officers also fumigated the council's rooms whenever Boorde's patron, Howard, was intending to visit Norwich.[37] In 1542, the chamberlain recorded a payment:

> for perfume to make the cownsell chambyr swete ageynst my lord of Norffolk's coming to the citie 3 severall days; that is to saye, every day a perfume panne made with damast water and clows 12*d*., and for perfume candyles every day, 2*d*.[38]

Two years later, when the duke was due to make an appearance that was, in fact, postponed due to a bout of ill health, the procedure was repeated. An 'ownce of perfume brent in the cownsell chambyr to heyer the howse' was accompanied by another sprinkling of damask water and cloves. When Howard finally did arrive, a second consignment of perfume pans was purchased and, for good measure, the building was thoroughly swept and re-perfumed.[39] Civic rooms were also fumigated when large meetings left the atmosphere stuffy and stale. In 1542, after the aldermen (the city's senior elected officials) had gathered to watch an interlude in the assembly hall, the chamberlain

[36] Boorde, *Dyetary of Helth*, sig. C3r.

[37] 'Norwich Cathedral Priory Gardeners' Accounts, 1329–1530', ed. C. Noble, in *Farming and Gardening in Late Medieval Norfolk*, ed. C. Noble, C. E. Moreton and P. Rutledge, NRS 61 (Norwich, 1997), pp. 1–93 (p. 9). Cuningham's patron, Robert Dudley, earl of Leicester (d. 1588), would appear to have been equally perturbed by the thought of encountering pockets of bad air, if his financial accounts are a good guide. In the course of the epidemic year 1558–59, Dudley – then the intimate of Queen Elizabeth I – spent an extraordinary amount of money on perfumes and a perfume pan, perfumed gloves, pomanders and nosegays, musk, cloves, fragrant strewing herbs, flowers and rose water, whilst his favourite perfumer, one Cooke, accrued payments to the extraordinary value of £72 for his services: *Household Accounts and Disbursement Books of Robert Dudley, Earl of Leicester, 1558–1561, 1584–86*, ed. S. Adams, Camden 5th series 6 (Cambridge, 1995), pp. 48, 52, 54, 57–8, 61–5, 70, 82, 84, 97, 102, 119. On Dudley as a patron to astrologers, see B. Capp, *Astrology and the Popular Press: English Almanacs 1500–1800* (London, 1979), p. 180.

[38] NCR 18a/7 CA 1541–49, fol. 71^{v}.

[39] NCR 18a/7 CA 1541–49, fol. 174r–v. On one occasion, the chamberlain also ensured that the marketplace was swept in advance, lest ordure and rubbish there should offend the health-conscious aristocrat *en route* to the guildhall: NCR 18a/6 CA 1537–47, fol. 85v. Similarly, alderman Augustine Steward had the guildhall swept and perfumed in honour of a visit by the collectors of a royal subsidy in 1546: NCR 18a/7 CA 1541–49, fol. 252r.

spent 1*d*. on perfuming the rooms which 'savoured sore', whilst the guildhall's 'jakes' (latrines) were also cleaned.[40]

Countering cosmological influences: exerting control through prediction and observation

Taking precautions for health at the most local level – that is, within the four walls of one's own house – was relatively straightforward, at least for those with the resources in time, cash or labour to fulfil the requirements of good hygienic practice. However, in a universe where even the elements themselves were apparently mutable and fickle, the body also seemed vulnerable to a wide array of seasonal, meteorological and cosmological influences which could not be so easily circumvented. To begin with, the circuit of the planets through the twelve houses of the zodiac seemingly precipitated damaging climatic changes and turbulences. The sign of Cancer, for example, was believed to rule over some particularly perilous dates including the *canicular* days of summer when the atmosphere was deemed especially mutable, and the body, therefore, especially susceptible.[41] Meanwhile, less predictable 'accydentes and mutation of the ayre',[42] encountered alongside extreme meteorological conditions, comets, earthquakes and eclipses, also apparently caused, accompanied or foretold outbreaks of a wide range of devastating diseases.[43] The

[40] NCR 18a/6 CA 1537–47, fols. 114v, 121v; 18a/7 CA 1541–49, fol. 71r(b).

[41] Bartholomaeus Anglicus, *De proprietatibus rerum*, trans. Trevisa, fol. 123r (book 8, chapter 13); Hippocrates, *AWP*, ed. Lloyd, pp. 157–9.

[42] Cuningham [Kenningham], *A&P* 1558, 'Prognostication', sig. A3r.

[43] For a prediction that a lunar eclipse, visible from Norwich on 2 April 1558 at 10:42 pm would be followed by 'many strange diseases ... both in man and beast', see Cuningham [Kenningham], *A&P* 1558, 'Almanacke', sig. A3r. See also S. J. Schechner, *Comets, Popular Culture and the Birth of Modern Cosmology* (Princeton, 1997), pp. 91–103. On meteorological causes of epidemics, see Hippocrates, *AWP*, ed. Lloyd, p. 150, and see the heavy emphasis upon changeable weather, comets, falling stars, thunder and lightning in prognostications for pestilence in Pickett, 'A Translation of the "Canutus" Plague Treatise', pp. 270–1 (a text rendered into English at some point in the second half of the fifteenth century): 'The tokens of pestilence of the pronosticacion be 7 ... The furste ys whan in a sommer day, the aer often tymes chyaunge, as in the mornyng yt appyereth as yt wolde raen, then after yt ys cloudy, and after wyndy, and namely of sowthern wynde. The 2nd token ys whan often tyme in summer the days sheod derke, as yt wil raen and raen not, and yf thys contynue longe, yt ys for to drede of gret pestilence. The 3rd token ys whan yt appyereth many flyes

threats were such that the author of the 'Pageant of Knowledge' (citing Galen) wondered how a man could maintain a stable course through life when beset by 'all weathers', 'contrary winds', 'variable seasons' and the movements of heavenly bodies.[44] The moralists' answer, of course, was to firmly fix one's eyes on the certainties of eternal life. But pragmatists tried to categorize the likely outcomes of particular types of astronomical or meteorological events in order to take suitable precautions.

During the last third of the fifteenth century, Robert Reynes – a constable and churchwarden of the parish of Acle, which is situated about twelve miles west of Norwich in the Norfolk Broads – jotted down in his commonplace book several rules for health maintenance in which events in the worldly and heavenly spheres featured heavily. Reynes is perhaps indicative of what a pious, literate man of relatively modest standing may have understood about his body's place in the cosmos.[45] Alongside facts and material of general interest – statutes of the realm, weights and measures, notes about local and national geography, prayers and saints' lives, recipes for ink, and the histories of his family and parish – Reynes recorded the zodiac signs that related to each season, and the likely destinies of individuals born under

upon the yerth, and this betokeneth that the aer ys enffect and venemouse. The 4th token ys whan the sterrys often tymes yt symeth that they falle adoun, and also yt ys a token that the aer ys enffect, and that many venemouse vapours be in the aer. The 5th token hys whan you sye the Sterre Cometta, yt symeth that yt dow flye, as it ys hade in [*De*] *Methauris* ... yt ys a token of mens deth in battelys, etcetera. *Unde* this verse: *Mors furit, urbs rapitur/ Seuit mare, sol operitur/ Regnum mutatur, plebs peste fame cruciatur.* The 6th token ys whan moche lyttyngs and tounderyng beth, and namely whan yt cummeth on the south syde. The 7th token ys whane moche wynde and ventosite cumme of the south syde, for they be stynkyng and unclenly.'

44 Lydgate, *Minor Poems*, II, 732. The poet noted that autumn was a season in which the human body was especially liable to experience rapid changes, predisposing it 'to many uncouthe [and] straunge infirmitees'. John Paston III was likewise chary about the effects inclement weather might have on his health: 'the wedyr is siche that I wyll not jopart [risk] to ryde as yet, for I am not best at ease and a lytill colde myght mak me worse': *Paston Letters and Papers*, ed. Davis, I, 629 (*c.* 1500).

45 For Reynes's biography, see T. Kohnen, 'Commonplace-Book Communication: Role Shifts and Text Functions in Robert Reynes's Notes Contained in MS Tanner 407', in *Communicating Early English Manuscripts*, ed. P. Pahta and A. H. Jucker (Cambridge, 2011), pp. 13–24 (pp. 15–16).

particular constellations.[46] He also copied calculations of the distances between cosmic entities,[47] and movable dates, in addition to charms against fever and toothache, sudden death and falling sickness, information about the best times to phlebotomize, and rules for forecasting the weather.[48] For this last, Reynes reproduced a system derived from the position of Sunday in the first week of any given year (the annual 'dominical letter').[49] For example, Reynes (echoing Metham's prognostications referenced below) noted down troubling predictions for when Sunday fell on the sixth day of January:

> Whanne the domincall lettyr fallyth upon the *F*, than shall be a blakke wynter and also a scharppe colde; a drye somer; plente of oyle; gret sekenesse of eyne [eyes] be but comon; deth of yonge people; gret werre in dyvers placys and erthe qwawghe [earth quakes] etc.

Sunday falling on the seventh day of January could bring troubles as well:

> Whanne the domincall lettyr fallyth upon the *G*, than xal be a warme wynter and a dyvers [changeable] somer; gret plente of corn; gret tempest of fyer of howsys; grete sekenesse of the apcesse [abscess]; plente of be[a]n; gret fellyngges of tymber; deth of olde people; and gret plente of heyres.[50]

Two generations later, William Cuningham devised more elaborate meteorological prognostications and phlebotomy charts based on similar principles. He published these in a series of printed almanacs

46 On the zodiac and the seasons, see Oxford, Bodleian Library, MS Tanner 407, fol. 34r. For a published edition see Robert Reynes, *The Commonplace Book of Robert Reynes of Acle: An Edition of Tanner MS. 407*, ed. C. Louis (New York, 1980), and see C. L. S. Linnell, 'The Commonplace Book of Robert Reynys of Acle', *NA* 32 (1962), pp. 111–27.

47 That is, the distance in leagues between the earth and the firmament of the stars, and of all of the planets in between.

48 MS Tanner 407, fols. 11v–13r, 15r, 19v, 34v, 54r, 64v; Linnell, 'Commonplace Book', 113–17, 126.

49 If the letters A to G are assigned iteratively to the first seven days of the year starting with 'A' for the first of January, the letter assigned to the first Sunday of the year (and thus to all subsequent Sundays) is the dominical letter. 29 February is generally skipped. For an explanation of this and related calendric conventions, see S. Kusukawa, 'Andreas Nolthius's *Almanach* for 1575', *Journal for the History of Astronomy* 42 (2011), 91–110 (p. 92).

50 MS Tanner 407, fol. 53r–v.

which constitute some of the earliest examples of this type of literature to survive in English. Judging by their content, they were probably intended to appeal to a diverse readership including professional phlebotomists, apothecaries and domestic readers, as well as Cuningham's professional colleagues. The first in his series of publications is now lost.[51] The second (calculated for the Norwich meridian) gave guidance on the changing aspects of the moon, 'the varietie of the ayre, also of the windes throughout the whole yeare', and listed propitious times to make commercial exchanges and begin journeys.[52] Cuningham went on to produce subsequent editions calculated for London between 1559–63 and 1565–66, although most no longer survive.[53] Each of Cuningham's extant almanacs opens with an illustration of an astrological figure depicting the zodiac signs governing particular parts of the body. In his earliest surviving version, he also included a table which marked out not only the highlights in the liturgical calendar, but also the days in that particular year which were suitable for bloodletting, taking medicines or planting medicinal herbs (fig. 2).[54] He also noted the exact times of particular days at which the seasons would begin and end (according to the position of the sun on the ecliptic), and listed the diseases that were likely to predominate in each quarter according to the aspects and conjunctions of the planets.[55] For autumn 1558, for example, he made this alarming prediction:

> [T]his quarter shall not be but moderate in heate, geven unto rayne, and som thunder; victualles shall be reasonable sould ... [but m]any new and perilous diseases [there] shal be, and mortalitie. For both *Luna* [the moon], lady of this last quarter, is wyth the Dragons Tail [the constellation of Draco] in *sexta* [the sixth house] and also *Mercurius*, lord of thascendent is ther combust of [i.e. in conjunction with] the sunne,

[51] See Cuningham [Kenningham], *A&P* 1558, 'Prognostication', sig. A2r–v for evidence of its existence.

[52] Cuningham [Kenningham], *A&P* 1558. For the theoretical constructs underpinning this, see L. M. Matheson and A. Shannon, 'A Treatise on the Election of Times', in *Popular and Practical Science*, ed. Matheson, pp. 23–59 (pp. 24–5, 47–59); I. Taavitsainen, 'A Zodiacal Lunary for Medical Professionals', in ibid., pp. 283–300 (pp. 289–91, 293–300).

[53] Cuningham, *A&P* 1564; Cuningham, *A&P* 1566; Capp, *Astrology and the Popular Press*, p. 357.

[54] On these themes in other, similar pamphlets, see Kusukawa, 'Andreas Nolthius's *Almanach*', pp. 97–9.

[55] For example, Cuningham [Kenningham], *A&P* 1558, 'Prognostication', sigs. A8r–B2r, B6r–v.

> wherfore manye yonge persons and children shalbe in daunger: as in the spring time, there shall be pestilent fevers, *colica* passions, cold reumes, distillations of the humoures from the head, putrifaction of the lunges and other many [diseases].[56]

Cuningham justified his enterprise with reference to the ancient Hippocratic tract *Airs, Waters, Places,* which supposedly endorsed astrology and astronomy as appropriate tools for medical practice.[57] A celebrated passage of that work maintained that a physician should be able to gauge the rising and setting of the stars in order to 'foretell the progress of the year',[58] not least because seasonal changes purportedly altered bodily states.[59] Thus armed with a thorough understanding of the seasons, a practitioner could rest assured that:

> with the passage of time ... he would know what epidemics to expect, both in the summer and the winter, and what particular disadvantages threatened an individual who changed his mode of life [i.e., his regimen].[60]

Professionals like Cuningham tried to encourage people to leave prognostications to the experts. Accessing the advice of a specialist – in print or in person – was one thing, especially if one were taking laudable precautions to secure one's health. Meddling with more occult aspects of divining, however, was dangerous territory – as a group of Norwich practitioners found out to their cost. A deposition delivered to the Norwich justices of the peace in 1528 reported that a

[56] Ibid., sigs. B1v–2r.

[57] As reported in William Fulke, *Antiprognosticon* (London: Henry Sutton, 1560), sig. C6v. The author subverted Cuningham's position for his own polemical advantage. See also below, p. 64.

[58] Hippocrates, *AWP*, ed. Lloyd, p. 149. For the context in which the Hippocratic tract was written, see L. Taub, *Ancient Meteorology* (London, 2003), chapter 2; V. Nutton, *Ancient Medicine*, 2nd edn (Abingdon, 2013), pp. 274–5.

[59] See Hippocrates, 'The Nature of Man', ed. Lloyd, p. 264 where, for example, it is argued that 'the quantity of phlegm in the body increases in winter because it is that bodily substance most in keeping with the winter seeing that it is the coldest'. Symptoms reflected this humoral imbalance: 'people spit and blow from their noses the most phlegmatic mucus in winter; swellings become white ... and other diseases show phlegmatic signs'.

[60] Hippocrates, *AWP*, ed. Lloyd, pp. 148–9. Prognostications could then be made accordingly, as the following aphorism demonstrates: 'If the summer is rainy with southerly winds and the autumn similar, the winter will necessarily be unhealthy': ibid., p. 158.

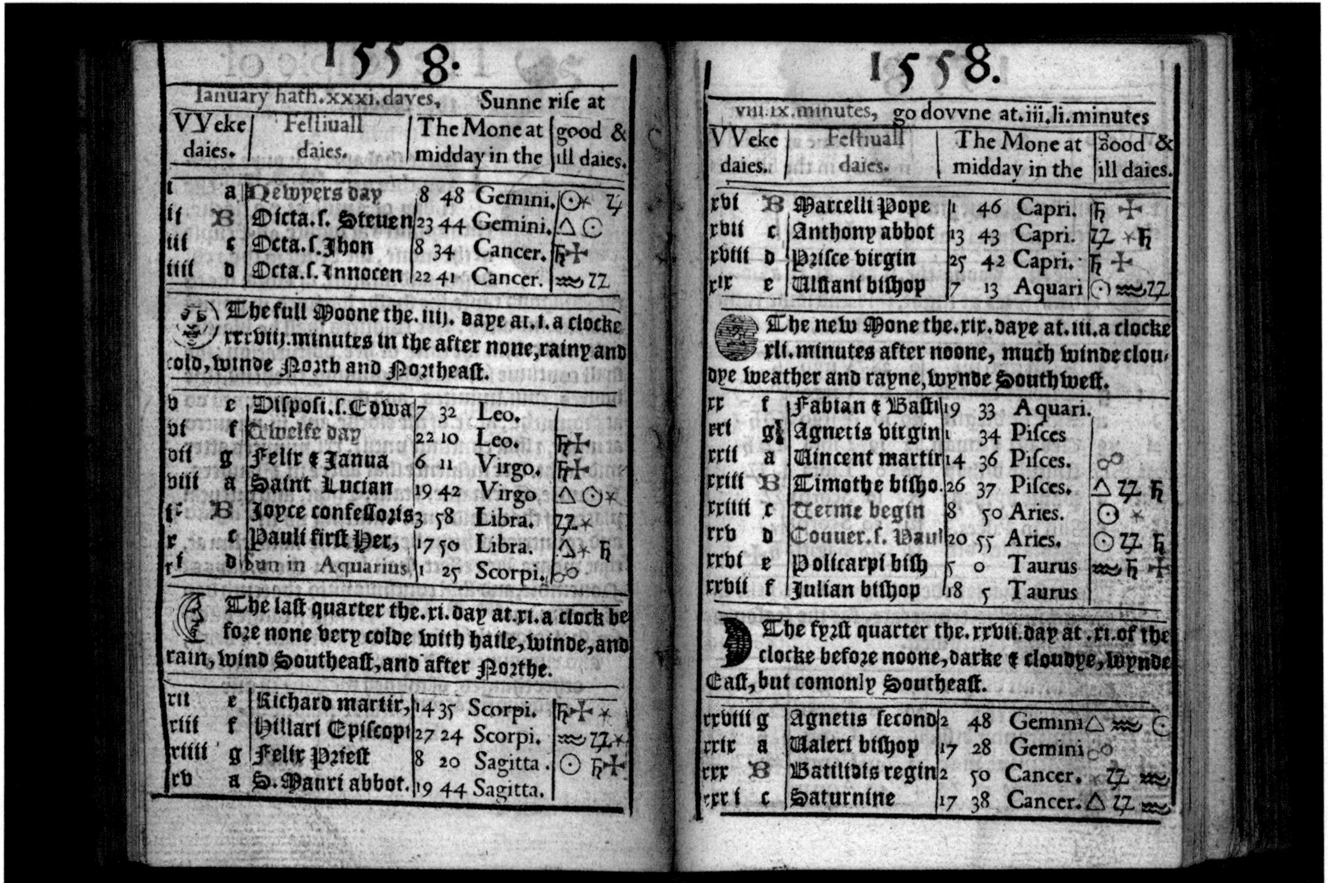

1558.

January hath.xxxi.dayes, Sunne rise at viii.ix.minutes, go dovvne at.iiii.li.minutes

VVeke daies.		Festiuall daies.	The Mone at midday in the			good & ill daies.
i	a	Newyers day	8	48	Gemini.	
ii	B	Octa.s. Steuen	23	44	Gemini.	
iii	c	Octa.s.Jhon	8	34	Cancer.	
iiii	d	Octa.s.Innocen	22	41	Cancer.	

The full Moone the.iiij. daye at.i.a clocke xxxviij.minutes in the after none, rainy and cold, winde North and Northeast.

v	e	Disposi.s.Edwa	7	32	Leo.	
vi	f	Twelfe day	22	10	Leo.	
vii	g	Felix & Janua	6	11	Virgo.	
viii	a	Saint Lucian	19	42	Virgo	
ix	B	Joyce confessoris	3	58	Libra.	
x	c	Pauli first Her,	17	50	Libra.	
xi	d	Sun in Aquarius	1	25	Scorpi.	

The last quarter the.xi.day at.xi.a clock before none very colde with haile, winde, and rain, wind Southeast, and after Northe.

xii	e	Richard martir,	14	35	Scorpi.	
xiii	f	Hillari Episcopi	27	24	Scorpi.	
xiiii	g	Felix Priest	8	20	Sagitta.	
xv	a	S.Mauri abbot.	19	44	Sagitta.	

1558.

VVeke daies.		Festiuall daies.	The Mone at midday in the			good & ill daies.
xvi	B	Marcelli Pope	1	46	Capri.	
xvii	c	Anthony abbot	13	43	Capri.	
xviii	d	Prisce virgin	25	42	Capri.	
xix	e	Wlstani bishop	7	13	Aquari	

The new Mone the.xix.daye at.iii.a clocke xli.minutes after noone, much winde cloudye weather and rayne, wynde Southwest.

xx	f	Fabian & Basti	19	33	Aquari.	
xxi	g	Agnetis virgin	1	34	Pisces	
xxii	a	Vincent martir	14	36	Pisces.	
xxiii	B	Timothe bisho.	26	37	Pisces.	
xxiiii	c	Terme begin	8	50	Aries.	
xxv	d	Conuer.s. Paul	20	55	Aries.	
xxvi	e	Policarpi bish	5	0	Taurus	
xxvii	f	Julian bishop	18	5	Taurus	

The fyrst quarter the.xxvii.day at.xi.of the clocke before noone, darke & cloudye, wynde East, but comonly Southeast.

xxviii	g	Agnetis second	2	48	Gemini	
xxix	a	Valeri bishop	17	28	Gemini	
xxx	B	Batilidis regin	2	50	Cancer.	
xxxi	c	Saturnine	17	38	Cancer.	

Figure 2: Table from Cuningham's almanac for 1558. The symbols in the right hand column indicate (according to a key set out earlier in the pamphlet) propitious and 'infortunate' days, good days for taking medicine, for travelling or planting out and sowing seeds.

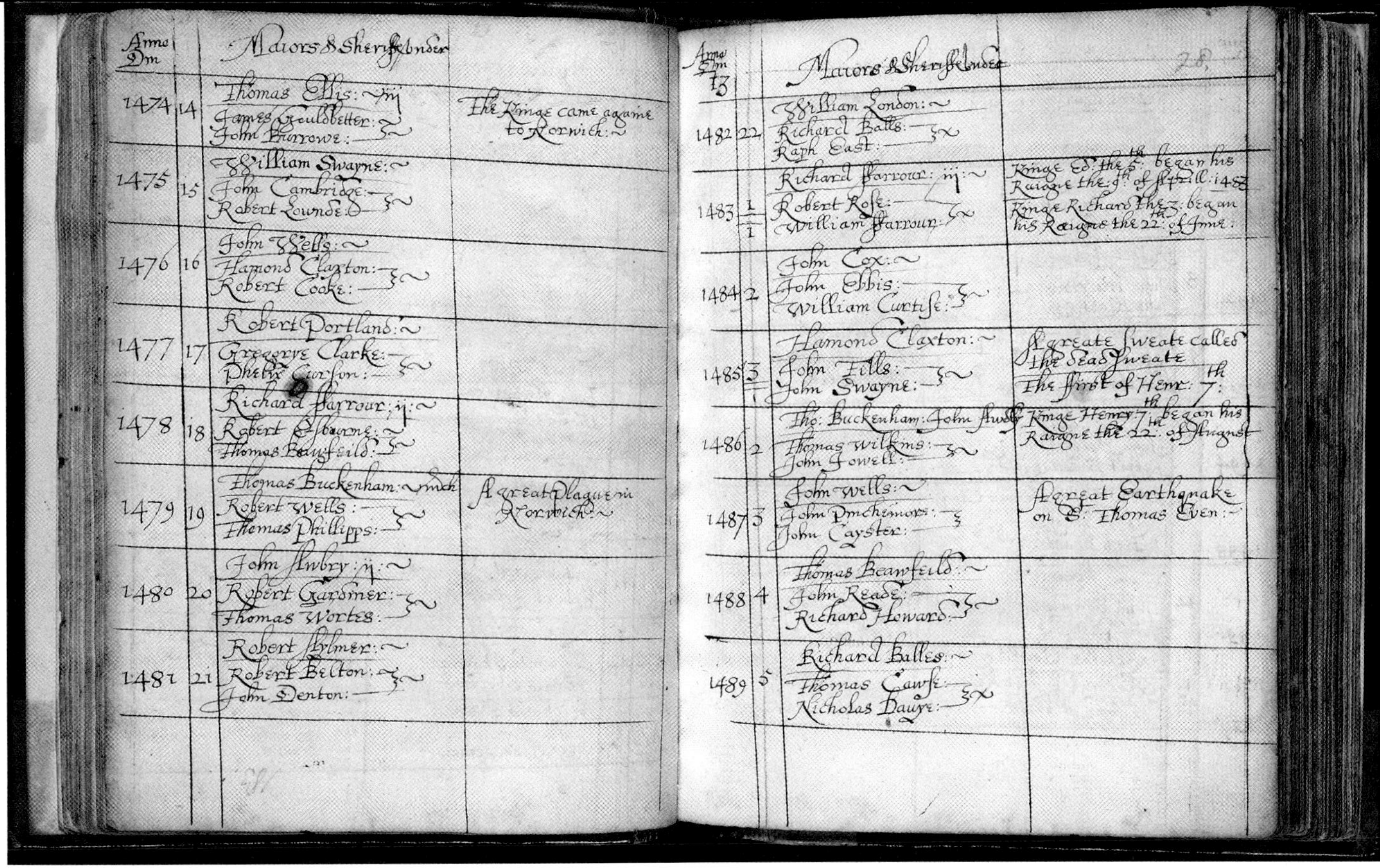

Anno Dom		Maiors & Sheriffs under	
1474	14	Thomas Ellis: mi James Geuldbetter: John Farrowe:	The Kinge came againe to Norwich:
1475	15	William Swayne: John Cambridge: Robert Lounde:	
1476	16	John Wells: Hamond Claxton: Robert Cooke:	
1477	17	Robert Portland: Greegorye Clarke: Phelix Curson:	
1478	18	Richard Farrour: ij: Robert Osborne: Thomas Bawfeild:	
1479	19	Thomas Buckenham: mck Robert Wells: Thomas Phillipps:	A great Plague in Norwich:
1480	20	John Awbry: ij: Robert Gardiner: Thomas Wortes:	
1481	21	Robert Aylmer: Robert Belton: John Denton:	

Anno Dom		Maiors & Sheriffs under	
1482	22	William London: Richard Balls: Raph East:	
1483	1	Richard Farrour: iij: Robert Rose: William Farrour:	Kinge Ed: the 5th began his Raigne the 9th of Aprill: 1483 Kinge Richard the 3: began his Raigne the 22: of June:
1484	2	John Cox: John Ebbis: William Curtise:	
1485	3	Hamond Claxton: John Fills: John Swayne:	A greate Sweate called the Sead Sweate The First of Henr: 7th:
1486	2	Tho: Buckenham: John Awb Thomas Wilkins: John Fowell:	Kinge Henry 7th began his Raigne the 22: of August
1487	3	John Wells: John Pmchemore: John Cayster:	A great Earthquake on St: Thomas Even:
1488	4	Thomas Beawfeild: John Reade: Richard Howard:	
1489	5	Richard Balles: Thomas Cawse: Nicholas Dawye:	

Figure 3: Table from Valentyne Bourne's commonplace book, showing chronological lists of the names of Norwich's ruling elite, outbreaks of disease and natural events.

small group of citizens from various backgrounds had been attempting to forecast future events. They were named as John Barbour, a resident of Tombland; Sir William, the chaplain of one Mr Halse and an active forecaster; Roger Coper; a worsted weaver called Robert; and William Harlokke, a former lodger with a Dr Austyn of Colchester (an astronomer and doctor of physic). Harlokke, who had previously borrowed a calendar of prognostication from his physician-landlord, had at least three books of prophecies in his possession.[61] He must have known that they were dangerous, as he endeavoured (unsuccessfully) to keep them secret. Tensions soon erupted within the group. Sir William accused Harlokke of using his divinations in an attempt to locate lost or buried treasure. Harlokke tried to exact revenge by telling the sheriffs of Norwich (Henry Fuller and Thomas Cranke) of the chaplain's forecasting. The sheriffs were dismissive of any sinister motives. Fuller reported: 'thys ys but a tryffyllinge mater'. Nonetheless, Harlokke's activities were subsequently brought to the attention of the central government, and he was interrogated in the Tower of London on the basis that certain of the group's activities smacked of treason.[62]

The activity of recording historical occurrences was much less dangerous than attempting to predict future ones. An effort to memorialize astral, meteorological and epidemiological phenomena after they happened was part of a wider endeavour to situate human experience within the observable changes and fluctuations of the cosmos.[63] A series of events of just this type constitutes part of the earliest civic historiography of Norwich inscribed into a handsome, sixteenth-century volume known as the Mayor's Book.[64] The memoranda included landmarks in the development of the corporation, as well as notable political occasions, epidemics, eclipses, earthquakes and floods.[65] The

[61] Thomas, *Religion and the Decline of Magic*, pp. 476–7.

[62] *LP*, IV, 2997–8.

[63] For context, see G. Pomata and N. G. Siraisi, 'Introduction', in *Historia: Empiricism and Erudition in Early Modern Europe*, ed. G. Pomata and N. G. Siraisi (Cambridge MA, 2005), pp. 1–38 (pp. 4–8, 10), in which *historia* is identified as an endeavour rooted in observations of places, physical features and natural events, as well as of human actions.

[64] It is described in *Records of Early English Drama: Norwich*, ed. Galloway, p. lviii.

[65] The table from NCR 17b Mayor's Book (Book of Oaths) is transcribed in 'Chronological Memoranda Touching the City of Norwich', ed. G. Johnson, *NA* 1 (1847), 140–66. The list included, amongst other things, the death toll in Norwich due to plague in 1351 (erroneously inflated to 57,474); a total eclipse of the sun in 1432; and an earthquake on 20 December 1456.

book was given to the city by alderman Augustine Steward (d. 1571) who also caused the opening pages to be inscribed with the names of Norwich's early bailiffs, sheriffs and mayors – a tradition which, thus established, continued until 1889.[66] Later, another similar table recording many of the same events was inscribed in a different type of text: a medical commonplace book created by a Norwich-born pharmacologist called Valentyne Bourne (b. 1566, fig. 3).[67] Bourne began his volume prior to 1610 and continued to write in it until 1646. His large compendium additionally included a list of weights used in medicines; a glossary of medical terms; and aphorisms on pain (attributed to Avicenna and Johannes de Vigo), as well as on nourishment and fatness, afternoon sleep and temperance. It also contained five rules for preserving health attributed to Asclepiades; a list of 'comforts for the brain'; a small number of experiments in natural magic (for example, on how to make a dog follow you, and the bestowing of toad or frog bones on friends and foe);[68] a guide to judging urines taken from 'divers authoures and practicioneres in phisicke both Du[t]ch and French';[69] recipes for medicines for a wide range of diseases in humans, horses, cattle and pigs, as well as for ink, wax, stain-remover, rat poison, perfumes for clothes and for rooms, dyes, preserves, jellies

[66] NCR 17b Mayor's Book (Book of Oaths), pp. 1–42, cf. Tittler, *The Reformation and the Towns in England*, pp. 284–6; R. Tittler, 'Henry Manship: Constructing the Civic Memory in Great Yarmouth', in *Townspeople and Nation: English Urban Experiences 1540–1646*, ed. R. Tittler (Stanford, 2001), pp. 121–39 (p. 127, on 'the need of contemporary governing authorities ... for a relevant and legitimising history'); and compare 'Norvicus', in Alexander Neville, *De furoribus Norfolciensium Ketto duce, liber unus; eiusdem Norvicus* (London: Henry Binneman, 1575).

[67] Oxford, Bodleian Library, MS Tanner 397, fols. 17r–37v (reverse pencil foliation). Bourne spent the early part of his life in the Norwich parish of St Andrew. The family also had property in London.

[68] The latter derives from Pliny's *Natural History*, XXXII.xviii.

[69] MS Tanner 397, fol. 10r–v (reverse pencil foliation). This reflected the presence of Dutch and Walloon refugees in the city, who were invited to settle in Norwich by the corporation in 1565 in order to help revive its flagging textile manufacturing sector: Pound, 'Government to 1660', p. 40. One such refugee, Anthony de Solemne, set up a printing shop and produced the first almanac to be published in Norwich itself (rather than in London). This included a perpetual calendar and historical notes, and was issued in Solemne's native language for the benefit of the growing Dutch community: Anon, *Eenen Calendier Historiael* (Norwich: Anthony de Solemne, 1570), described in P. Valkema Blouw, *Dutch Typography in the Sixteenth Century: The Collected Works of Paul Valkema Blouw*, ed. T. Croiset van Uchelen and P. Dijstelberge (Leiden, 2013), p. 776, cf. Kusukawa, 'Andreas Nolthius's *Almanach*', pp. 100–2; and see below, Epilogue.

and candies, and for the health-restoring 'Ipocras' wine (which he had apparently learned from 'an expert apothicary'). He also copied out extracts of Galen's *De alimentorum facultatibus* ('On the properties of foodstuffs').[70] Bourne tackled the connectedness of calendar dates, astral movements and a person's regimen rather more succinctly than his predecessors when he noted these ominous aphorisms:

> If you misdoubt that you shall not have proffitt or good successe [with healing] then meddle with nothinge in the first of Auguste, the 14th of September and the 11th of March,

and

> Theise 3 dayes beware of too much eating and drinkinge: the first of August, the first of December and the 16th daye of Aprill, for theis be dismall dayes and maye cost a man's life.[71]

*

Having established a framework of ideas concerning the body and its relationship to the wider environment – that is, of the significance of clean domestic accommodation, of sweet or noxious smells and putrefying substances, of precautionary self-care, of the interrelationships between food and medicine, of exercise and rest, of good and bad times of the year, and of the movements of the heavenly bodies – it is now possible to probe in further detail the mechanisms which sustained the circulation of these ideas in pre-modern Norwich. What other local authorities regularly accessed sources of medical or hygienic information? How did they learn it? And what resources did men and women require in order to access it themselves?

[70] On this, see E. Leong, 'Collecting Knowledge for the Family: Recipes, Gender and Practical Knowledge in the Early Modern English Household', *Centaurus* 55 (2013), 81–103 (p. 99, n. 24); MS Tanner 397, fols. 205v–201v (reverse pencil foliation; the manuscript was turned upside down, and information was entered from the back of the volume).

[71] MS Tanner 397, fol. 3r.

Networks of knowledge: medical authority, practice and learning in pre-modern Norwich

Tens of healing specialists, including several Norfolk men, are cited in another medical recipe book,[72] this time dating to the 1560s, which was held in the possession of Thomas Butts – probably he of that name who died in 1592, a gentleman whose extensive holdings in Norfolk included houses and land in nearby Catton.[73] The father of our Thomas, if he was indeed the owner of this text, was Dr William Butts (d. 1545), an illustrious son of Norwich and physician to none other than Henry VIII. It is interesting to note, however, that the first local authority cited in the volume was not a medical practitioner but a civic official, the Norwich mayor, Nicholas Norgate (d. 1568). Norgate had purportedly not only used his signature recipe ('an especyall good medycyn for the collyck') to good effect on himself, but had also 'easyd and helpen many otheres therwyth'.[74] Even more distinguished people donated their favourite cures to the compiler. A second remedy – for toothache – was copied out of a book owned by Master Robert Talbot, an antiquarian and a prebendary of Norwich cathedral (d. 1558).[75] Lastly, a cure for 'the stone' which is dated 1565, was supplied by Dr Thomas Thirlby (d. 1570), bishop of Ely near Cambridge, a friend of William Butts and the former (albeit, absentee) bishop of Norwich (1550–54).[76] The exchange of books and ideas between learned friends was, therefore, one way in which forms of knowledge about healing were generated.

The cathedral priory itself was a repository for medical, astronomical and astrological knowledge. The medieval library held a range of relevant titles: *Questiones physicorum*; *Secreta secretorum*; Avicenna's *Canon* and the pseudo-Galenic *De passionibus puerorum*; *De proprietatibus*

[72] Oxford, Bodleian Library, MS Rawlinson C 816. The endpaper is inscribed 'Thomas Buttus me possidet', and the flypaper 'Buttus me possidet'.

[73] On the Butts family and their connections (including the master of the grammar school in Norwich, Stephen Limbert), see K. J. Höltgen, 'Sir Robert Dallington (1561–1637): Author, Traveler and Pioneer of Taste', *Huntington Library Quarterly* 47 (1984), 147–77 (pp. 149–53).

[74] MS Rawlinson C 816, fol. 32r (pencil foliation).

[75] MS Rawlinson C 816, inserted leaf at fol. 73r (pencil foliation). The recipe was copied in 1569.

[76] MS Rawlinson C 816, inserted leaf at fol. 66r (pencil foliation).

rerum by Bartholomaeus Anglicus;[77] as well as a manual on horoscopy (replete with diagrams); another on constructing a planetary equatorium; a set of astronomical tables; advice on diet and prophylactics for use against the plague; and Latin–English glossaries of medical terms.[78] It was also a locus for the creation of original ideas and content. One manuscript – probably compiled at Norwich cathedral and added to at various points between 1450 and the late fifteenth century – included medical recipes, a uroscopy treatise and herbal lore, as well as an apparently unique toothache charm.[79] At a slightly earlier date, one monk, William Bokenham, bent his efforts towards making therapeutic and diagnostic practices more easily accessible to the infirmary's staff: he compiled two further, simple guides in the vernacular on the art of uroscopy – a means to gauge a person's humoral state.[80]

[77] Concepts and knowledge extracted from this Franciscan's text may have reached the wider Norwich population via a different conduit: like similar encyclopaedias produced by the Dominicans Thomas of Cantimpré and Vincent of Beauvais, Bartholomaeus's first purpose was to supply materials usable in sermons by orders of preaching friars. Indeed, surviving catalogues of English friary libraries point to its possession: *The Friars' Libraries*, ed. K. W. Humphreys, Corpus of British Medieval Library Catalogues (London, 1990), pp. 68, 69, 144, 145, identifies three copies (with a probable fourth held at the Austin friars in York), viz.: a copy with Carmelite friars at Hulne, Northumberland (p. 172), and (regionally) a copy with Dominicans in Cambridge (p. 196), and a copy with Franciscans at Ipswich (p. 196). Norwich was home to convents of each of the four great orders of friars, with the *studium* of the Franciscan friary (Greyfriars) in particular attaining an international reputation: Tanner, 'The Cathedral and the City', pp. 270–3; Soden, EAA 133, p. 53. In these circumstances, it seems a reasonable conjecture that Norwich friars also had access to the text. See also M. C. Seymour, 'Some Medieval English Owners of *De proprietatibus rerum*', *Bodleian Library Record* 9 (1974), 156–65.

[78] J. Greatrex, 'Horoscopes and Healing at Norwich Cathedral Priory in the later Middle Ages', in *The Church and Learning in Later Medieval Society: Essays in Honour of R. B. Dobson*, ed. C. M. Barron and J. Stratford, Harlaxton Medieval Studies 11 (Donington, 2002), pp. 170–7; C. Rawcliffe, 'On the Threshold of Eternity: Care for the Sick in East Anglian Monasteries', in *East Anglia's History: Essays in Honour of Norman Scarfe*, ed. C. Harper-Bill, C. Rawcliffe and R. G. Wilson (Woodbridge, 2000), pp. 41–72 (pp. 58, 65); and see: 'Gardeners' Accounts', ed. Noble, p. 9; H. C. Beeching and M. Rhodes James, 'The Library of the Cathedral Church of Norwich', *NA* 19 (1917), 67–116 (p. 110); W. T. Bensly, 'St Leonard's Priory, Norwich', *NA* 12 (1895), 190–227 (pp. 210–11).

[79] C. F. Bühler, 'A Middle English Medical Manuscript from Norwich', in *Studies in Medieval Literature in Honor of Albert Croll Baugh*, ed. M. Leach (Philadelphia, 1961), pp. 285–98 (pp. 287–8); Keiser, *Manual*, p. 3847.

[80] Bokenham was resident in the region in *c.* 1430–55: J. Greatrex, *Biographical Register of the English Cathedral Priories of the Province of Canterbury, c. 1066–1540*

Another vehicle for knowledge exchange was the interactions that took place in the crucibles of Norwich schools and, by extension, in university colleges. The sons of Norwich merchants and craftsmen were provided with a basic education at the episcopal school (later a free grammar school) and the Benedictine almonry school.[81] Elementary tuition was also available at the hospital of St Paul, known as Norman's Spital (map 3).[82] Scholars in pursuit of a higher education do not seem to have been deterred from attending the University of Cambridge by a difficult journey across the fens. Before the Dissolution of the Monasteries, Norwich supplied a steady stream of students from the ranks of the Benedictine order and also, occasionally, from the aldermanic class.[83] At least two of the medieval infirmarers at the priory had university educations and would thus have been familiar with the principles of Aristotelian natural philosophy.[84] Medical graduates (as opposed to students of theology) are also sometimes to be glimpsed in the service of the cathedral. For example, Master Conrad (a Cambridge MB) rented rooms and a garden at the almonry for use whilst he was

(Oxford, 1997), p. 485; Rawcliffe, 'Threshold of Eternity', p. 65.

[81] J. Greatrex, 'The Almonary School of Norwich Cathedral Priory in the Thirteenth and Fourteenth Centuries', in *The Church and Childhood*, ed. D. Wood, Studies in Church History 31 (Oxford, 1994), pp. 169–81; Greatrex, *Biographical Register*, pp. 470–1; Rawcliffe, *MFTS*, pp. 20, 60, 220–1, 234.

[82] Rawcliffe, 'The Eighth Comfortable Work: Education and the Medieval English Hospital', in *The Church and Learning in Later Medieval Society: Essays Presented in Honour of R. B. Dobson*, ed. C. M. Barron and R. Stratford, Harlaxton Medieval Studies 11 (Donington, 2002), pp. 371–98 (p. 394). See also N. P. Tanner, *The Church in Late Medieval Norwich, 1370–1532*, Studies and Texts 66 (Toronto, 1984), p. 34.

[83] Greatrex, *Biographical Register*, p. 471; B. Cozens-Hardy and E. A. Kent, *The Mayors of Norwich, 1403 to 1835, Being Bibliographical Notes on the Mayors of the Old Corporation* (Norwich, 1938), p. 36 (Henry Caus).

[84] J. Greatrex, 'Monk Students from Norwich Cathedral Priory at Oxford and Cambridge, *c.* 1300 to 1530', *English Historical Review* 106 (1991), 555–83: John de Fornsete, D.Th., a friend of the Pastons, graduated from Oxford and became the Norwich infirmarer in 1455/56 (p. 572). Another long-term student at Cambridge, who did not graduate, was Geoffrey de Totyngham, infirmarer 1309/10 to 1312/13 (pp. 569–70). See also Greatrex, 'Horoscopes and Healing', p. 172. Financial accounts surviving from the early fourteenth century until the Dissolution testify to a very significant expenditure on medicines in the infirmary: see Greatrex, *Biographical Register*, *passim* for expenditure recorded in NRO, DCN 1/10.

treating the priory's brethren in 1471, a time of plague in the city.[85] Such individuals, when returning to or visiting Norwich, could hope to build a base of affluent clients and their friends. Margaret Paston was alerted to the presence of one such individual (a 'ryght ... konnyng [knowledgable] man and a gentyll [man]') who was attending Lady Isabel Morley in Foulsham, north Norfolk, in case she wanted to make the most of the opportunity to confer with him (*c.* 1450).[86] Similarly, associates of the Pastons, Sir Miles and Lady Katherine Stapleton, commissioned several manuscripts from John Metham, a former Cambridge scholar (*fl.* 1448–49). The commissions touched upon aspects of meteorological prognostications (including the effect on health of different weather events), physiognomy (derived from the *Secretum secretorum*) and astrology, and outlined propitious days for bloodletting as well as the likely outcome of any sicknesses befalling a man on each day of the lunar month.[87]

One alumnus, however, stands out as especially illustrious. John Caius (1510–73), an active president of the college of physicians in London (an elite, professional body founded in 1518), and the second founder of Gonville and Caius College, Cambridge,[88] was born in

[85] Rawcliffe, 'Threshold of Eternity', p. 48. On plague in Norwich in November 1471, see *Paston Letters and Papers*, ed. Davis, I, 355, 440. On connections between Norwich and the university in the sixteenth and seventeenth centuries, see *A History of the University of Cambridge*, ed. D. R. Leader, V. Morgan and P. Searby, 4 vols. (Cambridge, 1988–2004), II, 181–240.

[86] *Paston Letters and Papers*, ed. Davis, II, 338; on the dynamics of the relationships between the actors involved, see V. Creelman, '"Ryght Worchepfull Mastres": Letters of Request and Servants' Scripting of Margaret Paston's Social Self', *Parergon* 26 (2009), 91–113 (pp. 100, 102). Margaret later displayed antipathy towards *London* physicians: *Paston Letters and Papers*, ed. Davis, I, 291 (to John Paston I, 8 June 1464: 'fore Goddys sake be ware what medesynys ye take of any fysissyanys of London. I schal neuer trust to hem be-cause of yowre fadre and myn onkyl').

[87] Keiser, *Manual*, pp. 3603, 3622, 3624, 3782 and references given there, and see p. 3606 for a further version of the *Secretum secretorum* commissioned by Stapleton. Although they were residents of Ingham in the Broadlands of north-east Norfolk, some sixteen miles from Norwich, both Sir Miles and his wife had regular opportunities to mix with the aldermanic and ecclesiastical elite in the city, as they were members of St George's guild: *Records of the Gild of St George in Norwich, 1389–1547*, ed. M. Grace, NRS 9 (Norwich, 1937), p. 23.

[88] On this, see *History of the University of Cambridge*, ed. Leader, Morgan and Searby, II, 25–32.

Norwich, probably in the parish of St Etheldreda.[89] His early education in the city served him well, providing him with preliminary tuition in Greek, and it was no doubt owing to his local connections that he secured not only the patronage of William Butts[90] but also the friendship of Thomas Thirlby. Caius went on to complete his MD at the university of Padua, where he became acquainted with the celebrated anatomist, Vesalius, and subsequently lectured. On his return to England, after a tour of Italian libraries, he was heralded as a 'second Linacre': that is, as a humanist practitioner of the greatest ability and honour.[91] He continued to move in the very highest circles, acting as personal physician to successive Tudor monarchs, and enjoyed a literary friendship with Archbishop Parker.[92] As we will see in more detail in a later part of this book, Caius affirmed his early and continuing ties to Norwich in the introduction to his *Boke or Counseill Against the Disease Commonly Called the Sweate or Sweatyng Sicknesse* (1552), a small handbook of advice printed in black letter type which gave information on avoiding infection based on environmental and regimenal principles.[93] This text was almost certainly read by members of the ruling elite in the city who – when Caius's text was published – were already engaged in enacting new hygienic measures of the kind endorsed by the physician in an attempt to improve the state of Norwich's streets and watercourses.[94]

The connection between the London college of physicians and Norwich was further strengthened by the activities of Marten Corembeck, MD (Bologna), who died in 1579. Under Caius's reforms, the college attempted to exert its exclusive control in the capital over what it

[89] J. Venn, 'Memoir of John Caius', in *The Works of John Caius, M.D.* ed. E. S. Roberts (Cambridge, 1912), p. 1.
[90] V. Nutton, *John Caius and the Manuscripts of Galen* (Cambridge, 1987), p. 11.
[91] His 'learned lectours' and 'secrete anothomies' at Barber-Surgeons' Hall (the home of the Barber-Surgeons' company of London) reportedly laid open the 'hidden juelles, and precious threasours of Cl[audius] Galenus, shewyng [Caius] to be the seconde Linacar': William Bullein, 'A Little Dialogue Betwene Twoo Men, the one called Sorenes and the other Chyrurgi', in *idem, Bullein's Bulwarke of Defence Againste all Sicknes, Sornes and Woundes* (London: John Kyngston, 1562), sig. Aa4r; Venn, 'Memoir', pp. 6–8; Nutton, *John Caius*, pp. 1–2. On Thomas Linacre, see C. Webster, 'Thomas Linacre and the Foundation of the College of Physicians', in *Essays on the Life and Work of Thomas Linacre, c. 1460–1524*, ed. F. Maddison, M. Pelling and C. Webster (Oxford, 1977), pp. 198–222.
[92] Venn, 'Memoir', p. 8. On Caius's friendship with Parker, see *History of the University of Cambridge*, ed. Leader, Morgan and Searby, II, 29.
[93] See below, introduction to Part III.
[94] 'River and Street Accounts', ed. Fay, pp. 109–10, and see below, chapter 5.

characterized as a cabal of ignorant, disorderly, unqualified empirics. A native Dutchman, Corembeck himself initially ran into trouble with the college in 1553 for practising medicine in London without a licence. But as soon as he satisfied the prerequisites, Corembeck became a fellow of the college. Moving to Norwich, he was asked to track down unlicensed local empirics in 1570 on behalf of the institution.[95] By about this time, Corembeck had purchased two properties in the parish of St Michael Coslany, and his connections with Norwich were further augmented by his role as physician to Thomas Howard, 4th duke of Norfolk (the son of Andrew Boorde's patron).[96] His impressive network of supporters and contacts also included William Bullein (d. 1576), a native of Ely, and the author of a variety of textbooks on medicines including the popular *Governement of Healthe* (1558).[97]

No doubt as a response to the pressure of the London college's drive to raise standards, Norwich's medieval guild of barbers and barber-surgeons was supplanted by a new company of physicians and barber-surgeons in 1561.[98] This fraternity also sought to distinguish itself from the practice of what it chose to deem 'ignorant' laymen and women. Walter Haugh, a member of the company who possessed a licence to engage in physic, acted as an agent for the college of physicians in the same manner as Corembeck.[99] In 1559, he was given a commission to seek out unlicensed practitioners in the region after two 'empirics' from Norwich had been reported to, and fined by, the college in 1558. A much larger body of less distinguished healers was also resident in the city. Exact figures are difficult to extrapolate, but the names of over 80 surgeons, apothecaries and physicians living or owning property in the city are known for the period 1260–1560, as

95 Pelling and Webster, 'MP', pp. 215–16; and for context, see M. Pelling, *Medical Conflicts in Early Modern London: Patronage, Physicians and Irregular Practitioners, 1550–1640* (Oxford, 2003); John Caius, 'Annalium Collegii medicorum Londini Liber', in *Works of John Caius*, ed. Roberts, pp. 64, 66.

96 *Landgable*, ed. Rodgers and Wallace, pp. 21, 132–3; Pelling and Webster, 'MP', p. 215.

97 Bullein wrote for the 'good gentleman reader': Wear, *Knowledge and Practice*, pp. 56–60; R. W. Maslen, 'The Healing Dialogues of Doctor Bullein', *The Yearbook of English Studies* 38 (2008), 119–35 (pp. 122–8). For other men who may have undergone formal medical training and who settled in the city towards the end of our period, see Pelling and Webster, 'MP', p. 210.

98 The new company's regulations are printed in *The Barber-Surgeons of Norwich*, ed. C. Williams (Norwich, 1896), pp. 7–10.

99 Caius, 'Annalium Collegii medicorum', p. 50.

well as about 160 barbers.[100] The actual number of individuals claiming healing ability was almost certainly much greater.

The civic government also chose to employ a range of other healers when the need arose, specifically for charitable purposes, and these men and women constitute the final elements in our network. The choices might not always have pleased the college, but officers clearly felt it was within their remit, and their knowledge, to make their own health care contracts on behalf of the corporation. In September 1570, for example, the sum of 3*s.* 7*d.* was paid from the civic coffers to the wife of one William Clementes who lived in the Conesford area of Norwich.[101] She had apparently tended to a child resident at the Norman's hospital who had some kind of complaint relating to his or her head. Another, unnamed woman was similarly paid the following March for healing two children with 'skalde heade' (a scalp complaint).[102] Officers were on safer ground when they contracted the aptly named surgeon William Fever to cure a labourer of some unknown affliction. It seems likely that the labourer in question had worked for the corporation at some point, but was now (owing to his illness) too poor to work to pay for his own treatment.[103]

In this chapter, we have glimpsed a network of individuals who drew on a shared ideology concerning the body, its care and its allotted place in the cosmos. The occasions and places in which such knowledge was created and sustained were not only varied but were specifically *urban* in nature, dependent upon the demographic, organizational and economic circumstances of city life. Several of the men and women mentioned here were, of course, not representative of the majority of the residents of Norwich with regard to their resources and social or educational attainments. On the other hand, some – Robert Reynes, the city's financial administrators and perhaps the prognosticator William Harlokke – may more fairly represent the ideas accessible to a person possessing a basic or solid local education.

100 See Pelling and Webster, 'MP', *passim*; F. M. Getz, 'Medical Practitioners in Medieval England', *Social History of Medicine* 3 (1990), 245–83 (*passim*); I. Fay, 'Health and Disease in Medieval and Tudor Norwich' (unpublished PhD thesis, University of East Anglia, 2007), pp. 115–26, table 3.

101 NRO, NCR 18d, Clavors' Book 1 [Hamper] 1550–1601, fol. 66v.

102 NCR 18d, Clavors' Book 1 [Hamper] 1550–1601, fol. 66v.

103 Ibid., fol. 75v. On the context, see Pelling, 'Healing the Sick Poor', in Pelling, *CL*, pp. 79–102 (esp. p. 98).

Throughout our discussion, prestigious texts have been indicated as a vehicle for conveying concepts. But we have also glimpsed a wider phenomenon: behind the creation of texts themselves frequently lay a process that hinged either upon verbal exchanges, or a variety of less formal scribal processes, including letter writing, commonplacing or the recording of financial transactions. Those processes involved the solicitation of patronage or endorsement (as with Andrew Boorde and Thomas Howard, or John Halle and William Cuningham), the making of commissions (as with the Pastons or Stapletons), and the compilation of other people's medical recipes (by Thomas Butts and Valentyne Bourne). In later chapters we will expand our network of actors still further to assess how not only magistrates and surgeons but also guildsmen, parish sextons and householders developed ideas about health, the landscape and healing that were conditioned by, and appropriate to, civic life. Now it is time to turn to one particular (sumptuous and expensive) text written by a Norwich-born man, and discover the artful, nuanced way in which it encoded aspects of the ancient, enviro-medical tradition for readers already familiar with the precepts, but who wished to master recent advances in allied sciences.

2

An Epitome of Hygiene: William Cuningham's Prospect Plan

> [The] wholesomeness [of a place] chiefly dependeth upon two elements – air and water; the one concerneth the vital, the other the natural, parts of the body, for what mortal creature can live without breathing, eating and drinking? So that, if the air be pure and subtle, the spirits be refreshed; but if impure and gross, the heart, which is the fountain of life, is soon stifled, whereby the whole body soon perisheth.[1]
>
> Henry Manship, 'History of Great Yarmouth' (1619), when reflecting on the salubrious nature of easterly towns

Cuningham's plan of Norwich (fig. 1), published in his *Cosmographical Glasse* (1559), has been called both a realistic reconstruction of Norwich as the surveyor 'actually saw it', and a manipulated and idealized image.[2] Alongside important institutions and facilities, such as the cathedral, parish churches and the city's water-driven corn mills (to the left of the panorama), the most striking elements of the image are the gardens, pastures and orchards, the width and order of the streets, and the relationship between the urban centre and the open countryside around it. The splendid architecture and lush vegetation were not simply devices to please the eye. Cuningham's image

1 Henry Manship, *The History of Great Yarmouth*, ed. C. J. Palmer (Great Yarmouth, 1854), p. 103.

2 B. Ayers, 'Norwich: A City and its Image', in *East Anglian Studies: Essays Presented to J. C. Barringer on his Retirement*, ed. A. Longcroft and R. Joby (Norwich, 1995), pp. 1–10 (p. 2), and J. Pound, *Tudor and Stuart Norwich* (Chichester, 1988), pp. 20–3. For a (much larger) metropolitan map of similar date, see the engraved plates of Frans Franken's map of London, 1553–59, which are held at the Museum of London.

conveyed a message: the quality of an urban environment determines its inhabitants' health.[3]

The plan of Norwich is now quite famous and it appears frequently in books on Tudor cartography and in histories of Norwich. But less is known about the man who created it. Indeed, the identity left to posterity by William Cuningham (or Kenningham, as he sometime spelled it)[4] is both shadowy and ambiguous. One historian recently identified him as an associate of a gang of notorious charlatans peddling fraudulent prognostications in Elizabeth London,[5] although his credentials as a skilled practitioner of technical arts and as a draughtsman have been noted by historians of navigation, cosmography and cartography.[6] What little is currently known of his career and persona can now be sketched out. William's early life in Norwich remains largely a mystery before he moved to Cambridge to read arts in 1548.[7] Enrolling as a pensioner of Corpus Christi, he matriculated in 1551, and was examined for his MB in 1557.[8] In November 1556, he had returned to Norwich where he was still stationed in March 1557 and July 1559.[9] During these times, he made astronomical calculations using an astrolabe, drew up the first of his almanacs and worked on his main text, *The Cosmographical Glasse*. His patron, Robert Dudley, earl of Leicester, gave him funds to travel to Heidelberg in May 1559, and he acquired

[3] Contemporary viewers of the plan would have been familiar with the ability of maps to carry a range of meanings, including references to political, social, moral, religious, literary or philosophical ideas: J. B. Harley, 'Meaning and Ambiguity in Tudor Cartography', in *English Map-Making, 1500–1650*, ed. S. Tyacke (London, 1982), pp. 22–45.

[4] William published under both spellings of his surname. The Latinized version was no doubt pleasing to him because of its English connotation of 'cunning', meaning wisdom, though his earliest surviving almanac gave the original form: Cuningham [Kenningham], *A&P* 1558.

[5] A. Ryrie, *The Sorcerer's Tale: Faith and Fraud in Tudor England* (Oxford, 2008), p. 155.

[6] Heninger, *The Cosmographical Glass*, pp. 1–4; D. W. Waters, *The Art of Navigation in England in Elizabethan and Early Stuart Times* (London, 1958), pp. 58–9, 98–9, 104, 244; and see the works by E. G. R. Taylor referred to below.

[7] His father may have been a tailor by the name of Mathew Kennyngham; a man of this description died in the parish of St Peter Parmentergate, Norwich, in 1545 (see Appendix IV): NRO, NCC will register Whytefoote, fols. 4v–5r.

[8] C. H. Cooper, T. Cooper and G. J. Gray, *Athenae Cantabrigienses*, 3 vols. (Cambridge, 1858–1913), III, 1.

[9] Cuningham, *CG*, 'Preface', sig. A6v, and see ibid., pp. 47, 92.

his doctorate in that city.[10] His religious outlook was clear. The decision to go to Heidelberg rather than to Italy, his working relationships with Protestant printers and the mention of 'Christ our saviour' in his works were unambiguous statements of his confessional stamp.[11]

On his return to England, Cuningham moved to Colman Street in London. In weak health during 1563 and 1565,[12] he was unable to pursue his plans to complete a promised programme of works: a *Chronographie* in which he intended to discuss the 'whole arte ... of calculating the motions of the planets, with the rising and setting of the fixed starres', seems never to have come to fruition.[13] Instead, he collaborated with the eminent royal naval surgeon, Thomas Gale, and Gale's close friend, John Halle, on surgical compendia.[14] At about this time he was lecturing to the Barber-Surgeons' Company in the capital,[15] and published a (lost) Latin composition on methods of prognostication.[16] However, his financial position was precarious. In 1566, he reportedly owed Richard Ferris, sergeant surgeon of Elizabeth I, the substantial sum of £30.[17] A final possible glimpse of Cuningham surfaces towards the end of the century. A William Keningham of the parish of St Mary Woolchurch, London (not far from Colman Street), declared in front of witnesses as he lay dying in February 1595 that, although he had 'no money to leave her', now that his two daughters were provided for, 'the litle that he had (naminge all his worldly goodes and chattles) he gave to his wife Joyce'. He added, 'yf he had a greate deale more, his wife was worthye of it and she shoulde have it'.[18]

[10] Cuningham, *CG*, p. 181. Dudley presented Cuningham with £6 13*s.* 4*d.* on his departure to Flanders: *Household Accounts*, ed. Adams, p. 66.

[11] Cuningham, *A&P* 1564, 'Prognostication', sig. A4r; Cuningham, *A&P* 1566, sig. C3r.

[12] Apparently, he had badly fractured his leg which left him in great pain: Bodleian, MS Bodley 178, fol. 34v.

[13] It is referred to in Cuningham, *A&P* 1566, 'Prognostication', sig. C2r–v.

[14] Gale, *Certaine Workes of Chirurgerie*, sigs. A4r–7v, *4v (in which Cuningham dismisses his 'apish' detractors and claims to have edited Gale's work); *A Most Excellent and Learned Woorke of Chirurgerie, called Chirurgia parua Lanfranci*, ed. John Halle (London: Thomas Marshe, 1565), sigs. ¶3v–*1v; and for Cuningham's correspondence with Halle, see n. p 37 above. On the role of the 'chyrurgicall phisicions' (Bullein, 'Dialogue', sig. Bb2r), cf. Wear, *Knowledge and Practice*, pp. 220–2.

[15] *Chirurgia parva Lanfranci*, ed. Halle, sig. ¶2v.

[16] See references in Cuningham, *A&P* 1566, 'Prognostication', sig. C2r.

[17] *The Annals of the Barber-Surgeons of London*, ed. S. Young (London, 1890), p. 524.

[18] London Metropolitan Archive, Guildhall Library MS 9171/18ff, fol. 307r.

Taking all of his published and unpublished works together, it becomes clear that Cuningham saw himself as something of a pioneer whose task it was to seek out the latest scholarly and technical advances in astrology, medicine, cosmography and draughtsmanship, and to report his findings in attractive printed volumes for readers outside university circles.[19] Cuningham's acquisitive mind and broad interests, however, became something of a liability to him as his career progressed. His whole-hearted engagement with medical astrology landed him in trouble at a time when the practices of learned and artisanal healers were often in conflict,[20] and when the 'hotter' sort of Protestants were staking out their ground. Though theoretically part of the mainstream, his activities could too easily be misinterpreted or conflated with judicial astrology, prophesying and magical healing. These latter, in the wrong hands, arrogantly seemed to anticipate – or worse subvert – divine will.[21] The puritan divine William Fulke (1538–89), in assuming Cuningham to be one of the principal representatives of English astrology and therefore potentially little more than a necromancer, attacked him in print and greatly imperilled his reputation.[22] Perhaps because of the notoriety he attracted, his publisher during the late 1550s – John Day – ceased collaborating with him, and his later almanacs were produced by other London printers. But even if Cuningham's methods were liable to upset convinced Puritans, he alienated few in the medical mainstream. His contribution to the dissemination of knowledge was lauded by William Bullein who ranked Cuningham

[19] On, for example, his use of the revised tables of planetary and astral positions by Nicolaus Copernicus (d. 1543) and Erasmus Reinhold (d. 1553), rather than the older and corrupt Alfonsine ones, see Cuningham [Kenningham], *A&P* 1558, sig. A2v; Capp, *Astrology and the Popular Press*, p. 180. Cuningham also made a claim for being the first writer in English to contribute to the relatively new and ill-defined discipline of cosmography: Cuningham, *CG*, 'Preface', sig. A6v.

[20] On this, see Pelling, *Medical Conflicts*, pp. 136–88; Murray Jones, 'Medical Literacies', pp. 38–43.

[21] Cuningham [Kenningham], *A&P* 1558, 'Prognostication', sig. A2v recognizes the risks of confusing legitimate astronomy with 'necromancie, socerie and witchcraft'.

[22] In other respects, he judged Cuningham to be 'learned and honest': Fulke, *Antiprognosticon*, sig. B1r, and see sigs. C2r, C6v–8r. In contrast, for the conciliatory attitudes of early Protestants to astrology, see S. Kusukawa, 'Aspectio divinorum operum: Melanchthon and Astrology for Lutheran Medics', in *Medicine and the Reformation*, ed. O. P. Grell and A. Cunningham (London, 1993), pp. 33–56.

along with John Caius and other notable authors, and praised him for his work in distinguishing the legitimate and illegitimate uses of prognostications and medical astrology. 'Like a good soldiour', Bullein reported, Cuningham had successfully fought 'against the ignoraunt enemie, setting forthe the commendacion, praise, and profite of astronomie, cosmographie and geographe'.[23]

Through *The Cosmographical Glasse*: Cuningham's agenda

Cuningham's *magnum opus* was intended to appeal not only to his medical peers and his audience at the London Barber-Surgeons' Company, but also to laymen.[24] Thus, his preface to *The Cosmographical Glasse* was addressed to the well-heeled fireside traveller who might, as Cuningham put it, seek to satisfy a taste for exploration and knowledge of mathematics, geography and physic without leaving the comforts of his own 'warme study'.[25] The volume was an extraordinarily lavish publication. In his survey of the medium, Daniel Berkeley Updike considered that 'as a piece of printing, nothing better had hitherto appeared in England'.[26] This favourable opinion rested upon the elaborate woodcuts, tables and decorated capital letters accompanying the text (fig. 4), many of which were attractive reproductions of diagrams from books by scholars working on the Continent.[27] In addition to an extremely beautiful title-page and the Norwich prospect, there were fifty illustrations and diagrams, as well as a large table of eclipse

23 Bullein, 'Dialogue', sig. Aa4r. The other men listed in Bullein's medical pantheon were: William Turner, Thomas Phayer, Sir Thomas Elyot, Andrew Boorde, Thomas Paynell and Robert Recorde.

24 Works in the same tone and tradition as Cuningham's text formed part of the chosen reading matter of a new generation of astro-medical consultants: see Kassell, *Medicine and Magic*, p. 46 n. 34, p. 78.

25 Cuningham, *CG*, 'Preface', sig. A5r.

26 D. B. Updike, *Printing Types: Their History, Forms and Use*, 2 vols. (Cambridge, 1922), II, 126.

27 Cuningham produced versions of diagrams that had appeared in works by, *inter alia*, Oronce Fine, Peter Apian and Robert Recorde. For examples, compare Robert Recorde, *The Castle of Knowledge* (London: Reginald Wolfe, 1556), pp. 9, 18, 29, 64, with *CG*, pp. 13, 15, 26, 64; Oronce Fine, *Protomathesis* (Paris: Gerard Morrhy and Jean Pierre, 1532), fols. 102v, 103r, 108v, 110v, 144r, 155r–v with *CG*, pp. 10, 13, 30, 33, 42, 76, 114, 116; Oronce Fine, *De mundi sphaera, sive cosmographia* (Paris: Michel de Vascosan, 1555), fols. 3v, 8v with *CG*, pp. 13, 33; and Peter Apian, *Cosmographicus liber* (Landshut: Johann Weissenburger, 1524), pp. 9, 10, 12, 26–9, 35, 60 with *CG*, pp. [40], 62, 64, 74, 98–102, 121.

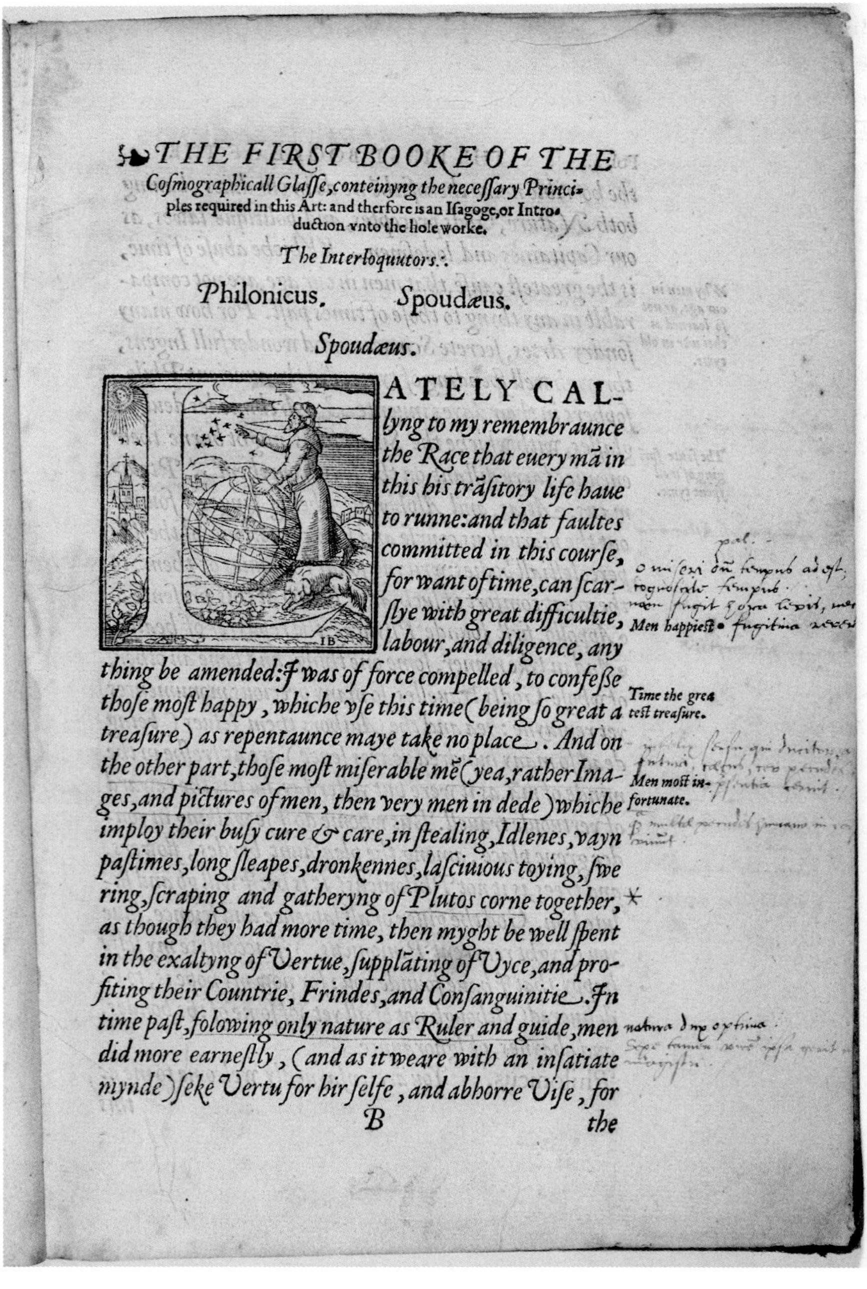

THE FIRST BOOKE OF THE Cosmographicall Glasse, conteinyng the necessary Principles required in this Art: and therfore is an Isagoge, or Introduction vnto the hole worke.

The Interloquutors.

Philonicus. Spoudæus.

Spoudæus.

LATELY CALlyng to my remembraunce the Race that euery mā in this his trāsitory life haue to runne: and that faultes committed in this course, for want of time, can scarsly with great difficultie, labour, and diligence, any thing be amended: I was of force compelled, to confesse those most happy, whiche vse this time (being so great a treasure) as repentaunce maye take no place. And on the other part, those most miserable mē (yea, rather Images, and pictures of men, then very men in dede) whiche imploy their busy cure & care, in stealing, Idlenes, vayn pastimes, long sleapes, dronkennes, lasciuious toying, swering, scraping and gatheryng of Plutos corne together, as though they had more time, then myght be well spent in the exaltyng of Vertue, supplāting of Vyce, and profiting their Countrie, Frindes, and Consanguinitie. In time past, folowing only nature as Ruler and guide, men did more earnestly, (and as it weare with an insatiate mynde) seke Vertu for hir selfe, and abhorre Vise, for the

B

Men happiest.

Time the great treasure.

Men most infortunate.

Figure 4: Initial letter by John Bettes showing an armillary sphere, opening Book One of *The Cosmographical Glasse*, which deals with the principal circles of the heavens. Each book of the *Glasse* opens with a decorated letter that reflects the main subject discussed within.

figures calculated for the meridian of Norwich (itself composed of almost forty small woodblocks) and thirteen further tables, in addition to purely decorative elements. Cuningham gratefully recognized John Day's skill and expense in producing them.[28] The large format of the work – a folio edition of over two hundred pages – indicates that it was intended to be a prestigious item of a quality fit to bear Robert Dudley's arms. Before *The Cosmographical Glasse* the only other books of this size produced by Day's press were the Latin missal and the Bible. Conversely, all of Day's previous or concurrent medical publications – Turner's herbal, a work on chiromancy and physiognomy, William Bullein's *Governement of Healthe* – were pocket-sized volumes of octavo or duodecimo proportions.[29] As a result, Cuningham's book was very expensive and only a limited number were ever printed.[30]

In the text, Cuningham took on the vast subject of 'the heavens with her planets and starres, the earthe with her beautifull regions, and the seas with her merveilous increse'.[31] The opening section constituted a primer in cosmographical theory. In it, Cuningham tackled such questions as the composition of the heavenly and elementary regions, and the size and rotundity of the earth. He also defined the great circles of the heavens and the terrestrial zones, and considered the use of various instruments including the quadrant, astrolabe, cross staff and Ptolemy's rulers. In accordance with his original working title for the volume (The *Geographicall Glasse*)[32] Cuningham went on to discuss the problem of calculating longitude, and explained how map-makers

[28] Cuningham, *CG*, 'Preface', sig. A6v. The printer's achievements and aims are discussed in E. Evenden, *Patents, Pictures and Patronage: John Day and the Tudor Book Trade* (Aldershot, 2008), pp. 59–61, 95.

[29] In the same year that *The Cosmographical Glasse* was produced, Day also printed Nostradamus's predictions on infirmities for 1559/60 and a tract on medicinal distillations: J. Ames, W. Herbert and T. F Dibdin, *Typographical Antiquities: The History of Printing in England, Scotland and Ireland*, 4 vols. (London, 1810–19), IV, 51, 70–1, 75.

[30] Evenden, *Patents, Pictures and Patronage*, p. 60.

[31] Cuningham, *CG*, 'Dedication', sig. A2r. E. G. R. Taylor, *The Mathematical Practitioners of Tudor and Stuart England* (Cambridge, 1967), pp. 26–8, and E. G. R. Taylor, *Tudor Geography, 1485–1583* (London, 1930), pp. 26–7, give digests of the methods, instruments and themes addressed by Cuningham. On the Germanic cosmographical tradition, the varying agendas of different 'cosmographers', and the use of the term cosmography in works – like Cuningham's – that were largely, in fact, geographies based on Ptolemaic principles, see McLean, *Cosmographia of Sebastian Münster*, pp. 111–26.

[32] Cuningham [Kenningham], *A&P* 1558, 'Prognostication', sig. A2v.

learn simple triangulation. These latter subjects he discussed in relation to surveying expeditions in Norfolk.[33] A thorough grounding in cosmography was essential, Cuningham argued, for both the physician and the anxious patient. Indeed, he went further, claiming that 'mannes helth ... can not be conserved in perfite estate, or once lost be recovered and restored *without* [an understanding of] cosmographie'.[34] Elaborating, he explained that, with such knowledge, a practitioner could advise the long-term sick to move to more salubrious places where it was possible to recuperate in healthier air. Cuningham referred his reader back to the ancient medical tradition for justification of his claims, stating:

> For howe greatlye herein it profiteth, to consider the temperature of regions, cities, townes, in what zone and under what clymate and parallele they are situated, Hippocrates dothe plainlye set out.[35]

The Hippocratic work to which Cuningham gestured was that known in English as *Airs, Waters, Places*,[36] a didactic and empirical manual for practising physicians based upon simple logic and observation. Written in Greek during the second half of the fifth century BC, *Airs, Waters, Places* comprehensively defined how a town's or district's environment (its aspect, climate, the nature of the prevailing winds and

33 He demonstrated how to perform triangulation using the towers of Norwich cathedral, Wymondham abbey and Swardeston church: Cuningham, *CG*, p. 140. Perhaps it was upon one of these expeditions that Cuningham also conducted his observations of oak galls, which he reported were not only 'growyng about Norwich' but were 'in certayne wooddes, very plentifull': this medically inspired interest was recorded by John Halle in the latter's edition of the *Chirurgia parua Lanfranci*, p. 42.

34 Cuningham, *CG*, 'Preface', sig. A6r.

35 Cuningham, *CG*, 'Preface', sig. A6r, my emphasis. See also ibid., p. 63 for the statement that it is important to know which parts of the earth are within a *habitable zone* 'for the conservation, and also reperation and restoring a man unto health lost; for by that invention the temperature of the aere is easely founde out'.

36 On the political use to which the same text was being put, contemporaneously, by Andrea Marini (d. 1570) in Venice, see J. Wheeler, 'Stench in Sixteenth-Century Venice', in *The City and the Senses: Urban Culture Since 1500*, ed. A. Cowan and J. Steward (Aldershot, 2007), pp. 26–38 (pp. 31–2). For the original context of its production, see J. C. Kosak, '*Polis nosousa*: Greek Ideas about the City and Disease in the fifth century BC', in *Death and Disease in the Ancient City*, ed. V. M. Hope and E. Marshall (London, 2000), pp. 35–54, and V. Nutton, 'Medical Thoughts on Urban Pollution', in ibid., pp. 65–73.

the quality of its water) impacted on its inhabitants' health. It opened with an exhortation that the successful physician must first understand the 'effect of each of the seasons of the year and the differences between them' (that is, the degree of heat, coolness, dryness and moisture characteristic of each season, and its influence upon the body's complexion). Secondly, 'he must study the warm and the cold winds, both those which are common to every country and those peculiar to a particular locality'. Lastly, he should be familiar with the impact of water upon health. These meteorological and environmental factors had then to be analysed in conjunction with the particular lifestyle of the inhabitants. The physician should, for example, consider whether his patients were prone to overindulgence, or if they willingly worked and exercised. A practitioner who understood these principles 'could not fail to observe what diseases are important in a given locality as well as the nature of the inhabitants in general', even if the district was unfamiliar to him.[37]

The Hippocratic author further elaborated on the distinct qualities credited to the each of the four cardinal winds. Cold winds blew from the northerly quarter and were the reputed cause of drying diseases such as constipation, abscesses and pleurisy. The warmer winds from the south caused moist, phlegmy conditions: vaginal discharges, miscarriages and diarrhoea. People living in towns exposed to the wet, westerly winds were victims of the worst, most unhealthy circumstances, owing to the persistently damp and impure air.[38] Conversely, towns which faced the east and which, therefore, had an easterly prevailing wind, were believed to be the healthiest.[39] Cuningham made a pictorial reference to the quality of the winds and their significance for health when illustrating his text (fig. 5).[40]

[37] Hippocrates, *AWP*, ed. Lloyd, p. 148.

[38] Later commentators differed in their assessment of the particular qualities of the winds: the southern wind, and not the westerly one, was generally described as the least healthy in medieval and sixteenth-century medical literature.

[39] Hippocrates, *AWP*, ed. Lloyd, pp. 149–52. See also Hippocrates, *Regimen* II.xxxviii, cf. *Hippocrates: Volume IV*, trans. W. H. S Jones (Cambridge MA, 1931) pp. 301–5, esp. p. 305 which suggests that extremes of wind temperature and air turbulence are key factors in causing disease.

[40] The image drew on an existing iconography of the correspondences between the winds, elements and seasons: see S. E. Holbrook, 'A Medieval Scientific Encyclopaedia "Renewed by Goodly Printing": Wynkyn de Worde's English "De proprietatibus rerum"', *Early Science and Medicine* 3 (1998), 119–55 (pp. 147–52), and (for the deeper history) see B. Obrist, 'Wind Diagrams and Medieval

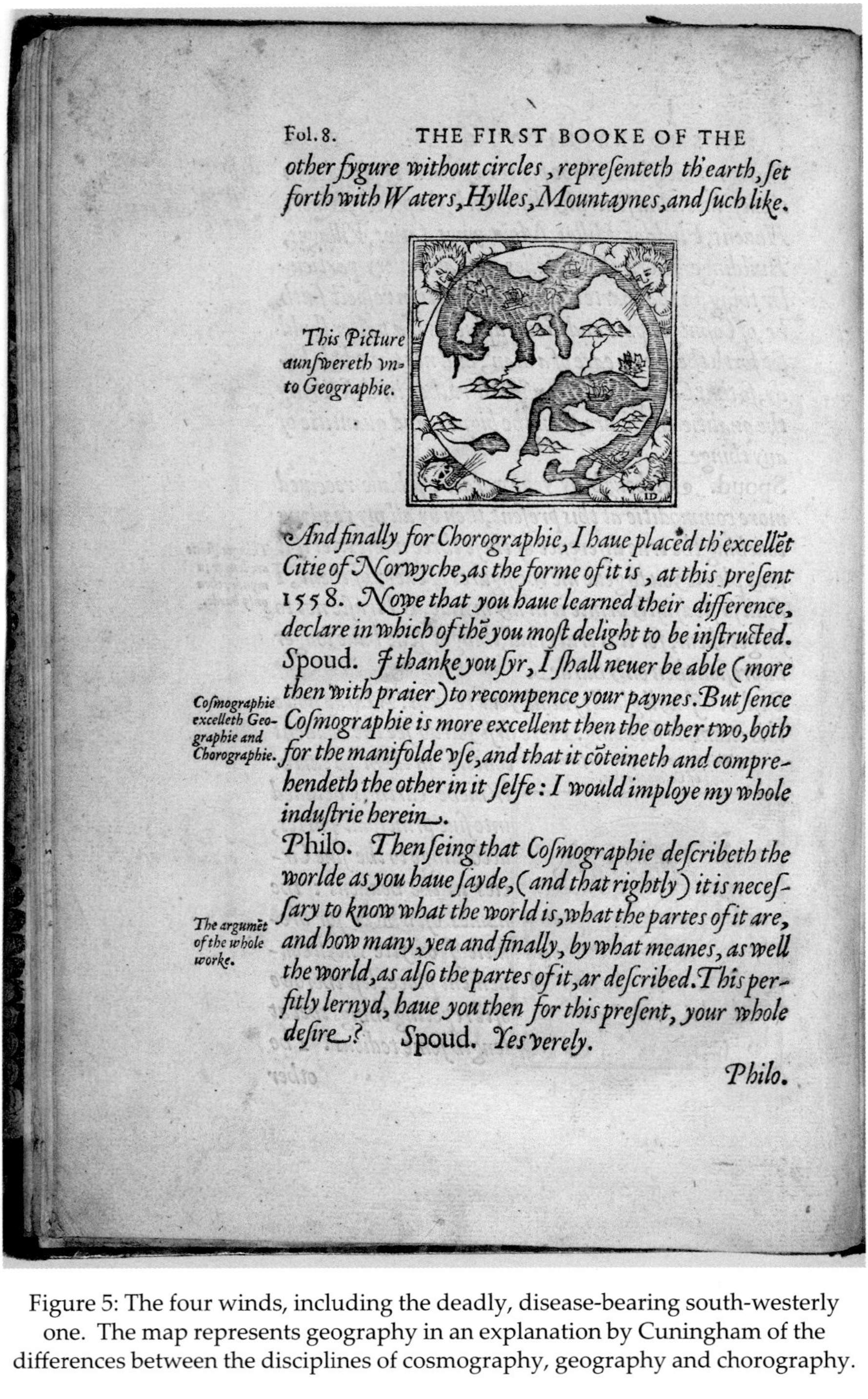

Fol. 8. THE FIRST BOOKE OF THE

other fygure without circles, repreſenteth th'earth, ſet forth with Waters, Hylles, Mountaynes, and ſuch like.

This Picture aunſwereth vnto Geographie.

And finally for Chorographie, I haue placed th'excellẽt Citie of Norwyche, as the forme of it is, at this preſent 1558. Nowe that you haue learned their difference, declare in which of thẽ you moſt delight to be inſtructed.

Spoud. I thanke you ſyr, I ſhall neuer be able (more then with praier) to recompence your paynes. But ſence Coſmographie is more excellent then the other two, both for the manifolde vſe, and that it cõteineth and comprehendeth the other in it ſelfe: I would imploye my whole induſtrie herein.

Coſmographie excelleth Geographie and Chorographie.

Philo. Then ſeing that Coſmographie deſcribeth the worlde as you haue ſayde, (and that rightly) it is neceſſary to know what the world is, what the partes of it are, and how many, yea and finally, by what meanes, as well the world, as alſo the partes of it, ar deſcribed. This perfitly lernyd, haue you then for this preſent, your whole deſire? Spoud. Yes verely.

The argumẽt of the whole worke.

Philo.

Figure 5: The four winds, including the deadly, disease-bearing south-westerly one. The map represents geography in an explanation by Cuningham of the differences between the disciplines of cosmography, geography and chorography.

Much of the second half of *Airs, Waters, Places* comprised an extended gazetteer which described the climate and topography of Asia and Europe on a country-by-country basis. In each case, the Hippocratic author demonstrated how the local environment shaped the physiology and character of the inhabitants.[41] Cuningham drew inspiration from this too when, in the fifth and final book of *The Cosmographical Glasse,* he interspersed a Ptolemaic table of longitude and latitude with observations on the difference between the peoples of different countries[42] and their medical practices, and descriptions of the landscape.[43] In tabulating the principal towns of England in this way, he referred the reader back to the depiction of his birthplace at the very beginning of the volume, stating: 'Norwiche [is] an healthfull and pleasant citye' with 'a faire [i.e. clean] river ... ronning thorow it'.[44]

Cuningham was well placed to understand the nuances of *Airs, Waters, Places.* He claimed to have produced commentaries on the tract,[45] and he chose to quote directly from it in his almanac for 1564.[46]

Cosmology', *Speculum* 72 (1997), 33–84. On Cuningham's understanding of the relationship between air, health and medicine more broadly, see *CG*, pp. 81–2 (where he cites Avicenna and Hippocrates on the changeability of air temperature as a cause of disease), and p. 158 (on the study of the heat or coldness of the winds being a subject belonging to physic rather than to navigation).

41 Hippocrates, *AWP*, ed. Lloyd, pp. 159–69.

42 Cuningham, *CG*, pp. 169–202. One of Cuningham's sources, Peter Apian, had done the same thing in his *Cosmographicus liber*, pp. 70–104.

43 These observations were heavily influenced by Cuningham's prejudices. For example, he described the Irish as, 'savage, wilde, and beastly; [and] given to sorcerie, superstition and witchcraft'. Yet, whilst disparaging of its people, Cuningham praised Ireland's situation, which generated 'very many herbes necessarye for the healthe of man': Cuningham, *CG*, p. 172, and see (for the 'precious drugges' of America) p. 201.

44 Cuningham, *CG*, p. 174.

45 This he must have done at some point prior to mid-1559: his *magnum opus* gives the *terminus ante quem*. Cuningham, *CG*, 'Preface', sig. A2v.

46 Cuningham, *A&P* 1564, 'Prognostication', sigs. A3v–4r. The passage detailed the dire consequences for reproduction caused by a wet and mild winter dominated by southerly winds if it was followed by a cold spring: 'mulieres quae uterum gestant, et partus ipsis ad ver instat, abortum facturas verisimile est, quae vero pepererint, impotentes ac morbosos parere, ita ut aut statim pareant [*r.* pereant] aut tenues, imbecilli, et morbosi vivant: reliquis vero dissenterias, et lippitudines siccas, aliquibus, defluxiones a capite in pulmonem senibus autem propter raritatem, et eliquationem venarum, ita ut nonnulli phrenites de subito pereant, alii vero dextra aut sinistra parte resoluantur, etc.' (Women who are carrying in the womb and whose offspring are due in spring will probably induce abortion; those, however, who do give birth, give birth to weak and

The first, revised Greek and Latin printed editions of the work itself were produced in Italy and Basel in the latter half of the 1520s.[47] Cuningham's medical colleagues would thus have fully understood the concepts behind his allusions. But other readers of *The Cosmological Glasse* need not have been as familiar as Cuningham with the Hippocratic text in order to understand the basic premise. The same ideas were accessible in a digested form in recently published printed health manuals. For example, Andrew Boorde (who we have already encountered as the beneficiary of the patronage of the duke of Norfolk) echoed Hippocrates when he stressed the importance of an easterly aspect to anyone choosing to build or to improve his house.[48] A gentleman should, he wrote:

sickly <children>, such that they either die immediately or live on weak, fragile and sickly. As to other people, <they have> dysenteries and dry inflammations of the eye; some old people experience flows from the head into the lung, on account of the sparseness and draining off of the veins, such that some of them <become> frenzied <and> die suddenly, while others are paralysed on the right or left side, etc). Cf. Hippocrates, *AWP*, ed. Lloyd, p. 157 and, for a different Latin translation from the Greek, see Hippocrates of Cos, *Hippocratis coi medicorum omnium longe principis, opera quae ad nos extant omnia,* trans. Janus Cornarius (Basel: Hieronymus Froben and Nicolaus Episcopius, 1546), p. 110. (On this translation, see J. Jouanna, *Airs, eaux, lieux* (Paris, 1996), pp. 157–8.)

47 In addition to the Latin collected works published in 1525 (in a translation attributed to Calvius) and the Greek Aldine edition of 1526, Janus Cornarius produced a Greek edition with a Latin translation in 1529 (Basel) and 1542 (Paris), the Latin version of which was widely published in 1546 (in the *opera omnia,* see n. 46 above). Adrien L'Alemant's commentary on the text was printed in 1557, in Paris. These editions are catalogued in *Cinq cents ans de bibliographie Hippocratique 1473–1982*, ed. G. Maloney and R. Savoie (Quebec, 1982). On the pre-modern transmission of *Airs, Waters, Places* more broadly, see Hippocrates, *Airs, eaux, lieux*, ed. J. Jouanna (Paris, 1996). On the channels of direct and indirect transmission of Latin versions of the text during the high Middle Ages, see P. Biller, 'Proto-Racial Thought in Medieval Science', in *The Origins of Racism in the West*, ed. M. Eliav-Feldon, B. Isaac and J. Ziegler (Cambridge, 2009), pp. 157–80 (pp. 160–4). The medieval *Ars medicinae* did not normally contain the text; C. O'Boyle, *The Art of Medicine: Medical Teaching at the University of Paris, 1250–1400* (Leiden, 1998), p. xiii, n. 12 notes two manuscripts containing it, but these are exceptional. A reduced Latin translation was incorporated in Pedro Pomar, *Articella* (Lyons, 1515), fols. 77r–82v. The concepts were, nonetheless, available to medieval readers: book I, part II, thesis II, chapter 11 of Avicenna's *Canon* included material on healthy and less healthy situations drawn from the Hippocratic text.

48 See above, p. 39–40. For the Italian tradition of similarly marketed texts on the same theme as Boorde's, see Cavallo and Storey, *Healthy Living*, esp. pp. 70–112,

ordre and edyfy the howse so that the pryncipall and chefe prospectes may be Easte and West ... for the South wynde doth corrupte and doth make evyll vapours. The Est wynde is temperat, fryske and fragrant.[49]

Visualizing the ancient Greek tradition: Cuningham's plan of Norwich in focus

Cuningham introduced his Norwich plan in a passage of his text which discussed the ancient Ptolemaic distinction between the disciplines of chorography, geography and cosmography.[50] As he conceived it, the purpose of chorography was to illustrate 'the qualitie and figure [form]' of a place such as a town, city, harbour or building. Geography, on the other hand, delineated the whole earth and the things contained within it, and thus treated such subjects as the sizes and quantities of hills, mountains and seas. Finally, cosmography described the surface of the earth in relation to heavenly coordinates, specifically the five principal parallels (or equidistant circles) of the heavens. The Norwich plan served to illustrate the aims of chorography: in other words, it is an image which represents the *quality* of a place.

The year before Cuningham's map was published, William Bullein (d. 1576), with characteristic humour, discussed the current state of knowledge about good air and safe locations to build. Despite the generally temperate climate, he claimed, England's variegated topography of 'fennes, marisses, wodes, heythes, valleis, playnes, and rockie places' was subject to frequent outbreaks of 'pestilence, horrible fevers, and sweeting sickenes', not only because of the influence of 'infortunate' stars, but also, by implication, because of the presence

which also discusses diachronic developments in medical thought regarding wind and air quality.

49 Boorde, *Boke for to Lerne A Man*, sig. B2v, and Boorde, *Dyetary of Helth*, sigs. C1v–2r.

50 On these differences, see Cuningham, *CG*, pp. 5–8, and see figure 5 in the present volume. For the tradition upon which he drew, see *Ptolemy's Geography: An Annotated Translation of the Theoretical Chapters*, ed. J. L. Berggren and A. Jones (Princeton, 2000), pp. 57–8, and Apian, *Cosmographicus liber*, pp. 1–4 (with thanks to Nick Jardine and Sachiko Kusukawa). For the wider context, see A. Mosley, 'Early Modern Cosmography: Fine's *Sphaera mundi* in Content and Context', in *The Worlds of Oronce Fine*, ed. Marr, pp. 114–36, and K. A. Vogel, 'Cosmography', in *The Cambridge History of Science*, ed. K. Park and L. Daston, 7 vols. (Cambridge, 2003–), III, 469–96.

on these shores of particular *loci insalubres*. These he listed as follows: places with 'multitudes of people dwelling to together (sic)',[51] 'foull houses' or 'houses invironed with standing waters wherinto jakes or sinkes have issues', and grounds where 'dead carions be cast' and swine wallow.[52] Each caused the air to become 'distempered', which in turn corrupted human blood. Cuningham's plan provided a striking contrast to such a downbeat appraisal; his Norwich was a model of a salubrious city, drawn upon Hippocratic lines.

However, in signalling the quintessentially healthy features of Norwich, Cuningham had to apply a cosmetic gloss to his subject matter. He devised a number of techniques which emphasized health-promoting features whilst minimizing or obscuring those aspects of Norwich's appearance that damaged his case. The most significant of these devices was his decision to orientate the map on an east–west axis, with east (and thus the gentle sweep of the river Wensum) at the top of the page (fig. 1).[53] This seems odd to modern viewers accustomed to the convention of placing north at the top of maps, but Cuningham was able to exercise free choice in the matter.[54] He used the opportu-

[51] That is, in excessive proximity or density.

[52] William Bullein, *The Governement of Healthe* (London: John Day, 1558), fols. 41r–42v.

[53] A fact that would not have been lost on readers of *The Cosmographical Glasse*, even those unfamiliar with Norwich. In the version reproduced here (fig. 1) a compass indicator has been included in the foreground. This addition, absent from an earlier version of the plan, supplemented the pointing arms of Philonicus and Spoudaeus (the two characters who conduct the book's dialogue) who also serve in the plate to indicate north: Frostick, *Printed Plans*, pp. 2–3. When a near contemporary reproduced Cuningham's map, he incorporated a lettered compass showing north to the left and east to the top, ensuring that the message could not be missed: William Smith, *The Particular Description of England, 1588*, ed. H. B. Wheatley (London, 1879), plate xxvii.

[54] For example, in a slightly earlier map of Norwich, the Norwich Sanctuary Plan, north was placed at the bottom of the page. On the Sanctuary Plan, see P. D. A. Harvey, *Maps in Tudor England* (London, 1993), p. 69; NCR 18a/6 CA 1537–47, fol. 61v (for the commission of the plan). On the fluid conventions relating to orientation in map-making in this period (where the most significant direction for a given purpose is placed at the top), see S. Tyacke, 'Introduction', in *English Map-Making 1500–1650*, ed. S. Tyacke (London, 1983), pp. 13–18 (pp. 15–16), and E. G. R. Taylor, 'The South-Pointing Needle', *Imago Mundi* 8 (1951), 1–7 (p. 1). The latter essay, incidentally, comments in passing on a diagram of a 'geographical plain sphere' as represented by Cuningham on p. 136 of *The Cosmographical Glasse*. In that image – as with a mariner's compass or theodolite – east and west are transposed, and so it reads (in a clockwise direction from the

nity to reference the aforementioned Hippocratic theory (elaborated upon by Andrew Boorde) that easterly situations, aspects and winds were most healthy. The issue at stake was laid out in an important passage in *Airs, Waters, Places*:

> [Towns] that face east are likely to be healthier than those facing north or south even if such places are only a furlong apart ... The water to the easterly side must necessarily be clean, sweet-smelling, soft and pleasant. This is because the early morning sunshine distils dew from the morning mist. The inhabitants are generally of good and healthy complexion ... They have loud clear voices and ... they are of better temperament and intelligence ... The climate in such a district may be compared with the Spring in that there are no extremes of heat and cold. As a consequence, diseases in such a district are few and not severe.[55]

Norwich – as the most easterly city in the country – was, therefore, healthy by force of its location. As we have already seen, Cuningham could reasonably expect his readers to make the association; the idea was in vogue. Bullein summarized the passage in *Airs, Waters, Places* very neatly: a city or town 'placed toward the east' owing to the more 'temperat aire or wynde' found in that region, was bound to suffer from few outbreaks of sickness (especially when compared to the 'townes builded towardes the north').[56] After his death, Cuningham's theme was revisited by a new generation of topographical writers.[57] For example, the antiquarian Henry Manship testified to the vitality of the theory in his 'History of Great Yarmouth', a manuscript chronicle of the borough, which he completed in 1619. Manship argued at length that the port's situation and bracing climate generated unusually 'wholesome air' (map 1). In direct emulation of 'cosmographers' since Cuningham, Manship noted Yarmouth's latitude and longitude before launching into a long digression which emphasized the port's easterly

top) S, E, N, W. This configuration assists a user in the field: the letter pointed to by the compass needle signifies the direction in which the operator is facing.

55 Hippocrates, *AWP*, ed. Lloyd, p. 151, cf., for example, Cornarius's translation in the 1546 edition of Hippocrates, *Opera*, p. 106.

56 Bullein, *Government of Healthe*, fol. 43r.

57 On the importance of situation and air in the mature tradition of urban panegyric (and for the ways in which the same symbolism was conscripted for polemical purposes), see M. Jenner, 'The Politics of London Air: John Evelyn's *Fumifugium* and the Restoration', *The Historical Journal* 38 (1995), 535–51 (p. 537).

situation and prospect.[58] Again echoing Hippocrates and citing Constantine the African (d. 1087), Manship declared that:

> the air of east lands and countries is clear and pure, and also dry and temperate between cold and moist; ... such a wind maketh waters clear and of a good savour, and they keep and save bodies in health ... also rivers and streams that run eastward and enter into the east sea be better and more wholesome and more clear than the others ...[59]

To add dignity to his subject, Manship was not afraid to draw biblical parallels:

> But to ground [the point] neither upon astrologers, astronomers or cosmographers, the very word of God approveth it: for Paradise, or the garden of Eden ... and the land of promise which did flow with milk and honey, are said to be seated in the east.[60]

Manship concluded that Yarmouth, which lay at the most easterly point in the country, could not be outdone in matters of health by any other town (implicitly, not even by its bigger cousin, Norwich):

> this town of Yarmouth being built north and south, in the whole longitude thereof, doth spread itself directly alongst the east, taking therby, as it were, a full possession of the benefit before remembered. It must needs, therefore, be concluded that Yarmouth is a town as wholesome for situation as any in this kingdom.[61]

In addition to air, the element of water also features prominently in Cuningham's image in the form of the river Wensum and the gathering rain clouds. Although later visitors were rather disparaging of the river's actual appearance (which they judged to be too narrow and sluggish), Cuningham portrayed the Wensum as wide and fast flowing.[62]

58 Manship, *History of Great Yarmouth*, p. 9. On Manship, who had been a town clerk of Yarmouth and a member of its civic council, see Tittler, 'Henry Manship'; 'The Cartulary of St Mary's Hospital, Great Yarmouth', ed. C. Rawcliffe, in *Poverty and Wealth*, ed. Bailey, Jurkowski and Rawcliffe, pp. 157–230 (pp. 171–8). Manship was educated first at a local grammar school and later at the prestigious Inns of Court.

59 Manship, *History of Great Yarmouth*, p. 104.

60 Ibid.

61 Ibid.

62 For Thomas Baskerville's disappointment with the river (recorded in 1681) see Rawcliffe, 'Introduction', p. xxiii.

His east–west configuration not only displayed the Wensum to its best advantage, but also hammered home the fact that the city's main water supply was mostly situated in the salubrious east.[63] In reality, Norwich had been regularly afflicted by flooding,[64] a situation that the informed would have feared on the basis that it was likely to generate unhealthy air. Worse still, extensive marshland and water meadows flanked the Wensum. In the Hippocratic tradition, marsh water was associated with 'an unpleasant smell', and was likely to cause an alarming catalogue of severe and fatal conditions including dysentery, diarrhoea, prolonged quartan fevers, pneumonia and madness. The inhabitants of such a place were likely to have obvious bodily and facial characteristics, including 'large and firm spleens', bellies that were 'hard, warm and thin', and a gaunt appearance around the face and clavicles 'because their spleens dissolve their flesh'.[65] Cuningham, then, had good reason to banish marshland from his depiction. Instead, lush greenery hints at a temperate climate and promising soil – again invoking the Hippocratic ideal of ground 'thickly covered with vegetation and well-watered'.[66]

Cuningham further manipulated the form and configuration of Norwich and its buildings in order to satisfy principles of order and harmony. Thus, he streamlined the layout of the streets in emulation of a grid pattern,[67] and he depicted the buildings as regular, sturdy constructions. In reality, certain areas of the city were in a very poor condition. In the autumn of the very same year that *The Cosmographical Glasse* went to press, the mayor and aldermen expressed concern about the number of dilapidated properties in the city. The minutes of a civic assembly held on or about 21 September 1559 lamented the appalling state of affairs whereby 'many commely and fayer howses ... in the whiche good howseholders and cittizens have heretofore dwelte' had been allowed to 'fall in rewin and decaye'. Some were altogether 'prostrate to the grounde'.[68] Even Cuningham was forced to admit in the

[63] A point that he further reinforced in the text, by mistakenly identifying the river's source as Great Yarmouth: Cuningham, *CG*, key to plan, before p. 9.

[64] There were serious floods in 1519, 1541, 1570: Fay, 'River and Street Accounts', pp. 108, 117; 'Chronological Memoranda', ed. Johnson, p. 143.

[65] Hippocrates, *AWP*, ed. Lloyd, p. 152.

[66] Ibid., p. 148.

[67] Viewers of the image might be forgiven for assuming that Norwich was a planned town; in fact it had grown organically over time. On the city's early development, see below, p. 131–3.

[68] *RCN*, II, 133.

accompanying text that his 'healthfull and pleasant citye' was 'much subject to fiers' which had 'not a little hindred the beuty' of his birthplace.[69] Nevertheless, in his plan, he took precautions to cover up the problem – and expunged damaged areas from it altogether.

Comparison of figures 7 and 8 with map 5 shows that Cuningham removed one centrally located street from his plan – the part of Pottergate east of St Lawrence's Lane – by filling it in with housing. The truncation of Pottergate was not due to any cartographical difficulty. Rather, it was part of Cuningham's sanitizing agenda. At least fifty-seven metres of buildings along the frontage here had been destroyed by the 1507 fire. In Cuningham's time, several plots on both sides of the street remained empty, and some were uninhabited into the mid-1600s (cf. map 4, site 149N).[70] This street was therefore in need of redevelopment (indeed, it may well have been one of those that the city fathers had in mind as they lamented the dilapidated state of the civic fabric). Cuningham employed a similar distortion in the south-east of the city. He depicted Ber Street – an important route into the city from the south – closer to the river Wensum than it truly ran, entirely omitting an area around King Street that had suffered particularly badly when insurgents ransacked the district in 1549.[71] Additionally, in reality, there was a concentration of lime-burning kilns situated on the tract of land between Ber Street and King Street, which would have belched out unpleasant fumes.[72] Comparison of figures 9 and 10 with map 6 shows how these alterations enabled Cuningham greatly to increase the amount of open space bordering onto the river, and also to exaggerate the size of St Catherine's croft in front. Health-promoting greenery thus displaced an area that was tainted with both physical corruption

69 Cuningham, *CG*, p. 174.

70 Atkin, Carter and Evans, EAA 26, pp. 72–4, 78–9. A civic land tax survey in 1568–70 indicates there were still a number of 'void' – that is, vacant – properties here, as well as others that (in the absence of population pressure) had been cultivated: *Landgable*, ed. Rodgers and Wallace, pp. 76–9. Indeed, there was a higher concentration of empty plots here than anywhere else in the city: see p. 168 n. 6 below. An act passed by the civic assembly in mid-April 1570 for new fire-prevention measures corroborates that plots, formerly graced with 'many goodly buyldinges and howses', had been turned into 'gardens and oretyards': *RCN*, II, 137.

71 NRO, NCR 18d, Landgable 1, fol. 3r, and see below, pp. 172–3.

72 B. Ayers, 'Building a Fine City: The Provision of Flint, Mortar and Freestone in Medieval Norwich', in *Stone, Quarrying and Building in England, AD 43–1525*, ed. D. Parsons (Chichester, 1990), pp. 217–27 (p. 220).

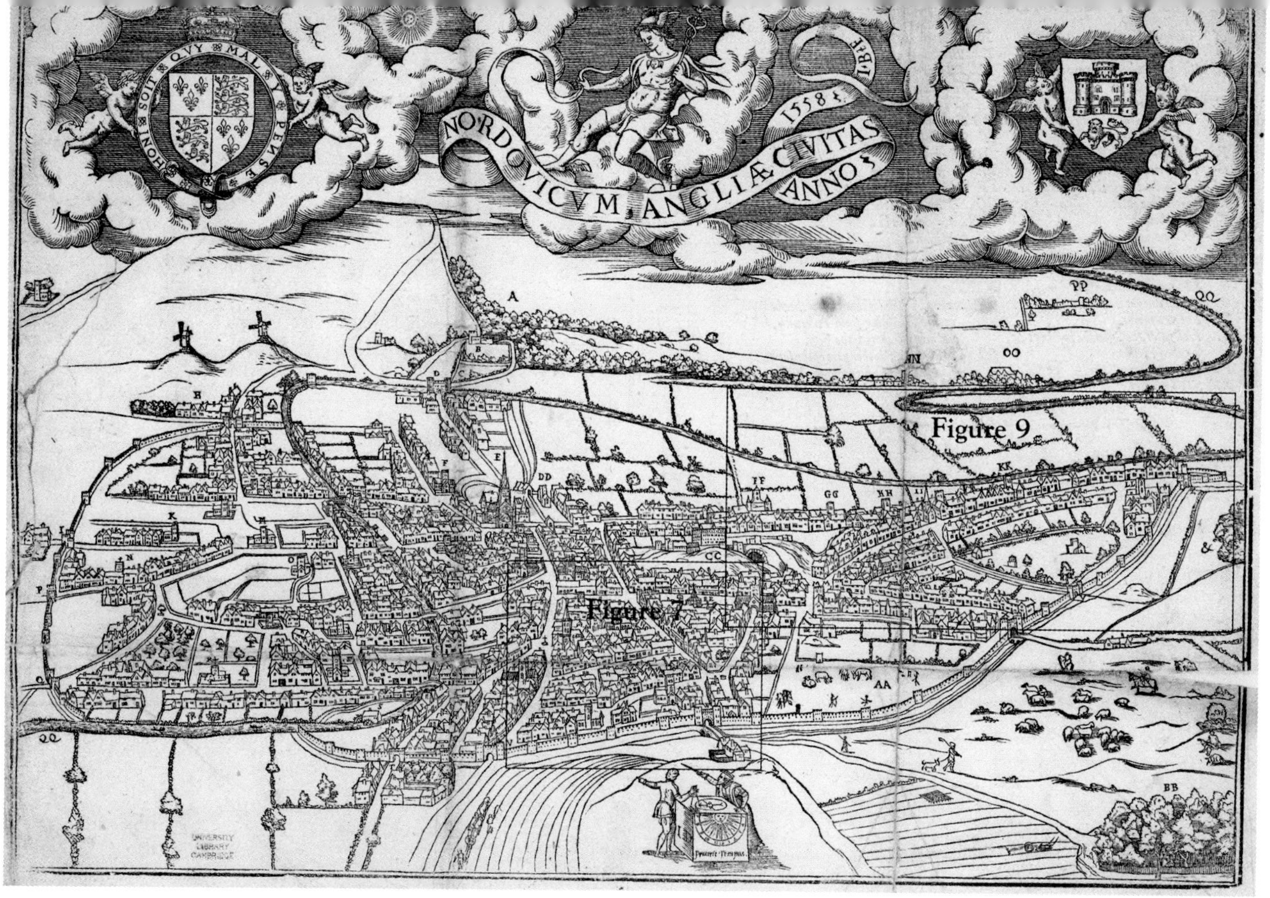

Figure 6: Cuningham's prospect showing the location of enlarged figures 7 and 9.

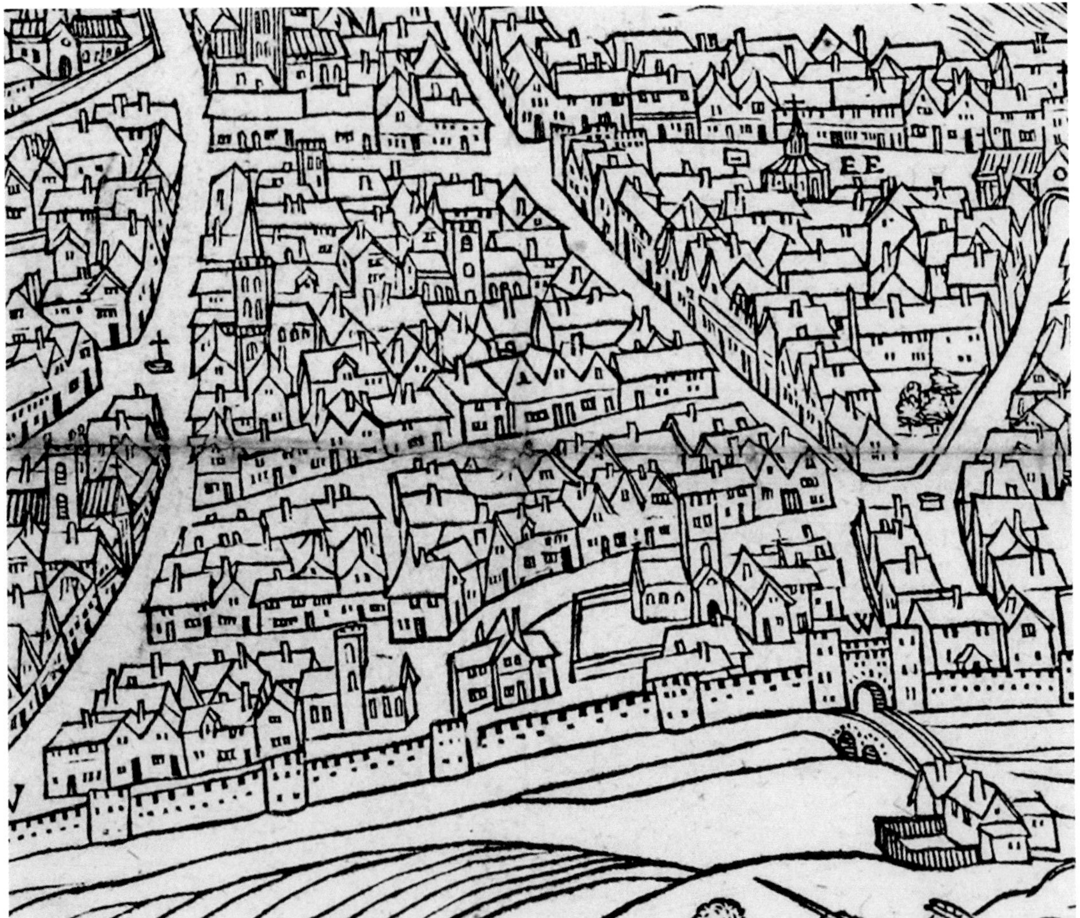

Figure 7: Cuningham's prospect: the surroundings of Pottergate.

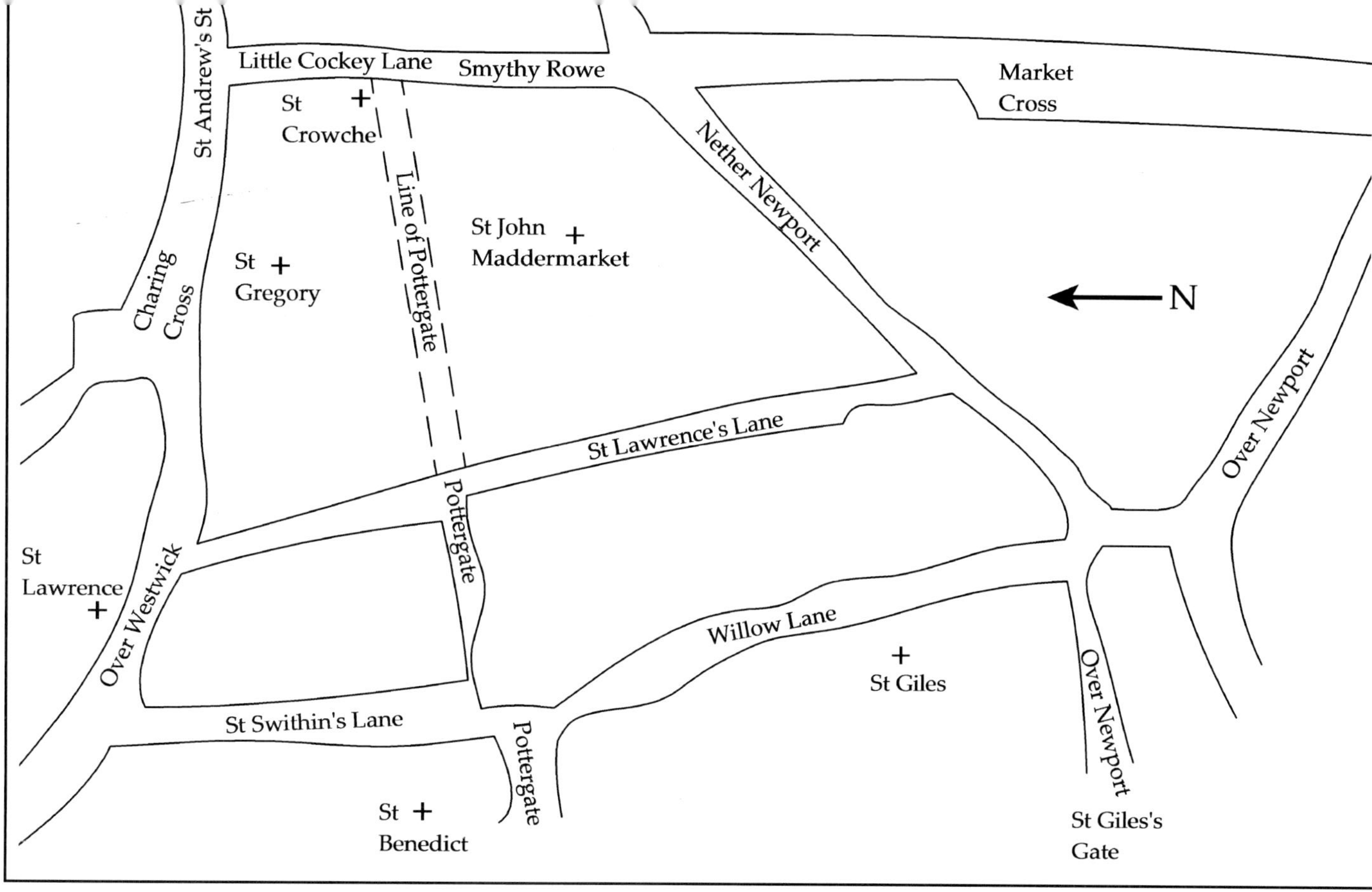

Figure 8: Outline of figure 7 showing street names and locations of churches.

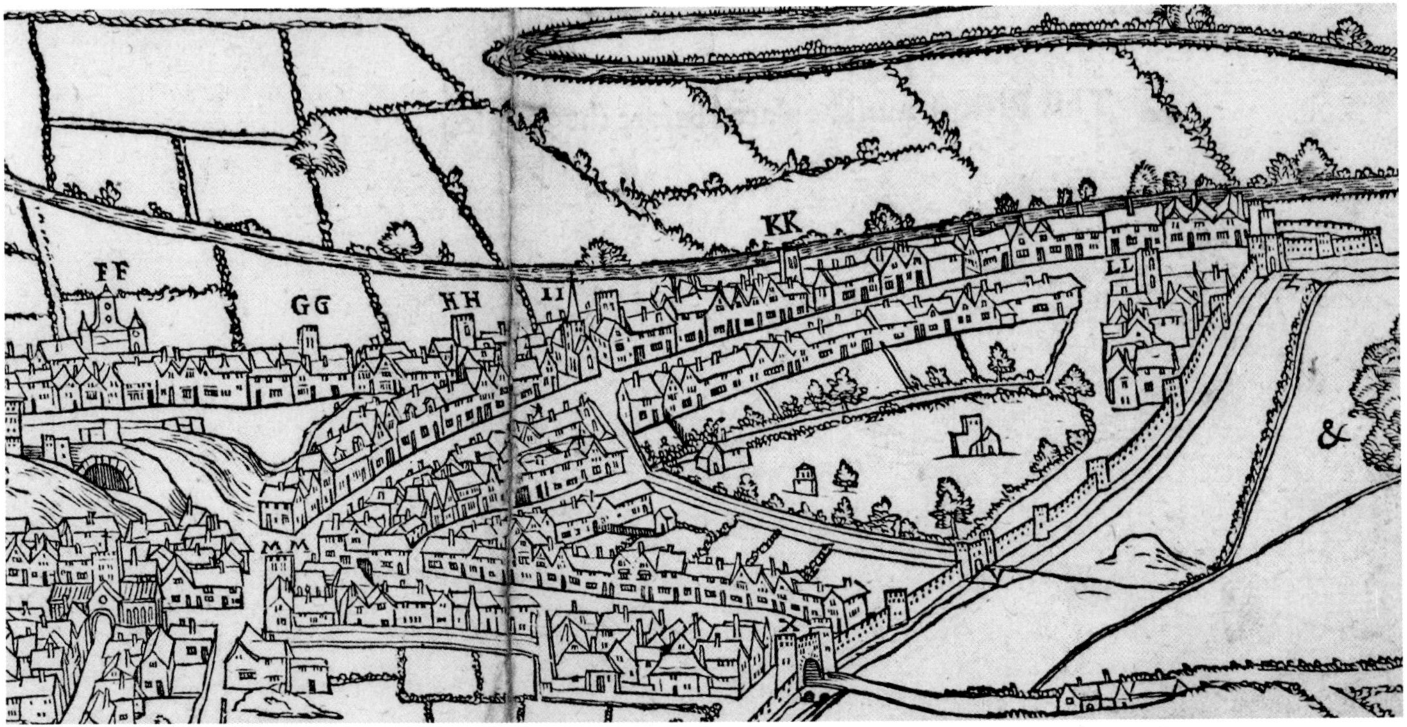

Figure 9: Cuningham's prospect: the surroundings of King Street (see figure 6 for location).

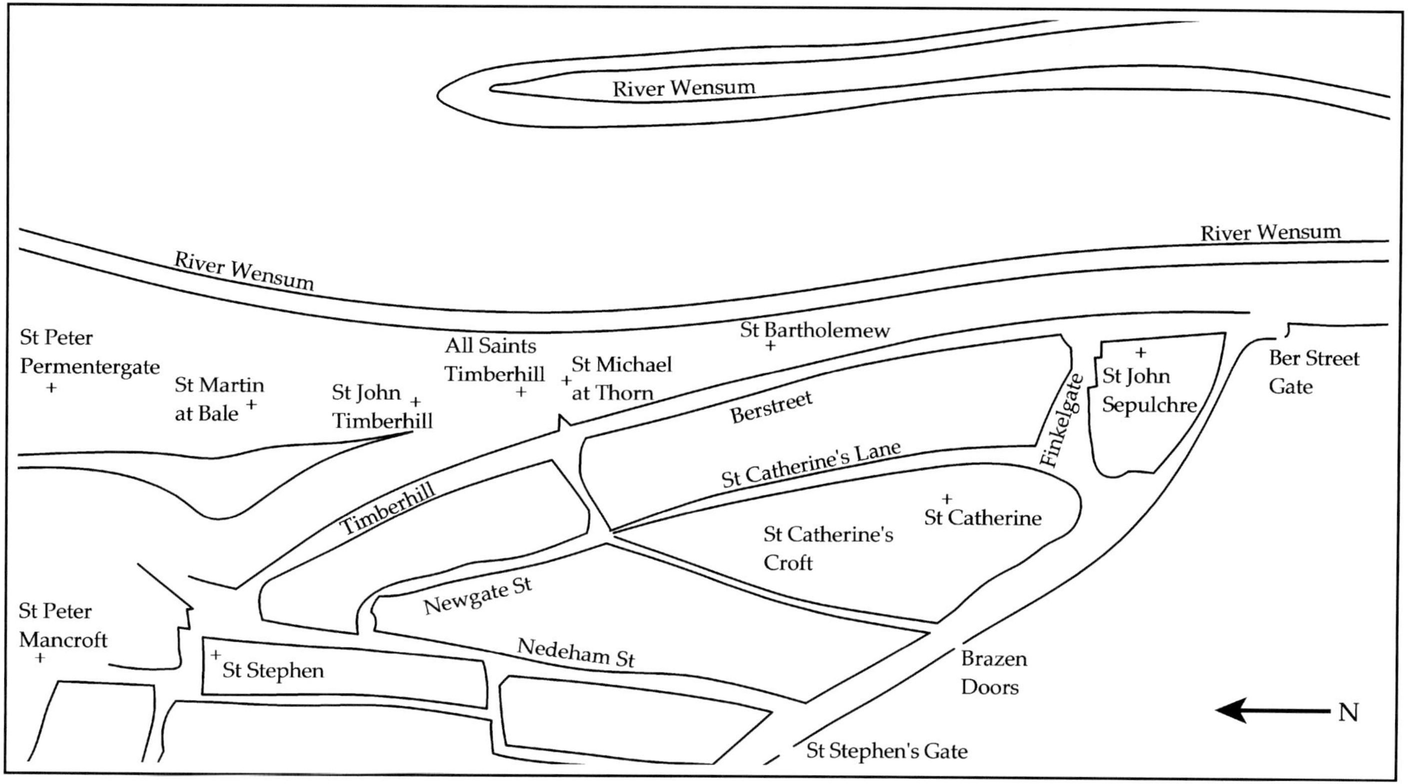

Figure 10: Outline of figure 9 showing street names and locations of churches.

and the memories of Kett's rebellion.[73] The result was an emphasis on the openness, symmetry and spaciousness of the city without any hint of the damage it had sustained.

Despite the setbacks which marked his later career, Cuningham made a favourable impression on some. Sir Martin Frobisher (d. 1594) thought *The Cosmographical Glasse* was of enough practical value to take a copy on his expedition to find a north-west passage to Cathay in 1576,[74] despite the volume's size and cost, and Cuningham's reassurance that the reader should not feel compelled to leave the comforts of his own hearth to see the world for himself. Most significantly, his 'prospect' held an enduring fascination for map-makers. One of several reproductions of it, a greatly simplified version of his plan published in Frankfurt in 1631 as part of a collection of emblematic European city scenes, played on Norwich's association with health and healing (fig. 11). Its Latin title referred to the divine gift of medicinal remedies: *Remedia ad sanitatem servandam creata sunt*.[75] Perhaps the chameleon in the image was a reference to Cuningham and his works; as noted above, the physician reportedly wrote a book on the subject of the *morbus gallicus* (or 'pox'), which he dubbed *chamaeleontiasis*, and as a result was apparently an authority on this disease.[76] Adepts who were familiar with the rules of decoding emblems may have drawn such a conclusion themselves.[77] Antiquarians in the early

[73] Similarly, the role of certain members of the city corporation in allowing the rebellion to take hold was blotted out of later written accounts of the event: A. Wood, 'Kett's Rebellion', in *MN*, ed. Rawcliffe and Wilson, pp. 277–99 (pp. 294–5).

[74] Waters, *Art of Navigation*, p. 99. Waters also notes that John Dee (d. 1609), the mathematician and royal astrologer, shared Cuningham's enthusiasm for maps and globes. For Dee's opinions on geography and chorography, see John Dee, 'Preface' to Euclid, *Elements of Geometrie*, trans. H. Billingsley (London, 1570), sig. A4r.

[75] The motto and derivative versions of the plan are discussed in Frostick, *Printed Plans*, esp. pp. 13–15. In the accompanying proverb, a raven mortally attacks a chameleon, and then medicates himself with bay leaves to counteract the lizard's poison.

[76] Gale, 'Treatise of Wounds made with Gonneshot', in *Certaine Workes of Chirurgerie*, fol. 9v, and see above, p. 37, n. 16.

[77] On medical emblems, see K. Ekholm, 'Anatomy, Bloodletting and Emblems: Interpreting the Title-Page of Nathaniel Highmore's *Disquisitio* (1651)', in *Observing the World Through Images: Diagrams and Figures in the Early-Modern Arts and Sciences*, ed. N. Jardine and I. Fay (Leiden, 2014), pp. 87–123, and references cited there.

eighteenth century persisted with Cuningham's basic message. The city's librarian, Benjamin Mackerell (d. 1738), a member of the 'Society of Icenians' (a learned group of local historians), declared in his own topographical survey that Norwich must be 'the most healthful city in England', owing to 'the goodness of its situation, the serenity of the air and the multitude of gardens in all parts'.[78] Another member of the group, Thomas Kirkpatrick, produced his own, beautiful 'prospect' of the city, which, when printed, spanned almost five feet.[79]

In tracing the filaments of the matrix of ideas concerning health and place, Part I of this book has taken us from the ancient world to the eighteenth century and across the boundaries of historical periodization and geography. Whilst the story is necessarily abbreviated here, we have glimpsed throughout how features from a substratum of common knowledge about the body and the environment were from time to time taken up in medical, civic, religious and domestic discourse. In the remaining circuits of our tour through Norwich, we will expand our methodology to incorporate the civic landscape itself. Part II of this book retains the theme of a city divided into healthy and unhealthy areas, but – instead of images and texts – it places behaviour, activities and objects at the forefront of enquiry.

[78] Rawcliffe, 'Introduction', in *MN*, ed. Rawcliffe and Wilson, p. xx, contextualized in pp. xxiii (on Norwich's gardens) and xxviii (on Mackerell).
[79] Frostick, *Printed Plans*, pp. 29–33.

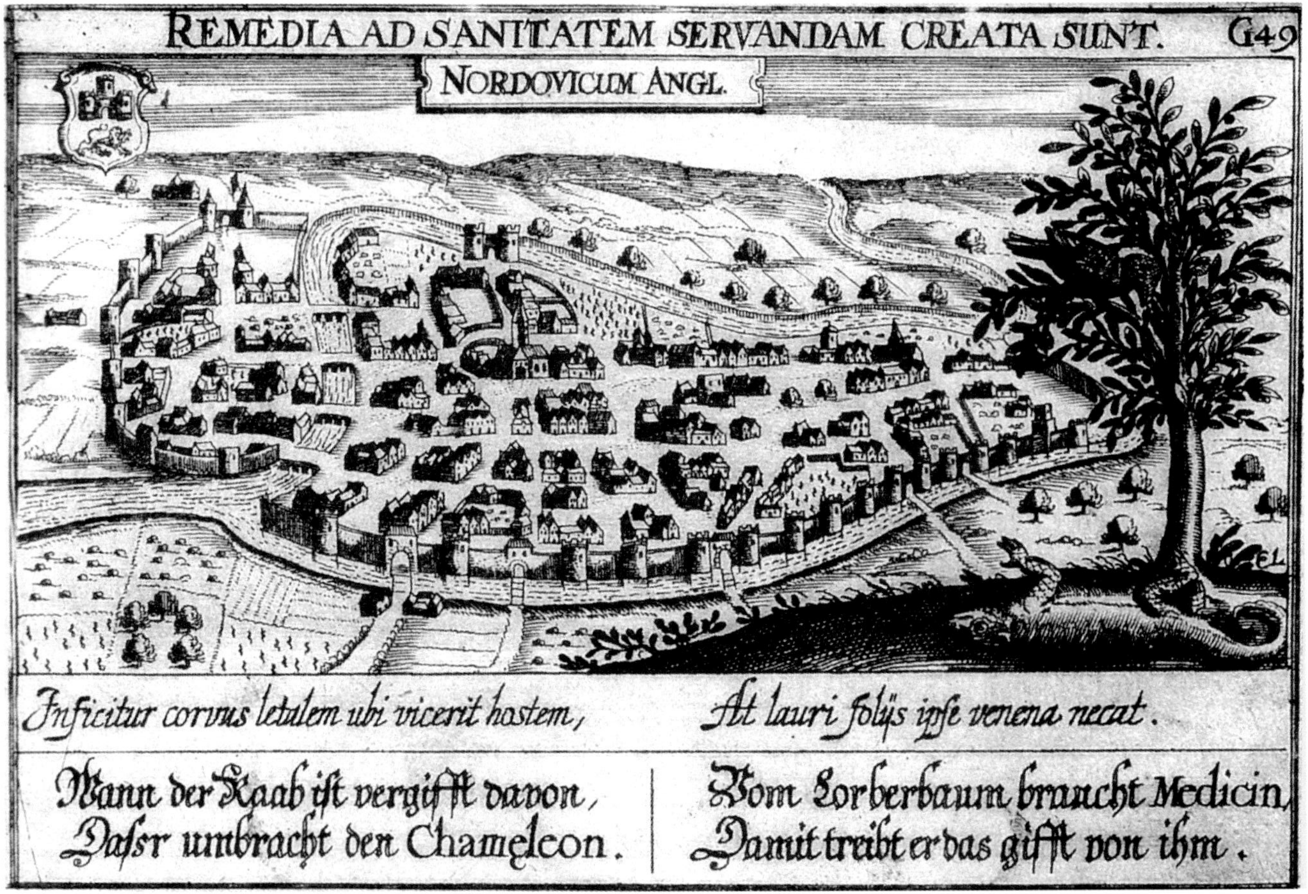
REMEDIA AD SANITATEM SERVANDAM CREATA SUNT.
G49
NORDOVICUM ANGL.
Inficitur corvus letalem ubi vicerit hostem,
At lauri foliis ipse venena necat.
Wann der Raab ist vergifft davon,
Dass er umbracht den Chameleon.
Vom Lorberbaum braucht Medicin,
Damit treibt er das gifft von ihm.

Figure 11: 'Medicines were created to preserve health': Norwich from Daniel Meisner's emblem book, *Thesaurus Philopoliticus VII* (Frankfurt, 1631).

Part II

Health and the Landscape

> In writing the history of health care, it is clearly important to respect indigenous categories ... A [broad] conception of the topic is called for: one that gives due weight to ritualism and symbolism, as we define them; and one that, equally, takes past conceptions of heath seriously ... The symbolic might be just as important as the material. That is, purity and community may be as desirable as health in a biomedical sense.[1]

What people think can be determined in two ways: firstly, from what they profess (write, depict or say), and secondly, from the evidence of what they do. Having established what men and women in Norwich and the region professed to believe about the interconnected nature of the human body and the wider environment, we can now determine how they actually used the space around them when prioritizing concerns about health and about disease. Part II of this book contrasts the idealized image of the city constructed by Cuningham with circumstances 'on the ground'. It brings together evidence from archaeology, osteoarchaeology and the documentary record to illustrate ways in which health culture was experienced and enacted in Norwich during our period. The resulting picture presents a philosophy of the body which is quintessentially civic. Although Norwich's native medical culture complemented, and encompassed, the ancient hygienic scheme, it was broader, and had particularly urban concerns at its heart: the differentiation of persons according to status, and the value

[1] P. Horden, 'Ritual and Public Health in the Early Medieval City', in *Body and City: Histories of Urban Public Health*, ed. S. Sheard and H. Power (Aldershot, 2000), pp. 17–40 (pp. 17, 19).

of property, of appropriate forms of corporate action and of individual responsibility. The following chapters offer two case studies on these themes. The first (which focuses predominantly on the initial 250-year period covered by this volume) takes people, disease and landscape as its leitmotifs; the second picks up developments from the fifteenth century onwards, and focuses on the city's healthy spaces. Both give us the opportunity to calibrate our notion of the constituent elements of pre-modern health culture; in both, the question of the nature and limits of the evidence is also kept in mind. Together, they locate sickness and pollution, poverty and salubrity in the city landscape: factors which throw light on the physical, economic and social categories at the heart of Norwich's 'indigenous' health culture. Our evidence base is composed of the rites and practices of pre-modern urban dwellers – of funerary customs, dramatic performances, recreations, therapeutic activities and pastimes. The particular physical setting in which such rites and practices were performed shaped their possible forms and limits; recursively, ideals about health and hygiene helped to determine how city space was used. Pre-modern city dwellers understood the capacity of urban space to shape and carry meaning in this regard;[2] they scanned it for significances, and interpreted the ways in which it was commonly manipulated. In what follows, therefore, we will ask: how did attitudes to health and disease help to shape the ways in which the urban environment was used and viewed?

[2] For more on this, see K. Giles, 'Framing Labour: The Archaeology of York's Medieval Guildhalls', in *The Problem of Labour in Fourteenth-Century England*, ed. Bothwell, Goldberg and Ormrod, pp. 65–83.

3

Placing Disease in the Urban Landscape: The Osteoarchaeological Evidence

> Space forms the arena in which social relationships are negotiated, expressed through the construction of landscapes, architecture and boundaries. The resulting spatial maps represent discourses of power based in the body.[1]

Entrenched in the Hippocratic tradition was the notion that the nature of a place determined the characteristics of people who lived there. This would have seemed self-evident to Norwich's residents who could observe at first-hand that more or less salubrious localities contained more or less healthy-looking individuals. In 1570, the civic authorities conducted a citywide census of the poor, that is, it made a house-by-house survey to identify all paupers who were apparently fit enough to work for a living and to distinguish them from those who were dependent, or might become dependent, on financial assistance from the community. The census demonstrated that some neighbourhoods contained dense concentrations of chronically crippled or bedridden residents, whilst others did not. For example, in the central part of the city closest to the economic hub, the rich and populous sub-ward of Mid Wymer – which housed the smallest proportion of sick poor of any district in Norwich – widowhood, old age and low-income employment accounted for cases of impoverishment, whereas

[1] R. Gilchrist, 'Medieval Bodies in the Material World: Gender, Stigma and the Body', in *Framing Medieval Bodies*, ed. S. Kay and M. Rubin (Manchester, 1994), pp. 43–61 (p. 43). Aspects of the present chapter revise the second part of Fay, 'Text, Space and the Evidence of Human Remains in English Late Medieval and Tudor Disease Culture: Some Problems and Possibilities', in *Social Archaeology of Funerary Remains*, ed. R. Gowland and C. Knüsel (Oxford, 2006) pp. 190–208.

debilitating disease in younger members of the community was rare.[2] A very different state of affairs prevailed in the city's margins.[3] In stark contrast to the relatively mobile residents of Mid Wymer, certain paupers (of all ages) living in the northern district 'Over-the-Water' were described as 'all together lame', 'deff', 'blynd', 'lunatick' or simply 'veri sick' (map 2).[4] One particular enclave housed a higher number of men and women with physical incapacities than anywhere else in the city.[5] That district was known as Fyebridge.

The association between poverty and disease in this area was very old: archaeological excavation from one of its parish cemeteries – St Margaret's Fyebridge – suggests a similar situation may have prevailed for up to 300 or 400 years (map 7, site 780N). Analysis of the skeletons removed from the site has indicated probable cases of tuberculosis and Hansen's disease (which used to be known as 'leprosy'), as well as other serious systemic infections, nutritional deficiencies, Paget's disease, physical trauma and a possible instance of paraplegia.[6] Why did the people buried in this enclave have such a distinctive pathological profile?[7] How were their deformities viewed by the community? And

[2] *The Norwich Census of the Poor, 1570,* ed. J. Pound, NRS 40 (Norwich, 1971), pp. 61–3.

[3] On the distribution of the poor across the city, see Pound, *Tudor and Stuart Norwich,* p. 127, table 10.1, and see Atkin and Evans, EAA 100, p. 156.

[4] *Norwich Census of the Poor,* ed. Pound, pp. 68–93.

[5] Fay, 'Text, Space and the Evidence of Human Remains', p. 194.

[6] Stirland, EAA 129, pp. 19–33; A. Stirland, 'Evidence for Pre-Columbian Treponematosis in Medieval Europe', in *L'origine de la syphilis en Europe: Avant ou après 1493?,* ed. O. Dutour, G. Pálfi, J. Bérato and J.-P. Brun (Paris, 1994), pp. 109–15, 300; A. Stirland, 'Patterns of Trauma in a Unique Medieval Parish Cemetery', *International Journal of Osteoarchaeology* 6 (1996), 92–100; A. Stirland, 'Care in the Medieval Community', *International Journal of Osteoarchaeology* 7 (1997), 587–90.

[7] I do not mean to imply with this question, or with the following discussion, that it is possible to reconstruct the total disease history of a population (or indeed of a single person) using skeletal evidence. This is in fact impossible for the following reasons: firstly, many serious and life-threatening diseases do not impact on the skeleton; secondly, bone has a propensity to heal and remodel itself (and thus remove evidence of injury and particular types of disorder); thirdly, (owing to factors governing funerary customs) an archaeological sample is unlikely to be representative of a live population. These issues are widely addressed in the palaeopathological literature, but for the *locus classicus,* see J. W. Wood, G. R. Milner, H. C. Harpending and K. M. Weiss, 'The Osteological Paradox: Problems of Inferring Prehistoric Health from Skeletal Samples', *Current Anthropology* 33 (1992), 343–70. My primary concern here,

what did that imply for the way in which the district was perceived in the wider civic landscape? Before attempting to try to answer these questions, it is worth pausing to consider the wider provision of cemetery space for the sick across Norwich at the time. This will help us to put the Fyebridge evidence – the main focus of this chapter – into its proper context.

Cemeteries for the sick in pre-modern Norwich

In pre-modern cities, parish churchyards, the cemeteries of religious houses and the burial grounds of hospitals all added to the local knowledge by which people classified the space around them; cemeteries were, in this regard, as important as commercial and judicial institutions or defensive structures for the identity of a locality, and for framing expectations of its use.[8] In Norwich, two large-scale, specialist cemeteries provided for the sick: the hospital of St Giles, and the *leprosarium* of St Mary Magdalen, Sprowston; each had its own burial grounds into which were placed the more or less decrepit or deformed bodies of their former residents (map 7). Both houses – which differed considerably in their remit, size and nature – provided spiritual care and a degree of physical succour, and, in return, the inmates were supposed to take an active part in the intercessory prayers offered there for departed benefactors.[9] Like St Margaret Fyebridge, both institutions also had their own characteristic populations: individuals who perhaps displayed evidence of stunted growth, scarred or altered faces, poor complexions, misshapen limbs, hands or feet, or whose respiration or mobility was compromised. No full-scale archaeological excavations have taken place in the precincts of either house to date,

however, is not with disease ecology (what diseases did the people of Norwich suffer from?), but to address the positive evidence of various ways in which the *manifestly disfigured or deformed* were treated after death in one particular locality, and, from this, to garner evidence of reactions to observable disease lesions in the urban milieu. For more on this approach, see Appendix I.

8 V. Harding, *The Dead and the Living in Paris and London, 1500–1670* (Cambridge, 2002), p. 3, which argues 'responses to death, in the form of burial practices and funeral rituals, are clearly bound up with issues of personal and family or community identity, geography and the use of space, control of the physical environment, and the ordering of society and social behaviour'. See also N. Whyte, 'The Deviant Dead in the Norfolk Landscape', *Landscapes* 1 (2003), 24–39.

9 At least prior to the dissolution of the chantries by act of parliament in 1547.

but we can nonetheless draw inferences about the kinds of conditions and illnesses suffered by the people accepted into each.

The ten-acre site of the hospital of St Giles possessed ample space for burial. Originally, the intention was to supply accommodation for at least thirty sick paupers, in addition to elderly, retired priests.[10] Other, comparable hospital sites indicate the kinds of disorders that may have affected the paupers admitted to St Giles's. A sample of thirty skeletons recovered from the cemetery at St Bartholomew's, Bristol, showed evidence of infected dental abscesses (a painful, even life-threatening condition owing to the potential complication of septicaemia); fractures; osteoarthritis of the shoulder, wrist and hip joints; periosteal new bone formation in the lower legs (suggesting a range of possible causes, including trauma, infection or vascular disturbances and, in one case, a probable chronic leg ulcer); and a long-term middle ear infection.[11] A comparable range of conditions has also been identified in excavated material from the large hospital and priory complex of St Mary Spital, London. The skeletons of the hospital's residents and the city's poor, taken from the hospital's main cemetery, demonstrated degenerative bone changes, impaired development, fractures and periosteal new bone formation.[12] Evidence of widespread defects in dental enamel[13] suggests that childhood illnesses disrupted the early growth of these individuals. The profile of the inmates offers a stark contrast to that of the long-lived, well-nourished clergy and lay benefactors who were buried in the St Mary's infirmary chapel. Widespread dental caries suggest that the latter group ate a richer diet, replete with sugar. Some attained an advanced age, and the skeletons from the

[10] On the population as envisaged by the institution's founder, Bishop Walter Suffield, see Rawcliffe, *MFTS*, p. 26. The dead, however, were likely to have included a wider sub-section of local people; the sick poor had the right to be interred in the precincts along with 'anybody else who [so] wished': C. Rawcliffe, 'The Seventh Comfortable Work: Charity and Mortality in the Medieval Hospital', *Medicina e Storia* 3 (2003), pp. 11–35 (p. 27). On similar themes, see also Harding, *The Dead and the Living*, p. 94.

[11] G. Stroud, 'Human Bone', in R. Price with M. Ponsford, *St Bartholomew's Hospital, Bristol: The Excavation of a Medieval Hospital, 1976–8*, CBA Research Report 110 (York, 1998), pp. 175–81.

[12] J. Conheeney, 'The Human Bone', in C. Thomas, B. Sloane and C. Phillpotts, *Excavations at the Priory and Hospital of St Mary Spital, London*, Museum of London Archaeology Service Monograp. 1 (London, 1997), pp. 225–31, and see ibid., pp. 111–12.

[13] Conheeney, 'The Human Bone', p. 225 (dental enamel hypoplasia).

chapel were also taller, implying that – unlike the hospital residents – they were not subjected to repeated periods of physiological stress as children and young adults.[14] Thus, medieval urban men and women could have distinguished people's status from the presentation of their bodies: differences were apparent in the skin and teeth, stature, girth and gait of the poor.[15]

At the Dissolution of the Monasteries, St Giles's hospital, Norwich, was purchased by the city government. The 'Great Hospital', as the refounded institution became known, provided a range of services for the education and welfare of Norwich residents. Its financial accounts provide evidence of the conditions suffered by the people then admitted, allowing glimpses of late Tudor diagnostic categories. 'Leprosy' and the 'pockes' apparently affected a very small number of people (both conditions required removal to one of the city's suburban 'spital houses' or almshouses, if confirmed). Tooth problems were recorded more often, and several people reportedly suffered with 'sore legs'. The hospital's surgeon was clearly capable of performing the very dangerous procedure of amputation; in 1575/76, one individual was provided with a 'stylt, after her legg was sawen of'. Sweats and fractured limbs were also mentioned.[16]

Conversely, the prestigious house of St Mary Magdalen in suburban Sprowston was founded exclusively for wealthier sufferers of 'leprosy'.[17] In the normal course of events, only manifestly disfigured or deformed people would expect to gain admittance at St Mary's as full-time residents.[18] This *leprosarium* had an important role in the ecclesiastical life of the city and, through its annual fair, in the rhythms of its economic

[14] Ibid., pp. 223, 229–31.

[15] On differences in growth and physiological stress (affecting stature and body shape) in medieval populations of contrasting socio-economic (and disease) status, see M. Schweich and C. Knüsel, 'Bio-cultural Effects in Medieval Populations', *Economics and Human Biology* 1 (2003), 367–77.

[16] Phillips, 'Charitable Institutions', pp. 252–3, 262–5.

[17] On the nature and diagnosis of medieval leprosy and its relationship to modern Hansen's disease, see the second part of Appendix I.

[18] On disfigurement as a determining factor in medieval diagnoses, see C. Rawcliffe, *Leprosy in Medieval England* (Woodbridge, 2006), pp. 158, 189, 195. A modern service trench excavated outside the infirmary at Sprowston revealed two partial skeletons. Unfortunately, because only a few bones were observed, we do not know whether there were any skeletal markers of deformity or disfigurement in these individuals. Substantial periosteal new bone growth was, however, noted: Norfolk HER 670NF.

and social cycles.[19] Its impressive two-storey infirmary and liturgical paraphernalia served as a testament to patrons' interest in the welfare of the inmates, whilst its location not more than a mile to the north of the city gates helped to promote the institution to potential sponsors.[20] Not all of Norwich's sufferers of 'leprosy' were, however, eligible for admittance at Sprowston. Either they were deemed unsuitable for monastic life, or they may not have wished to subject themselves to the rigours of the daily prayers and spiritual observances performed there.

What of lepers or paupers who did not access St Mary's or St Giles's? Some reputed lepers lived in the community, although in times of communal crisis they risked being reported to the authorities and ejected if they happened to upset their neighbours for any reason.[21] Others took up places in the five smaller, lowlier houses stationed outside Norwich's north and west gates (map 7). As leprosy declined from at least the sixteenth century if not before, these latter institutions began to diversify and to admit a wider range of sick individuals, including sufferers from the 'pox'.[22] The smaller *leprosaria* physically resembled another type of (often short-lived) hospice: the city's almshouses. These, since about the twelfth century, had provided respite for road-weary pilgrims, poor rural immigrants and (in steadily increasing numbers) the native aged and infirm of Norwich.[23] Only very

[19] On the reinstatement of civic processions to the chapel, see *RCN,* II, 120–1 (1532).

[20] R. Gilchrist, 'Christian Bodies and Souls: The Archaeology of Life and Death in Later Medieval Hospitals', in *Death in Towns,* ed. Bassett, pp. 101–18 (p. 115). The old historiographical assumptions about the universal stigma applied to, and the enforced isolation of, sufferers of 'leprosy' have been questioned. The identity of a leprous person might have been forged from a mixture of attributes depending on his or her circumstances: that is, out of appearances of vulnerability, weakness, impoverishment and dependency, and perhaps of dangerousness or sinfulness, but also (owing to connotations of forbearance and penance, and as a vehicle for the redemption of others) of increased religiosity and spirituality: C. Peyroux, 'The Leper's Kiss', in *Monks and Nuns, Saints and Outcasts: Religion in Medieval Society: Essays in Honor of Lester K. Little,* ed. S. Farmer and B. H. Rosenwein (Ithaca, 2000), pp. 172–88 (esp. pp. 185–8); Rawcliffe, *Leprosy,* chapters 3, 6 and 7 (esp. pp. 55–65).

[21] *LJ,* ed. Hudson, pp. 68, 71–2. On these kinds of reports, and their relationship to epidemic outbreaks and civil tension, see Rawcliffe, *Leprosy,* pp. 282–4.

[22] Pelling, 'Healing the Sick Poor', in Pelling, *CL,* pp. 91–101.

[23] For a similar evolution of purpose, see J. Magilton and F. Lee, 'The Leper Hospital of St James and St Mary Magdalene, Chichester', in *Burial Archaeology: Current Research, Methods and Developments,* ed. C. A. Roberts, F. Lee and J.

limited burial services, if any, were provided by either almshouses or the small *leprosaria*, as most lacked chapels or cemeteries of their own. For example, in 1582/83, the house known as St Clement's, which was situated outside St Augustine's gate, had to spend money on a bier, a spade to dig graves with, and a coffin before it could bury one female inmate who died there. It seems to have previously deposited its dead in the cemetery of the local parish church.[24] Similarly, in the absence of a burial ground of its own, Norman's hospital – a medium-sized Benedictine foundation dedicated to St Paul – probably had such an arrangement with the neighbouring parochial institution (map 7).[25] At its foundation, Norman's offered permanent assistance to enfeebled and impoverished inmates, as well as travellers to the city who failed to find a night's accommodation. During the fourteenth and fifteenth centuries it evolved from its original purpose and began to support a select group of twenty respectable almswomen, some of whom lived outside the institution and were fit enough to supplement their income with casual work.[26] After the Dissolution, it seems to have specialized briefly in providing care for bedridden patients until it was purchased by the civic authorities in the late 1560s and turned into a bridewell.[27] As with the other hospitals, leper houses and almshouses mentioned here, excavation of the graves of former residents of Norman's hospital (if they could be distinguished) would almost certainly reveal a distinctive demographic profile and a range of particular physical and disease characteristics.

Although they did not specialize in housing the sick or burying the sick dead, the four orders of friars also provided burial space for a significant minority of lay people and secular clergy.[28] Archaeological excavations have taken place in the cemeteries of two Norwich friaries to date, and the evidence extracted again indicates a particular catalogue

Bintliff, BAR BS 211 (Oxford, 1989), pp. 249–65 (p. 252, and see p. 264 for a list of conditions affecting sixteenth-century inmates).

[24] Phillips, 'Charitable Institutions', p. 254; Blomefield, *Norfolk*, IV, 461.

[25] C. Rawcliffe, *The Hospitals of Medieval Norwich*, Studies in East Anglian History 2 (Norwich, 1995), p. 70.

[26] Ibid., p. 72. For bequests to these women in the sixteenth century, see for example NCC will register Alblaster, fol. 116v (Webster, 1521).

[27] Rawcliffe, *MFTS*, p. 203.

[28] During the years 1370 to 1532, about thirteen per cent of Norwich testators sought interment at one of these institutions: Tanner, *The Church in Late Medieval Norwich*, p. 189 (I am combining Tanner's numbers of lay and ecclesiastical testators).

of diseases in the bodies disinterred. A sample of 136 skeletons dating from the thirteenth to the sixteenth centuries was recovered from the Greyfriars (the Franciscan friary) at site 373N (map 7). This group probably included the remains not only of the friars themselves but also of their secular benefactors. Indeed, the former were supposed to be strong, fit and free from infirmity in order to perform their pastoral duties.[29] Analysis of the excavated skeletal material suggests that, in life, the people inhumed at Greyfriars ate a refined diet; as at St Mary's Spital, London, large numbers of caries and also tooth-losses were recorded.[30] In contrast to the skeletons excavated from the burial grounds of another friary in the region,[31] and to those taken from parochial graveyards in Norwich, no examples of chronic or infectious diseases, nor of conditions associated with arrested growth, were seen in the recovered sample.[32] A small number of individuals were identified, however, who had clearly suffered painful conditions before their final, fatal illnesses, and they may have received physical assistance whilst at the friary. One adult, for example, seems to have endured excruciating bladder stones.[33] The sample also showed numbers of healed or partially healed fractured bones – over seventeen per cent of the skeletons were affected in this way.[34] A mature male had broken his left ribs and clavicle (collarbone), possibly during a serious fall compounded by a crushing injury.[35] Another had a chronically

[29] A. Montford, *Health, Sickness, Medicine and the Friars in the Thirteenth and Fourteenth Centuries* (Aldershot, 2004), chapter 1.

[30] Soden, EAA 133, pp. 24–5. The skeletons recovered were in a good state of preservation.

[31] Excavations at the Blackfriars' Ipswich found evidence of Hansen's Disease (1914, 1987, 2593, 2624), tuberculosis (2577), osteomyelitis, widespread *cribra orbitalia*, treponemal disease (1965), sharp-force trauma (1749, 2491), Paget's disease (0950) and a probable skin ulcer (1978): S. Mays, 'Part II: Appendix for the Medieval Burials from the Blackfriars Friary, School Street, Ipswich, Suffolk (Excavated 1983–85)' (unpublished Ancient Monuments Laboratory Report, 16/91, English Heritage, 1991), pp. 170, 180–1, 190, 195, 196, 198, 208, 212, 214, 217 and *passim*.

[32] This does not preclude the possibility that the individuals buried at the Greyfriars' suffered from diseases that are invisible to the palaeopathologist, nor that the chronic sick were buried in a part of the cemetery that was not excavated.

[33] Soden, EAA 133, p. 24 (sk 43); T. Anderson, 'A Medieval Bladder Stone from Norwich, Norfolk', *International Journal of Osteoarchaeology* 13 (2003), 165–7.

[34] Soden, EAA 133, p. 24.

[35] Ibid. (sk 67).

dislocating mandible (lower jaw).[36] A child suffered a femoral fracture, and the evidence for an excellent level of healing in this case suggests that sophisticated remedial treatment was available to him or her.[37] Norwich's civic rulers would later provide a free bone-setting service for poor men, women and children,[38] but this young person's treatment may have been provided by the friars themselves. The Carmelites' (Whitefriars') cemetery (site 26598N, map 7), situated in the north-east of the city, has to date yielded only a few, badly preserved skeletons from the medieval period. Even so, fractures of thoraxes and limbs have been recognized in the population buried here too.[39]

St Margaret's Fyebridge: a parish in a landscape

Each of the institutions mentioned above had some form of selective entry criteria: a person's familial, economic, religious status (or lack thereof), in addition to any disease they suffered determined whether they could successfully seek admittance. The majority of Norwich's sick residents, however, lived out their lives at home and were therefore interred in the graveyard of their parish church. One of the largest skeletal assemblages so far excavated in Norwich from such a context comes from the churchyard of St Margaret Fyebridge, which was in use from at least 1200 to about 1468.[40] The site was partially excavated in 1987, when 436 articulated skeletons were removed.[41] As we have

[36] Ibid. (sk 74).

[37] Ibid. (sk 30c). On fracture treatment, see A. L. Grauer and C. A. Roberts, 'Paleoepidemiology, Healing and Possible Treatment of Trauma in the Medieval Cemetery Population of St. Helen-on-the-Walls, York, England', *American Journal of Physical Anthropology* 100 (1996), 531–44 (pp. 540–2).

[38] *RCN*, II, 144 (1573).

[39] A. Caffell and M. Holst, 'Osteological Analysis Whitefriars Norwich' (unpublished archaeological report 0806 York Osteoarchaeology Ltd, 2007), pp. 21–2, 34.

[40] On the evidence for dating the early use of the site, see B. Ayers, 'Chapter 4. Archaeological and Historical Context', in Stirland, EAA 129, pp. 35–7. A small number of the skeletons has been radiocarbon dated. The earliest returned a calibrated date of AD 1088–1328; the latest, AD 1453–1644: Stirland, EAA 129, p. 35, cf. the appraisal of the reliability of this dating method by K. N. Harper et al., 'The Origin and Antiquity of Syphilis Revisited: An Appraisal of Old World Pre-Columbian Evidence for Treponemal Infection', *Yearbook of Physical Anthropology* 54 (2011), 99–133 (pp. 121–3).

[41] About 500 other individuals were represented in charnel and a further 100 were excavated under extreme salvage conditions: Bown and Stirland, 'CAP', n.p.

seen, the population included debilitated, deformed and disfigured people (site 780N, map 7). The chronic conditions evidenced by the extracted sample of skeletons imply that the personal histories of some of its parishioners were characterized by combinations of impoverished environmental circumstances, periods of pain and illness, and compromised physical ability. What factors contributed to this particular pathological profile? The nature of the parish itself provides an answer.

St Margaret's Fyebridge was situated on the economic, social and topographical margins of Norwich. Prior to *c.* 1100, the site was open land. Initially, the building of St Margaret's church at the outer limits of the settlement of the city may have appeared to augur well for the fortunes of the area; development in this northern district served as a counterpoint to building works south of the river, where the castle, cathedral, marketplace and new residential quarters were taking shape.[42] In fact, further development did not materialize on any scale in this northern enclave. The intramural lands to the west of the church comprised private and church-owned crofts, the precincts of St Augustine's church and a twelve-acre expanse of farmland known as the Gildencroft.[43] To the south-east of St Margaret's cemetery was the suburb around Norman's hospital, itself situated in open fields, and further south-east still, the precincts of the Whitefriars.[44] The area could, nonetheless, legitimately boast a wealth of institutional, spiritual and palliative services when it was first established. In addition to the main religious institutions, other parish churches were founded nearby at a similar date. But the district as a whole lacked the necessary economic

My very sincere thanks to Jayne Bown for allowing me to view this report, which is forthcoming in the EAA series. It includes data on the archaeological contexts of the graves, on burial practices and on the artefact finds, and complements the specialist human skeletal report for the site published in Stirland, EAA 129.

[42] Atkin and Evans, EAA 100, pp. 155–6; B. Ayers, 'The Urban Landscape', in *MN*, ed. Rawcliffe and Wilson, pp. 13–19.

[43] Ayers, *NAFC*, p. 104; Atkin and Evans, EAA 100, pp. 177, 182. The Benedictine priory and the hospital of St Giles, as well as the leper house of St Mary Magdalen, all had significant holdings of land in the area: Atkin and Evans, EAA 100, p. 156; *Landgable*, ed. Rodgers and Wallace, p. 110; Kirkpatrick, *Streets and Lanes*, p. 81; Rawcliffe, *MFTS*, p. 80 and map 5, p. 79.

[44] The friary was established in 1256, demonstrating that, at this time (a century and a half after St Margaret's cemetery came into use), large tracts of land were still available in the northern area of the city: Ayers, *NAFC*, pp. 71–2.

underpinnings to really flourish.[45] Symbolic of this, and as early as 1254, St Margaret's church was exempted from paying ecclesiastical taxation,[46] and, in the absence of a rector, it seems to have became a subsidiary chapel to the nearby parish church of All Saints'.[47] It was (probably) finally dissolved in the second half of the fifteenth century.[48]

The micro-landscape of the cemetery tells us even more about St Margaret's position in the city's wider social and economic scenery. The graveyard possessed a very singular nature; to contemporary eyes, it must have seemed an abject place. Medieval Christian cemeteries are generally laid out in a fairly uniform and predictable way. But a sense of disorder pervades St Margaret's. To begin with, the graveyard contained large numbers of group burials. A total of forty-nine graves housed between two and seven corpses each and, in one case, twelve bodies were packed into a single interment.[49] Thus, over forty per cent of the articulated skeletons recovered during excavation were found in graves containing more than one individual. More alarming still, within the group interments at St Margaret's, the remains of many individuals were treated with scant regard: they were either placed in a prone (face down) position or were not aligned on the normal east–west axis. Figure 12 (grave 480) illustrates an extreme incidence of the practices employed: the grave was oriented on a north–south configuration and held four bodies, one of which was deposited face down. The mound of excavated earth covering this grave, whilst it

[45] Stirland, EAA 129, p. 36.

[46] W. Hudson, 'The "Norwich Taxation" of 1254, so far as Relates to the Diocese of Norwich', *NA* 17 (1910), pp. 46–157 (pp. 76–7, 107).

[47] Blomefield, *Norfolk*, IV, 438 (All Saint's), 439–40 (St Margaret's Fyebridge). A rector was temporarily appointed to St Margaret's by the bishop of Norwich in 1453. In 1368, St Margaret's Fyebridge was valued at 13*s*. 4*d*., the same sum as St Olave's (which, like St Margaret's Fyebridge, was a rectory that became a chapel, being attached to St George Colegate in *c*. 1492), and the nearby chapel of St Margaret Newgate (also a satellite of St George's): Tanner, *The Church in Late Medieval Norwich*, p. 174.

[48] Blomefield, *Norfolk*, IV, 439. The church was not mentioned in Bishop Goldwell's visitation in 1492: Tanner, *The Church in Late Medieval Norwich*, p. 181. The building survived, however, for some time to come. The boundaries of the churchyard were still known in 1568–70: *Landgable*, ed. Rodgers and Wallace, p. 110. In 1661, a deed referred only to a plot of ground with a house 'that was previously called the chapel of St. Margaret': K. I. Sandred and B. Lindstrøm, *The Place-Names of Norfolk Part I: The Place-Names of the City of Norwich* (Nottingham, 1989), p. 44.

[49] Bown and Stirland, 'CAP', n.p.; and see Stirland, EAA 129, p. 37.

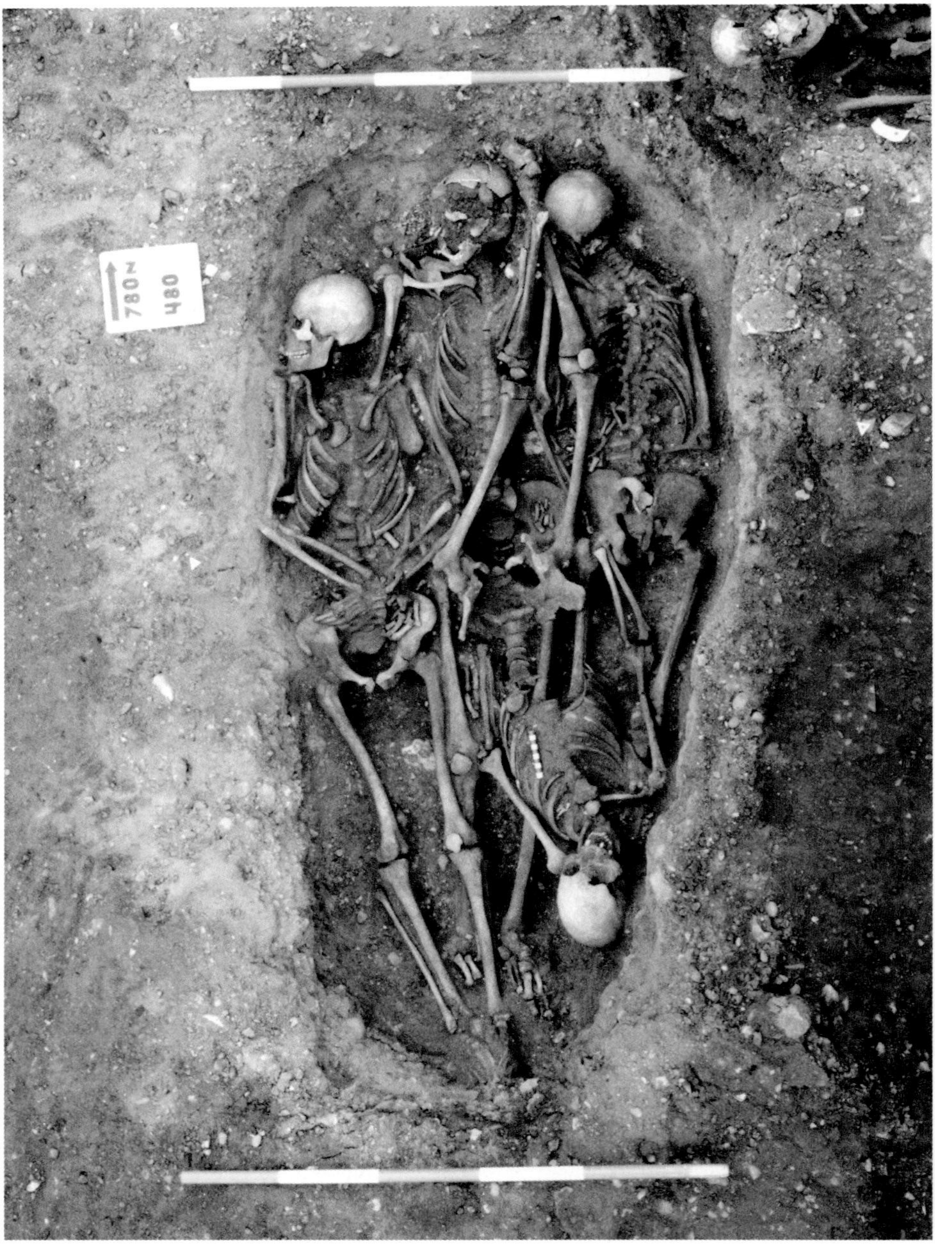

Figure 12: Grave 480, St Margaret's Fyebridge. Grave shows north–south alignment, prone and mal-orientated corpses.

remained visible, would have marked it out as both strange and unenviable. What reason did the sexton or cemetery manager have for treating a subsection of St Margaret's dead in this way?

We can see how far this burial fell from reaching the ideal standard by examining the observances most medieval men and women would have anticipated (or at least aspired to) after death at this time.[50] Normally, the length, format and content of a person's funerary arrangements depended upon his or her status and resources. A minority of people had the opportunity to stipulate what should happen to their body in a will. Some depended upon their spiritual fraternities or craft guilds to provide decent rituals.[51] But many people must have relied upon family and friends to oversee and care for their body between death and burial. Ideally, the processing of the corpse itself would follow a particular pattern. First, it would be stripped and washed. Then, either naked or dressed, it would be sewn into a shroud. Next came the arranging of the body for transportation to the church.[52] A number of clerics and intercessors would attend a funeral mass (according to the deceased individual's financial wherewithal and spiritual sensitivities) and many candles might be lit around the corpse. Finally, the burial would be performed, the relevant fee having been paid. Committal in the church building was a highly desirable option, but expensive. A stone-lined grave in the churchyard bought a degree of insurance against future disturbance at slightly less cost. Burial directly into the soil (with or without a coffin)[53] was more common, although the grave

[50] Funerary practices and rites are authoritatively discussed in Gilchrist and Sloane, *Requiem*, especially pp. 19–27. See also R. S. Wieck, 'The Death Desired: Books of Hours and the Medieval Funeral', in *Death and Dying in the Middle Ages*, ed. E. E. DuBruck and B. J. Gusick (New York, 1999), pp. 431–76; C. Gittings, *Death, Burial and the Individual in Early Modern England* (London, 1984), pp. 109–17; Hill, *Women and Religion*, pp. 150–60.

[51] On the functions of Norwich guilds at funerals, see 'The Hitherto Unpublished Certificates of Norwich Gilds', ed. J. C. Tingey, *NA* 16 (1907), 267–305.

[52] A case presented to the coroner of Norwich in November 1268 casts incidental light on the early stages of preparation for burial. It relates how the body of one Stephen Justice was prepared; his corpse was wrapped in an expensive sheet and was laid out on a bier in the hall of his house, overnight. A fine blanket, imported from Reims, hung over the bier as a pall. Unfortunately for his relatives, events then took a dreadful and unforeseeable turn; for an unreported reason, eight men broke into the hall and set fire to his body. See, *RCN*, I, 204–5. See also Gilchrist and Sloane, *Requiem*, pp. 23–4.

[53] On the use of coffins at the Norwich Greyfrairs, see Soden, EAA 133, p. 54.

had to be marked in some way if further weekly, monthly or annual commemorative services were expected.

The bodies in the disordered burials at St Margaret's were clearly not handled according to these protocols. Why did they not merit more care and attention? Other instances of prone and mal-aligned burials in English graveyards have been interpreted in a range of ways: that is, as evidence of penitential practice, or as a response to social 'deviancy', or to physical or mental disease, or as the result of accidental inversion caused by secondary or hurried burial.[54] In Norfolk's Anglo-Saxon settlements, for example, non-normative burials were used as a means to demonstrate social opprobrium.[55] Elsewhere, similar practices are associated with the burials of suicides,[56] excommunicates[57] and heretics.[58] Group burials, on the other hand, are normally associated with natural

[54] See the survey in Gilchrist and Sloane, *Requiem*, pp. 153–4.

[55] R. Hoggett, *The Archaeology of the East Anglian Conversion* (Woodbridge, 2010), pp. 138–41.

[56] *The Place of the Dead: Death and Remembrance in Late Medieval and Early Modern Europe*, ed. B. Gordon, and P. Marshall (Cambridge, 2000), *passim* and Gittings, *Death, Burial and the Individual*, p. 72; V. Harding, 'Whose Body? A Study of Attitudes Towards the Dead Body in Early Modern Paris', *The Place of the Dead: Death and Remembrance in Late Medieval and Early Modern Europe*, ed. B. Gordon and P. Marshall (Cambridge, 2000) pp. 170–87 (pp. 174–5); Whyte, 'Deviant Dead', p. 35.

[57] See E. Duffy, *The Voices of Morebath: Reformation and Rebellion in an English Village* (New Haven, 2001), p. 131, where a dissident, caught up in the disturbances of the West County in 1549, was interred on a north–south alignment. Similarly, in 1598, a former, unabsolved churchwarden of St John Timberhill, Norwich, was interred 'without the ordynarie course of sepulture' in response to his perceived spiritual crimes: *The Eastern Counties Collectanea*, ed. J. L'Estrange (Norwich, 1872–73), p. 170. For local archaeological examples of the mouths of the dead being stuffed with ash, which perhaps indicates a form of post-mortem penance, see Soden, EAA 133, pp. 54–5 (graves 87, 103, 132). (An alternative explanation might be that this was an aspect of mortuary presentation or hygiene.)

[58] Hostile reports suggested the Albanenses and others dealt 'most slightingly with human bodies after death', burying them 'secretly in pits here and there': *Heresies of the High Middle Ages: Selected Sources Translated and Annotated*, ed. W. L. Wakefield and A. P. Evans (New York, 1969), p. 274, and see ibid., pp. 24, 102–3, 235, 348. On the varied burial practices of Cathars (including pit disposal), see P. Biller, 'Medicine and Heresy', in *Religion and Medicine in the Middle Ages*, ed. P. Biller and J. Ziegler, York Studies in Medieval Theology 3 (York, 2001), pp. 155–74 (p. 171).

or civil catastrophes.[59] Why did these practices occur at St Margaret's? One plausible explanation was that the cemetery was used as a place to inter executed criminals. In 1254, a report on the value of local ecclesiastical property for taxation purposes referred to the church with the suffix *ubi sepeliuntur suspensi*, 'where the hanged are buried'.[60] (The gallows were situated within the parish on a stretch of land just outside Magdalen gate.)[61] As well as the parishioners, therefore, St Margaret's churchyard catered for individuals who – whilst remaining members of the Christian community – had placed themselves outside the bounds of acceptable behaviour.[62]

Factors of extreme exigency may also have played a part in determining the shape and form of the graves. An example of emergency mass burial has been recovered from elsewhere in Norwich, which may also help us to understand what was going on at St Margaret's. In 2004, a medieval well was discovered which had been used as a place to dispose of at least seventeen corpses. The well was located next to the boundary of the precinct of the college of St Mary in the Fields (site 51497N) on what is now part of the site of the Chapelfield Mall (map 7). Two-thirds of the dead were under twenty years of age, of whom

59 For a small group grave incorporating practices redolent of those seen at St Margaret's, and which has been interpreted as a response to famine or disease, see Gilchrist and Sloane, *Requiem*, p. 157; the grave in question contained three individuals: one prone (an aged male), one 'crouched' (a juvenile), and one 'strewn' (another aged male). Larger multiple burials have been associated with outbreaks of epidemic diseases, war and unrest. Pit burials were used, for example, in order to dispose of the bodies of forty-nine insurgents in Norwich after Kett's rebellion in 1549. The rebels were hanged at the market cross. The city government paid 3*s*. 9*d*. to have the pits dug and for the corpses to be conveyed thither: NCR 18a/7 CA 1541–49, fol. 304v. For the context, see Wood, *The 1549 Rebellions*, pp. 71–4, and see NRO, DN/Reg 30 'Tanner's Index' vol. I: Archdeaconry of Norwich and Archdeaconry of Norfolk, p. 29, for the reported burials of another thirty-five people at St Martin Timberhill (also known as St Martin at Bale). For a single mass grave containing about thirty-seven individuals, see *Blood Red Roses: The Archaeology of a Mass Grave from the Battle of Towton, AD 1461*, ed. V. Fiorato, A. Boylston and C. Knüsel (Oxford, 2000). On burial during a pandemic, see below, p. 115.

60 Hudson, '"Norwich Taxation" of 1254', p. 107; Stirland, EAA 129, p. 36.

61 Blomefield, *Norfolk*, IV, 440.

62 For cases of hangings at the Norwich gallows where the executed individuals revived and claimed sanctuary at St Margaret's Fyebridge, see Stirland, EAA 129 pp. 36–7, referring to a case in 1345, and R. B. Pugh, 'The Knights Hospitallers of England as Undertakers', *Speculum* 56 (1981), 566–74 (pp. 567–8), referring to a case in 1299 (also cited in Gilchrist and Sloane, *Requiem*, p. 73).

five were infants or small children.[63] The burial probably took place at some time during the twelfth or thirteenth centuries,[64] and it seems very likely that the excavated individuals all died within a short space of time – perhaps owing to infectious disease, famine or some other crisis.[65] It would appear that, in the absence of available man-power to convey the dead to a suitable resting place, the well shaft proved an expedient grave. In addition to any intrinsic, personalized factors in operation, happenstance, or the confluence of events, also played a role in determining the ways in which the dead were handled at St Margaret's Fyebridge. Across the churchyard as a whole, prone or mal-aligned burials were much more likely to occur when five or more corpses awaited burial (that is, when the task was difficult and exacting) than when only one individual was concerned.[66] St Margaret's was, after all, an outpost, located away from central businesses and facilities, and locked between the (largely undeveloped) landholdings of big institutions. Seemingly, under pressure, the mechanisms of oversight and decorum were liable to fail.

What other factors at St Margaret's might have prompted either cursory or differentiating treatment? Though it is offensive to modern mores, one post-medieval commentator assumed that the most seriously ill and deformed members of the community might receive distinctive burial treatment. The eighteenth-century Norfolk antiquarian

[63] G. Emery, 'A Medieval Mass Grave on the Site of the Chapelfield Shopping Centre, Norwich', Report (unpublished archaeological report 1562, NAU Archaeology, 2010), p. 15. My grateful thanks to Giles Emery and NAU Archaeology for allowing me to see this report.

[64] A fourteenth-century date cannot be excluded. The dating is inferred from carbon-14 analysis of skeletal samples and by pottery shards: Emery, 'Medieval Mass Grave', p. 25.

[65] Though we cannot be certain how the people buried in the well died, it is notable that interpersonal violence often causes characteristic patterns of trauma, yet no skeletal lesions of this nature were reported. On violent trauma, see S. A. Novak, 'Beneath the Façade: A Skeletal Model of Domestic Violence', in *Social Archaeology*, ed. Gowland and Knüsel, pp. 238–52; S. A. Novak, 'Battle-Related Trauma', in *Blood Red Roses*, ed. Fiorato, Boylston and Knüsel, pp. 90–102. At the time of writing, the possibility that these men, women and children were the Jewish victims of a pogrom (an idea raised in a BBC Two television programme, *History Cold Case: The Bodies in the Well*, 21:00 BST 23 June 2011, which presupposed a ritual form of murder such as throat slitting) continues to be investigated, but the DNA analysis evidence (used to determine ethnic identity) has so far proved inconclusive: Giles Emery, *pers. com.*

[66] Fay, 'Text, Space and the Evidence of Human Remains', p. 204.

Francis Blomefield related a local tradition in his *Essay Towards a Topographical History of the County of Norfolk* which united the themes of disease with religious and material 'pollution'. He described a tomb in the nearby churchyard of St Clement Fyebridge that was orientated on a north–south alignment – an obvious inversion of the Christian norm (map 7). It was, the legend went, the burial of a wealthy 'leper'.[67] According to Blomefield, the parish agreed to accept this individual for burial only after several others had refused to do so, on the proviso that it would gain substantial endowments of property in return. Blomefield suspected that some of the story's details were false; he suggested, for example, that residents at a leper house outside Augustine's gate had a parochial right to be interred in St Clement's churchyard because the house had no burial ground of its own. But he did not challenge the mode of inhumation. Features of Blomefield's vignette resonate with the kinds of funerary practices going on at St Margaret's in preceding centuries. However, as we will see, the relationship between medieval burial practice and disfiguring diseases was not, in fact, so clear cut and simplistic as his anecdote suggests. In order to understand this fully, we must step amongst the graves and dig down to the very bones, paying close attention to the form and manner of the burials we encounter. In this way, we can hope to get a firmer grasp on medieval urban attitudes towards the disfigured and deformed dead.

Death on the margins: deformity, violence and burial custom

Like the 'leper burial' described in Blomefield's legend, grave 624 at St Margaret Fyebridge (fig. 13) was aligned on a north–south axis. It contained a total of five individuals. There was no apparent practical necessity (such as the presence of a building) to account for the non-standard alignment.[68] Therefore, we are reliant on the 'osteobiographies' of the people buried in the grave in order to understand its nature.[69] It contained two individuals who suffered from types of diseases which can be identified in the surviving bone. The first, skeleton 694, an adult of unknown age and sex, had sustained a fracture of the mandible complicated by osteomyelitis (a suppurating infection

[67] Blomefield, *Norfolk*, IV, 459–61.
[68] Bown and Stirland, 'CAP', n.p.
[69] On osteobiographies, see Appendix I, n. 13.

of the bone cavity).[70] This would have caused the individual pain, and would have made eating difficult. He or she would also have felt feverish and ill as the infection took hold.[71] The other person, aged between about thirty and fifty (skeleton 695), had sustained a fracture of the right humerus (upper arm). This had healed in such a way that the two ends of the bone were poorly aligned; perhaps no one was available to treat – that is, reduce and immobilize – it. He or she also appears to have suffered from rickets during childhood, a condition which causes the malformation of long bones and has been associated with insufficient access to sunlight, nutritional deficiency (connected with maternal malnutrition) and infections during infancy.[72] Both corpses were buried in a prone position (face down), as was one of their three companions.

Another group was deposited in an equally undignified arrangement, although this time the grave at least had the proper east–west alignment.[73] Three skeletons were placed into a rectangular pit with a rounded base that had clearly been prepared by an inexpert gravedigger. Skeleton 684, a male of between nineteen and thirty years of age, was the first to be interred. His body formed an arc in the base of the grave as if he were 'lying in a hammock'.[74] A single destructive lesion, possibly associated with tuberculosis, was identified just above the right hip joint of this skeleton.[75] One of the others, a male adult of over fifty years of age (skeleton 356) had a mass of bone tissue within the anterior muscle of the right thigh (*myositis ossificans*),[76] a form of tissue growth often caused by an injury such as a muscle tear or as a consequence of (even quite minor) impact.[77] This corpse was buried on a 'reversed' orientation with the head to the east, but supine (lying on

[70] Stirland, EAA 129, p. 24, plate 8.

[71] B. J. Bailey, J. T. Johnson, and S. D. Newlands, *Head and Neck Surgery: Otolaryngology*, 2 vols. 4th edn (Philadelphia, 2006), p. 626.

[72] Stirland, EAA 129, pp. 18, 22; M. Lewis, *Urbanisation and Child Health in Medieval and Post-Medieval England*, BAR BS 339 (Oxford, 2002), pp. 24–6.

[73] Grave 664: Bown and Stirland, 'CAP', n.p.

[74] NAU Archaeology, 130–2 Magdalen Street Excavation Archive skeleton recording form 684.

[75] Stirland, EAA 129, p. 25.

[76] Ibid., p. 23.

[77] D. Resnick, *Diagnosis of Bone and Joint Disorders*, 3 vols. (Philadelphia, 1981), p. 3152. Such a mass reaches its full extent at about five to six months after injury, and then shrinks.

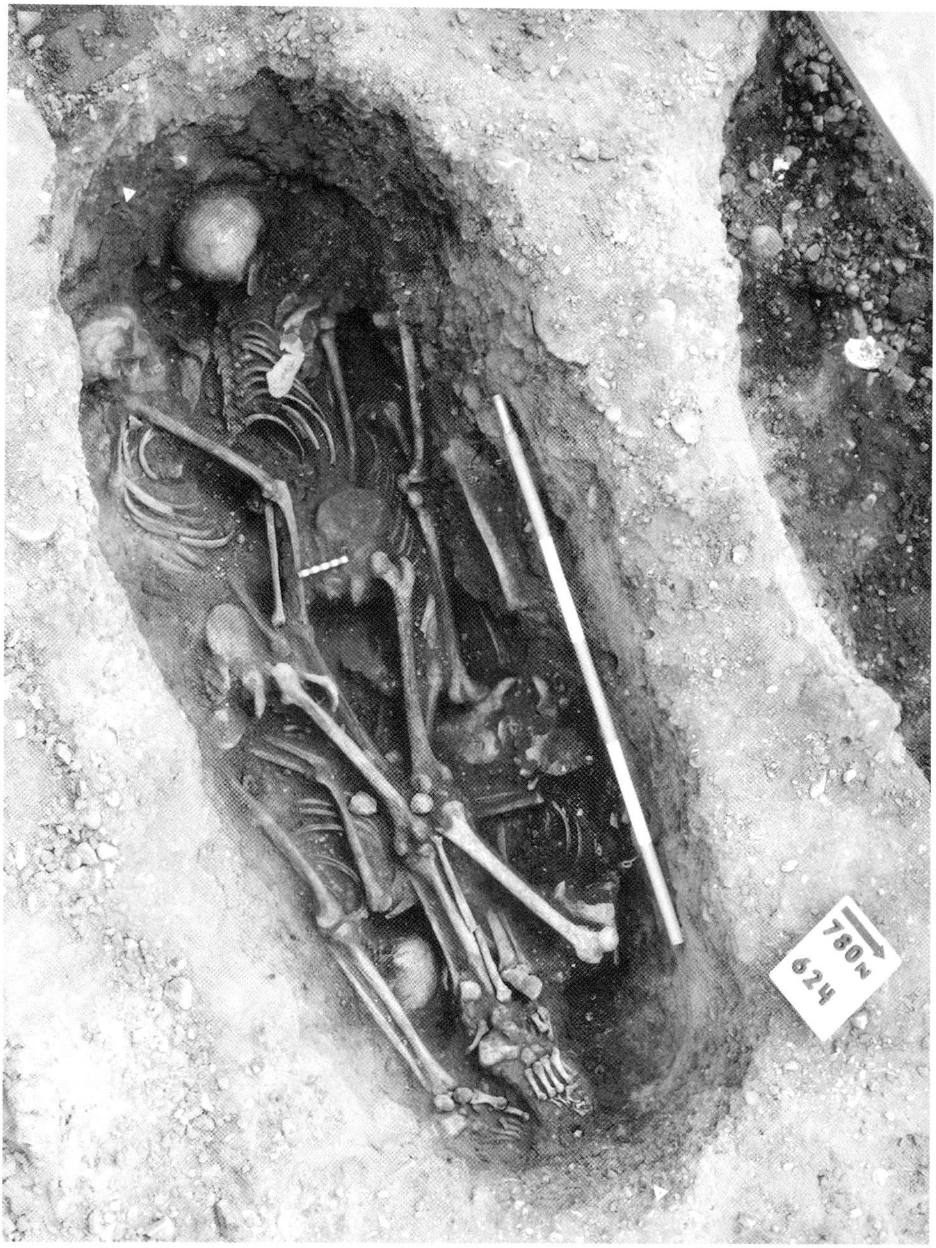

Figure 13: Grave 624, St Margaret's Fyebridge.

its back).[78] What can we conclude about these two graves? The picture is partial. But we might note the evidence for traumas and for compromised development in the groups.

Another east–west pit-burial at St Margaret's also seemed to imply a lack of regard for the dead (grave 276, fig. 14). This contained twelve individuals, nine of whom were buried face down. The grave was not wide enough to accommodate a single layer of corpses, and they were buried on top of one another. Three of the individuals had either one arm, or both hands, behind their backs.[79] The splayed limbs of several other individuals demonstrate that they were not put into shrouds, but were perhaps tipped or jettisoned into the grave.[80] At least one occupant of this unique grave met a sudden and forceful end: skeleton 374 sustained a blow from a sharp instrument which fractured his skull immediately before his death.[81] Another adult male (skeleton 618) showed bilateral changes to the feet and lower leg which indicate a serious systemic infection, and which match lesions seen on skeletons excavated from the graveyards of medieval *leprosaria*.[82] How do we account for the presence here of these individuals – that is, of a person killed by a blow to the head, and a person showing lower limb deformity?

[78] NAU Archaeology, 130–2 Magdalen Street Excavation Archive skeleton recording form 356.

[79] Bown and Stirland, 'CAP', n.p.

[80] Five were interred with their heads to the east.

[81] Stirland, EAA 129, pp. 19–20.

[82] There were lytic lesions in both feet (comprising the destruction of the fifth metatarsals) and periosteal new bone growth on the fibula and tibia (the lower leg bones): Stirland, EAA 129, p. 27. For comparison, see J. Magilton, F. Lee and A. Boylston, *Lepers Outside the Gate: Excavations at the Cemetery of the Hospital of St James and St Mary Magdalene, Chichester, 1986–87 and 1993*, Council for British Archaeology Research Report 158 (York, 2008), pp. 204–5 (for periostitis and remodelling of metatarsals), p. 209 (bilateral presentation of lesions), and see pp. 214–15 for a summary of the skeletons similarly affected in the Chichester sample. On the same lesions, associated with secondary infections arising from leg ulcers or foot sores in untreated cases of Hansen's disease, see K. Manchester, 'Infective Bone Changes in Leprosy', in *The Past and Present of Leprosy: Archaeological, Historical, Palaeopathological and Clinical Approaches*, ed. C. A. Roberts, M. E. Lewis and K. Manchester, BAR IS 1054 (Oxford, 2002), pp. 69–72 (p. 70). The facial skeleton was not well preserved and so we do not know if this man also displayed rhinomaxillary changes which are characteristic of *lepromatous leprosy*: NAU Archaeology, 130–2 Magdalen Street Excavation Archive skeleton recording form 618.

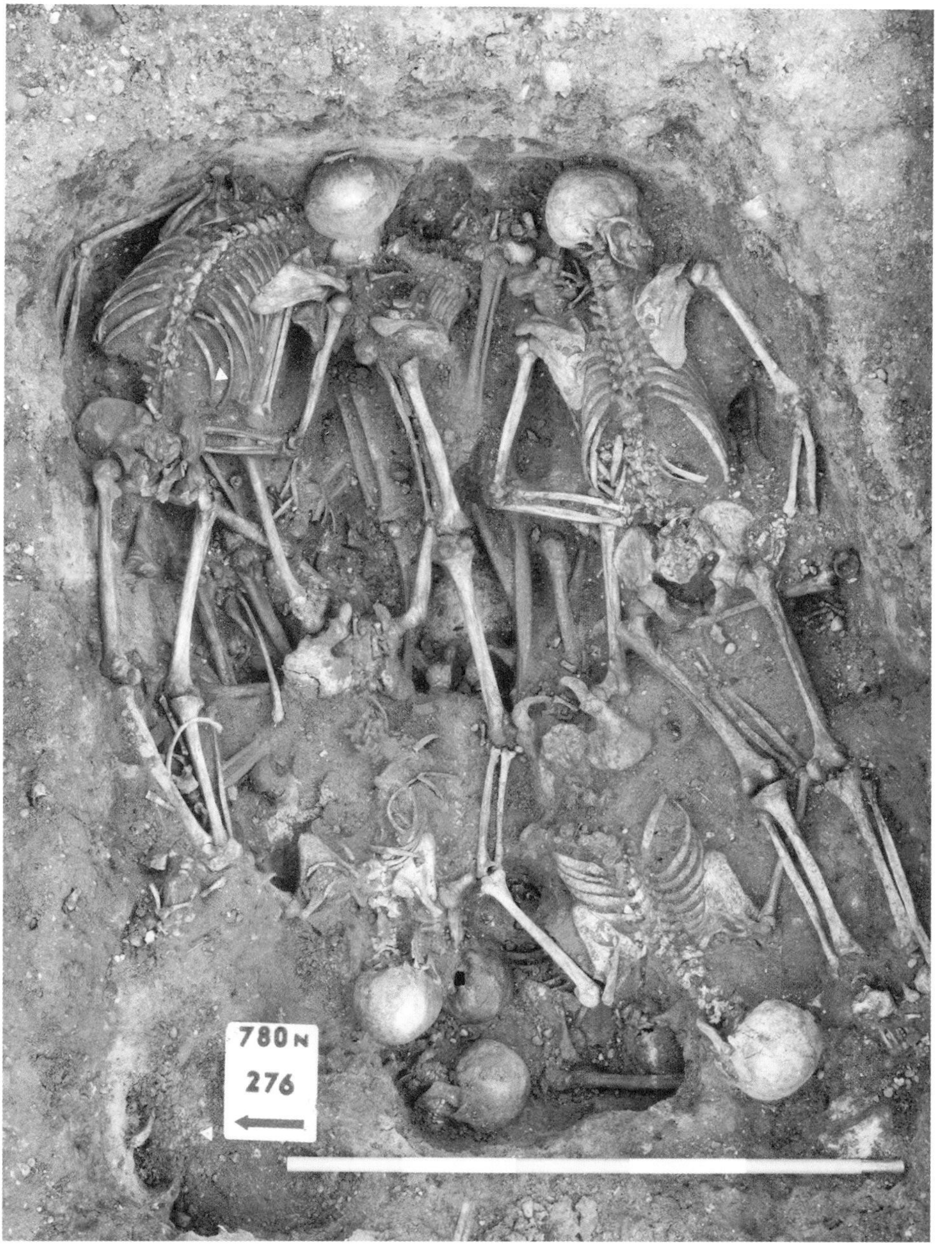

Figure 14: Grave 276, St Margaret's Fyebridge.

We do not need to look too far for a possible answer in the case of the second individual. A leper house – dedicated to St Leonard – was situated very close by, directly outside Magdalen gate on the other side of the city defences to this churchyard; he might have been a resident there.[83] Alternatively, he may simply have lived – and died – in the community. As for the individual who was killed with a blow from a sharp instrument, there is no evidence upon which to draw further conclusions. What is clear, however, is that both individuals died at a time when a number of other corpses were also awaiting burial. Indeed, such a high death rate – represented by the deposition of twelve bodies in one grave over a short period of time – in and of itself implies that an extraordinary situation prevailed. In a parish context, this would be a startling concentration of deaths.[84]

Lest we too readily assume, however, that the presence of the manifest sick and injured amongst these disordered burials implies a process of stigmatization of the kind suggested by Blomefield, we should note that there was no simple correlation between compromised burial status and either disfiguring disease or violence across the rest of the graveyard. Two skeletons displaying rhinomaxillary and post-cranial changes consistent with the lepromatous form of Hansen's disease, for example, were buried in individual graves, in a normal fashion,[85] as were three others showing similar levels of manifest disfigurement and/or digital deformities.[86] Similarly, other individuals who were the victims of sharp-force trauma, like skeleton 374 mentioned above,

[83] In fact, this house was situated on land that was part of the parish of All Saints Fyebridge on the opposite side of the road (which means that any resident ought, in theory at least, to have been buried in its graveyard, map 7). Two wills, made in 1448 and 1466 by residents of St Leonard's, requested burial at All Saints: NRO, NCC will registers Jekkys, fol. 43r (Richard Wellys) and Aleyn, fol. 9r (Henry Wellys).

[84] For context, the archaeologist Barney Sloane has calculated that the designated Black Death cemetery of Holy Trinity, London (which was set up to deal with the first disastrous outbreak of plague in England), hosted an average of about thirteen burials per day over a protracted period: B. Sloane, *The Black Death in London* (Stroud, 2011), p. 92.

[85] Skeleton 252 evidenced rhinomaxillary syndrome and a destructive lesion to one distal manual phalanx (fingertip); skeleton 633 also showed evidence of rhinomaxillary syndrome, as well as destructive, bilateral changes to the metatarsals and bilateral periostitis: Stirland, EAA 129, pp. 26–7.

[86] Skeleton 386 showed destructive remodelling and fusion in finger and toe bones, consistent with neuropathology; skeleton 637 showed destruction of the maxilla and bilateral periostitis of the lower limbs (to above the knee joint);

received normal funerary treatment at the site. One young man had endured repeated physical attacks, including receiving a penetrating wound to the skull.[87] At the point of death he had a severe ongoing infection of the left femur (thigh bone) which was suppurating pus into surrounding bodily tissues and causing a painful abscess.[88] In contrast to the dead man in the group burial, however, his grave suggested a degree of elevated personal status: it was one of a small number of cist (that is, mortar-lined) burials excavated along the street frontage of the cemetery, which conferred a measure of social distinction even after death.[89] Greater resources, or better standing in the community, seem to have made all the difference here.

Another startling instance of bizarre burial (associated, this time, with serious physical impairment) is rather more ambiguous in nature. Skeleton 253 displayed lesions and deformities which suggest that this person may have suffered from neuromuscular disease with paraplegia;[90] in addition, the body was deposited face down within the grave in a 'crouched' position (that is, the lower limbs were flexed underneath the torso).[91] But whether this configuration represented a lack of regard for the corpse – and by extension, for the person him or herself – is not clear. In life, this individual's right knee was in a state of permanent hyperflexion owing to muscular contraction, and this may have prevented the corpse from being manipulated into the normal burial position.[92] The burial, whilst peculiar, may not, therefore, represent an act of intentional denigration.[93]

and skeleton 396 showed either the congenital absence of the hard palate, or its destruction by infection: Stirland, EAA 129, pp. 26–7.

87 Skeleton 1075: NAU Archaeology, 130–2 Magdalen Street Excavation Archive, skeleton recording form 1075; Bown and Stirland, 'CAP', n.p.

88 Bown and Stirland, 'CAP', n.p.

89 Ibid. Cist burials, by preserving the skeleton as an articulated whole, seemed to promise a less fragmented amalgamation of body and soul at the Last Judgement.

90 Stirland, 'Care in the Medieval Community', p. 589; Stirland, EAA 129, p. 33.

91 This person was interred in close proximity to another (skeleton 252), who, like others mentioned above, showed lesions suggesting facial and digital disfigurement (consistent with a differential diagnosis of Hansen's disease). It is not clear, however, whether this was a double burial; rather the underlying grave may have been accidentally reopened when skeleton 253 was buried (*pace* Stirland, EAA 129, p. 35).

92 Stirland, EAA 129, p. 33.

93 Bown and Stirland, 'CAP', n.p.; cf. Gilchrist and Sloane, *Requiem*, p. 155 for another 'crouched' burial in a different context (the East Smithfield mass burial

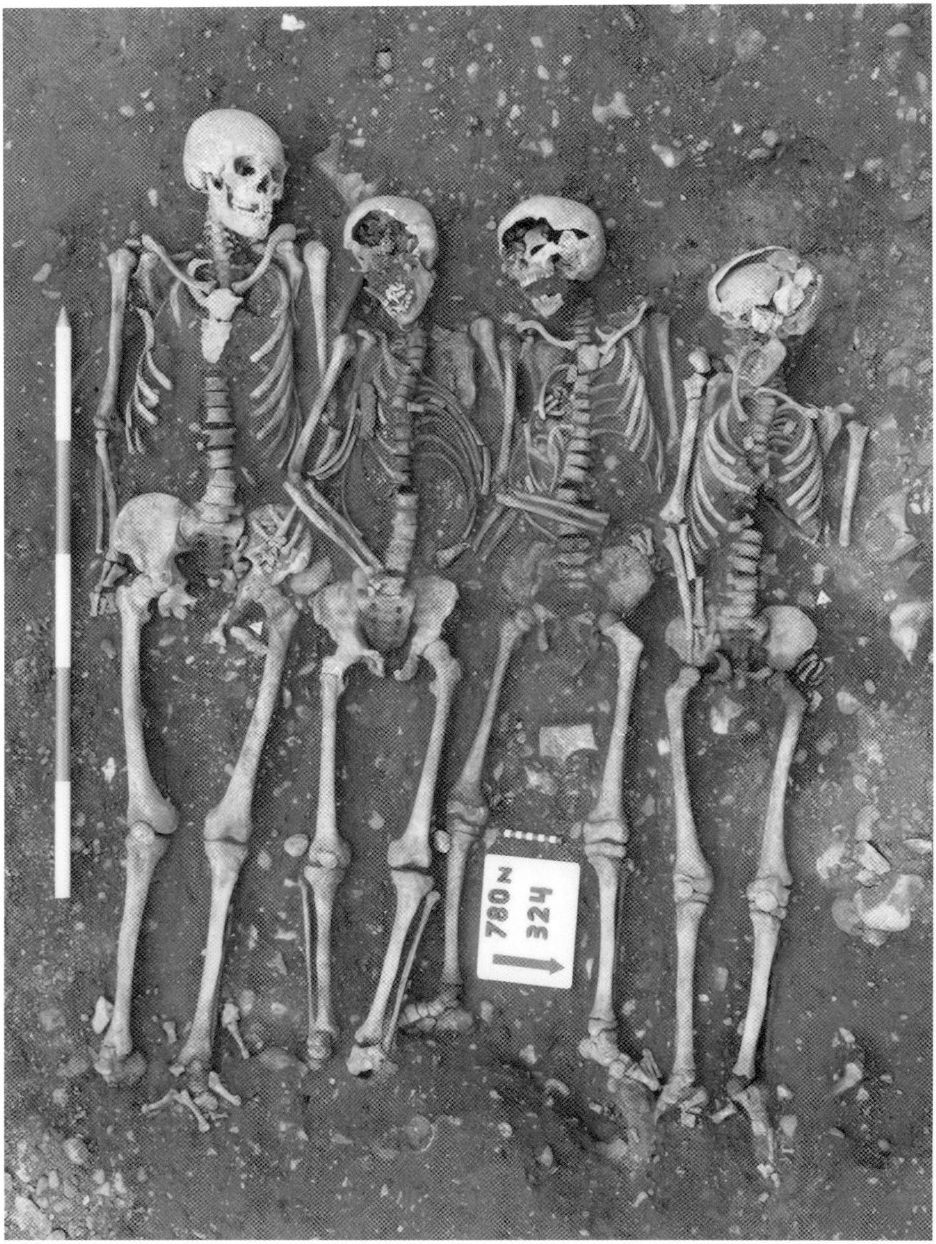

Figure 15: Grave 324, St Margaret's Fyebridge.

A concern to preserve order at St Margaret's despite apparently difficult circumstances is, in contrast, clearly demonstrated by yet another group interment. Grave 324 contained four skeletons laid out in the 'proper' fashion (that is supine, and interred east–west: fig. 15).[94] The dead comprised two adults (one male and one female) and two juveniles, one aged about nine to ten years and the other thirteen to fourteen years.[95] The wide, shallow grave suggests that the sexton was expecting all four individuals to arrive at once. Unlike other multiple graves at the site, where several corpses seem to have been placed in an area far too small to contain them all, this burial was well planned. One of the two adults displayed lytic lesions on the cranial bones, changes which in life would have shown as a grossly infected scalp. Other parts of her body indicate bony reactions, suggesting that she suffered from widespread and probably debilitating systemic infection (skeleton 305).[96] Three other individuals displaying similar lesions were also recovered from the site. Of these, one, a mature adult female, was buried in a group interment (skeleton 68).[97] The remaining two were placed in normal, individual graves.[98]

How should we interpret this varied evidence? We can be categorical in one respect: disfiguring disease was not the determining factor governing a 'bad burial'. The majority of people with facial

trench) where rigor mortis is implicated.

[94] The dead in this grave appear to have been buried in their clothes. Copper alloy lace tags were found with three of the skeletons, perhaps suggesting a rapid burial (i.e., with both adults and the youngest juvenile): Bown and Stirland, 'CAP', n.p. At St Margaret's more generally, lace tags and other evidence of clothing were more likely to be found in multiple and non-normative burials.

[95] NAU Archaeology, 130–2 Magdalen Street Excavation Archive.

[96] Consistent with widely accepted methods of palaeopathological differential diagnosis, this is interpreted as a case of treponemal disease in Stirland, EAA 129, p. 29. I am not concerned here with the debate over whether or not one form of treponemal disease – venereal syphilis – existed in Europe prior to 1493, but for a (pessimistic) account of the issues at stake, see Harper et al., 'The Origin and Antiquity of Syphilis Revisited'.

[97] She was buried in a narrow grave in an area that was already densely studded with earlier interments. Although the individuals were packed tightly into the available space, none of the occupants was arranged in a prone or mal-aligned position. It is likely that this arrangement reflected pressure on space as much as a lack of resources or care for the deceased. The composition of the grave is outlined in NAU Archaeology, 130–2 Magdalen Street Excavation Archive, skeleton recording form 68.

[98] NAU Archaeology, 130–2 Magdalen Street Excavation Archive, skeleton recording forms 129 and 412; Stirland, EAA 129, pp. 28–9.

or limb deformities and injuries excavated from the site were buried in a way that was entirely normative – that is, they were placed in their own grave, supine, and on the normal east–west axis. The indigenous health culture of medieval Norwich, as represented by the evidence of St Margaret's Fyebridge, does not fit into simple models of stigmatization and isolation. The finding is significant: it confirms the thrust in recent historiography which demonstrates that – whilst the tenor of comment on the subjects of deformity and disfigurement in literary, religious, natural philosophical and medical texts was on occasion both scandalized and febrile – urban community *practices* were graduated and nuanced.[99] Those who enjoyed greater personal agency and economic wherewithal, or who had access to religious and social support mechanisms in their lifetime, could expect better standards of funerary treatment than their disenfranchised neighbours, regardless of their disease status.

Nonetheless, aspects of some of the burials at the site clearly indicate ambivalence to the dead. The frequency and forms of the substandard graves imply that a clear lack of regard operated in relation to a substantial proportion of this population. As in death, so in life. Sickness, poverty and marginality coalesce in this parish. We might hazard a guess that the life experiences of the chronic sick subsisting in the environs of St Margaret's church bore little resemblance to those of either the quasi-religious inmates of the *leprosarium* of St Mary Magdalene, Sprowston, or of the respectable almswomen from Norman's hospital. When all eyes were turned towards mortuary provisions, better standards were met. As an analogue, we might observe (using the only evidence available to us) that the burials conducted within the *leprosarium* cemetery of St James and St Mary Magdalene, Chichester – the largest such site of its type thus far excavated on British soil – were remarkably well ordered in comparison to those of St Margaret's.[100]

[99] Indeed, such texts were themselves less straightforwardly condemnatory than earlier superficial readings would suggest: I. Metzler, *Disability in Medieval Europe: Thinking About Physical Impairment During the High Middle Ages, c. 1100–1400* (London, 2006), including pp. 38–64, 90 where the author refines the assumptions of historians concerning the connections between sin and disease in medieval natural philosophical and religious texts; and see Rawcliffe, *Leprosy*, chapters 2 and 6.

[100] Minor variations in grave orientation are accounted for by the presence of built structures, and no prone burials were seen: Magilton, Lee and Boylston, *Lepers Outside the Gate*, pp. 84–132. Also orderly and normative were the graves of

Visibility and a degree of community interest (or buy-in) clearly played a part in determining who did – and who did not – qualify for dignified treatment. This held true even in times of abject crisis: in at least one designated epidemic cemetery set up to cater for the urban poor during the Black Death, burial practice was also highly regular.[101] In St Margaret's parish, we might conclude, chronic disease was ghettoized.

There are other features of the site which are significantly harder to interpret. What, for example, is the true significance of the north–south burials? Do they provide a reliable datum line from which to measure moral censure? Is it simple chance that the diseases and deformities of the dead in the north–south grave were qualitatively different to those in east–west groups, or from those in individual graves?[102] What conclusions might we have drawn about health culture in Norwich if we could see the soft tissues and the skin of the St Margaret's dead, and not just the skeletal substructure? Indeed, what would we conclude if we could have viewed the whole population buried there, and not just a part? More broadly, we might like to know, did the sick poor of Fyebridge became sick owing to their poverty (and the associated physical deprivations that went with it)? Or were they rendered poor as a consequence of their sickness? These are probably unanswerable questions. Yet, the osteoarchaeologist might take heart from the fact that the limits of the evidence are not any more significant than those which commonly confront historians interested in the beliefs, attitudes and actions of the silent majority of people equally unrepresented in documentary records.

Finally, we should again note that the reduced physical and economic circumstances of the district's population – obvious to us through osteoarchaeological analyses – would have been equally apparent to observers passing through. In the landscape of the city, this northern enclave must have appeared as a distinctly insalubrious spot, replete

individuals from whose skeletal remains *mycobacterium leprae* DNA has been extracted at the pre-Conquest site of St John Timberhill, Norwich: Shepherd Popescu, EAA 132, p. 269.

101 I. Grainger, D. Hawkins, L. Cowal and R. Mikulski, *The Black Death Cemetery, East Smithfield, London*, Museum of London Archaeology Service Monograph 43 (London, 2008), pp. 12–22 (burials were carefully handled even in a small number of cases where the bodies were evidently already in an advanced state of decomposition: p. 13, context 6320).

102 That is, so far as can be ascertained from the surviving evidence, they related rather to trauma and to gait than to systemic diseases.

as it was with associations of liminality, criminality and disease. In the next chapter we will draw a contrasting picture: of a city divided into healthy zones. Again, the use to which land was put acts as our point of departure.

4

Placing Health in the Urban Landscape: The Gardens of Norwich

And of this pleasante garden that I have plant most goodlye
I wyll hym make the dresser for his good recreacion.
Therfor, Man, I gyve yt the, to have thy delectacion.[1]

God's prologue to the Norwich grocers' play (1565)

In the previous two chapters – whilst analysing both Cuningham's plan and the burial treatment of the scarred, deformed and injured – we have identified areas of Norwich that were fire-damaged, dilapidated and impoverished. But Cuningham's image of a 'pleasant and healthful' city could claim at least one basis in reality; the lush greenery depicted inside the mural defences of Norwich had actual counterparts. The city really *did* contain many gardens, orchards and open spaces. According to medieval medical culture, gardens (like clean water supplies and a wholesome situation) were a clear indicator of a place's sanitary credentials. What was their significance to the people of Norwich? This chapter considers the evidence of the extent and quality of green and open space in the city and traces its significance to Norwich men and women. As in the previous chapter, I continue to draw on evidence of topography in addition to objects and texts, but here our focus is trained upon the close relationship between gardens, food and well-being in local health culture.

[1] 'The Norwich Grocers' Play [text B]', in *Non-Cycle Plays and Fragments Edited on the Basis of the Edition of Osborn Waterhouse*, ed. N. Davis, EETS ES Supplementary Text 1 (London, 1970), p. 13, lines 3–5.

Health benefits of gardens

The literature on regimen and on healing in the fifteenth and sixteenth centuries invited men and women to meditate on the therapeutic properties of gardens and garden produce.[2] The herb bed, of course, supplied plants for inclusion in drugs and other therapies. Additionally, and in contrast to the alarmingly variable conditions of nature, a garden or a fruitful orchard constituted an environment that could be managed and controlled; specifically, the six non-naturals could be moderated within its bounds. Pleasure gardens, for example, were viewed as suitable arenas for gentle exercise or rest in sweeter, cleaner air.[3] The East Anglian poet John Lydgate toyed with this idea in his *Troy Book* in a passage that described the delight of witnessing dawn break over a garden:

> Aurora, of herte [sincere] and hool [wholesome] entente,
> With the swetness of hir sylver shoures,
> Bedewed hadde the fresh summer floures,
> And made the rose with newe bawme flete [overflow],
> The soote [sweet] lylye and the margarete,
> For to unclose theyr tender leves white,
> Oppressed hertes with gladnesse to delyte,
> That drery were afore of [n]ightes tene [hardship, sorrow],
> And hony souklys amonge the busshes grene,
> Embawmed hadde envyron all the eyre [Had perfumed the air all around].[4]

[2] C. Rawcliffe, 'Delectable Sightes and Fragrant Smelles: Gardens and Health in Late Medieval and Early Modern England', *Garden History* 36 (2008), 3–21, and 'Gardeners' Accounts', ed. Noble, pp. 11–12.

[3] On the therapeutic and corporeal benefits of walking in fragrant air and green spaces, see the discussion in F. Gage, 'Exercise for Mind and Body: Giulio Mancini, Collecting, and the Beholding of Landscape Painting in the Seventeenth Century', *Renaissance Quarterly* 61 (2008), 1167–207 (pp. 1177–86), which includes analyses of fifteenth- and sixteenth-century sources; and see e.g. Lydgate and John of Burgundy, *Governall of Helthe,* sigs. A3v–6r, which argues that exercise is one of the 'highest and noblest' things to be undertaken by man's body, as (unlike bathing or medicine) it costs nothing and (unlike phlebotomy) it is not frightening; rather it is 'pure recreacyon of body and of soule (so it be done in clene places)'. In such a way, 'sholde men shewe themselfe to the clene ayer and delyte in seynge ferre and nere, water and londe, heven and erth, grene and falowe' (sig. A4v).

[4] Lydgate wrote his text in the second decade of the fifteenth century. It was printed in the early sixteenth century: John Lydgate, *The Hystorye, Sege and*

A garden also acted beneficially on the body's senses. The colour green was considered to be particularly soothing, and viewing plants and resplendent lawns supposedly improved vision. With qualities situated midway between those of red and black, it was believed that green 'comforteth the eyen to loke theron, and restoreth and comforteth the syghte'.[5] One medieval encyclopaedist, Bartholomaeus Anglicus (*fl.* 1220–30), described why this was so:

> Grene [is the] colour ... mooste lykynge to the syghte for comyng togeders of firy parties and of erth: for brightnes of fyre that is in grene is temperat, and pleseth the sight; and dimnes of erth and blacknes (for hit is nyghe mooste blacke) gadereth menely [plucks slightly at] the sighte, and comforteth the visible spirite.[6]

In fact, many of the more impressive gardens evident in Cuningham's plan would have been hidden from the view of the general public by large enclosing walls or fences.[7] Access to salubrious space was not a privilege available to all. The boundary walls of the Benedictine cathedral priory, for example, screened a variety of green spaces which blended together different types of corporeal and spiritual therapy (map 7).[8] A pleasure garden, tended by the hosteller, and an orchard with a moat belonging to the prior were intended to impress the priory's most distinguished lay visitors and provided a place for quiet contemplation.[9] Less exalted guests were free to stretch their legs in the preaching yard and around the Carnary chapel. Meanwhile, a garden dedicated to St Mary was used by the brethren for meditation

Dystruccyon of Troye (London: Richard Pynson, 1513), sig. B4v (book 1, chapter 5).

5 Bartholomaeus Anglicus, *De proprietatibus rerum*, trans. Trevisa, fol. 358v (book 19, chapter 19). See S. Landsberg, *The Medieval Garden* (London, *c.* 1995), p. 36, for further references to this theory, and see J. Hawkins, 'Sights for Sore Eyes: Vision and Health in Medieval England', in *On Light*, ed. K. P. Clarke and S. Baccianti (Oxford, 2013), pp. 137–56 (pp. 143–7).

6 Bartholomaeus Anglicus, *De proprietatibus rerum*, trans. Trevisa, fol. 358v (book 19, chapter 19). Bartholomaeus's work also included a compendium of plants and their properties (book 17): *De proprietatibus rerum: Volume VI: Liber XVII*, ed. Ventura.

7 On this point, see E. Rutledge, 'An Urban Environment: Norwich in the Fifteenth Century', in *The Fifteenth Century XII: Society in an Age of Plague*, ed. L. Clark and C. Rawcliffe (Woodbridge, 2013), pp. 79–93 (pp. 80–3).

8 C. Noble, 'Aspects of Life at Norwich Cathedral Priory in the Late Medieval Period' (unpublished PhD thesis, University of East Anglia, 2001), pp. 91–178.

9 Ibid., pp. 140–5.

on spiritual health.[10] In addition to plots designed for recreation and prayer, there was also the infirmary garden. This was used strictly for the cultivation of medicinal herbs for the monks until the mid-fifteenth century when financial difficulties forced the infirmarer to diversify and grow cash crops, especially saffron.[11] That one and the same person might fill the offices of gardener and infirmarer nonetheless implies the transfer of appropriate knowledge between posts.[12]

Gentle, therapeutic exercise in green spaces also seemed to offer patients an opportunity to fight the natural and harmful urge to rest or sleep after bloodletting or a large meal: 'yf a body list to slepe', one author suggested, 'then suche lust shalbe forborn by a space walking in the gardyns or feldes'.[13] The fear was that, whilst resting following phlebotomy, the heart might draw poisonous air into itself. Quiet movement avoided such a potentially fatal state of affairs by dispersing heat. The monks of Norwich cathedral priory seem to have followed this advice with enthusiasm. They periodically retired to their garden to physically refresh themselves and to sip wine after having their blood let by the priory's resident barber; for wine – like gentle exercise – purportedly dispersed heat by warming the body.[14]

Plants for food and medicaments (including henbane) were produced in the gardens of the hospital of St Giles. The nursing sisters had their own walled garden, which they cultivated.[15] Likewise, in

[10] Ibid., pp. 205–12. For a similar practice in the social circle of the Pastons, see *Paston Letters and Papers*, ed. Davis, I, 39, where Agnes Paston relates the story of Sir Jon Henyngham, who, having announced his intention to 'sey a lytyll devocion in hese gardeyn', was taken ill. The situation did not end well for Henyngham: '... forth-wyth ... [he] felt a [f]eyntyng in hese legge and syyd doun. Thys was at 9 of the clok, and he was ded or none [ere noon]' (to John Paston I, 6 July 1453).

[11] Noble, 'Aspects of Life at Norwich Cathedral Priory', pp. 147–9.

[12] Ibid., p. 83, table 1.12c.

[13] Knutsson, *A Litill Boke … Agenst the Pestilence*, fol. [6v]. Cf. Bengt Knutsson, *A Moche Profitable Treatise Against the Pestilence*, trans. Thomas Paynell (London: Thomas Berthelet, 1534), sig. A8r.

[14] 'Gardeners' Accounts', ed. Noble, pp. 31–2, 36; on wine's various salutary effects, see Lydgate, 'The Nine Properties of Wine', *Minor Poems*, II, 724. For evidence that the monks' barber lived, with his wife, in the precincts of the cathedral, see Gilchrist, *Norwich Cathedral Close*, p. 15. On exercise and innate heat, see *Galen's Hygiene*, trans. Green, p. 40; Lydgate and John of Burgundy, *Governall of Helthe*, sig. A4v.

[15] C. Rawcliffe, 'Hospital Nurses and their Work', in *Daily Life in the Late Middle Ages*, ed. R. Britnell (Stroud, 1998), pp. 42–64 (p. 59).

the sixteenth century, John Porter – Norwich's first civic barber-surgeon at the institution – was provided with a garden as part of his contract. This was probably used primarily for recreational purposes; but it may also have supplemented a few staple ingredients alongside the imported oils, salts, resins, clays and waxes that formed the majority of the active constituents and bases of surgical ointments and plasters.[16] The last will and testament of Thomas Reynolds (d. 1558), a Norwich surgeon, is suggestive – but inconclusive – on this score. It demonstrates that he lived in a house with a garden attached in St James's parish. An inventory of his household goods survives and mentions some of the tools of his trade, including surgical irons and a mortar ('morther'). Reynolds *could*, therefore, have made up his own unguents with the produce of his land, but we do not know whether he did.[17] The evidence for medicinal gardening elsewhere in Norwich is even more uncertain. A basic distribution map, if drawn from legal records such as enrolled property deeds and wills, would show that a number of other Norwich physicians, apothecaries and surgeons owned tenements with gardens and lands during the period 1285 to 1500.[18] However in most cases – Norwich having had a thriving rental market – it is difficult to know whether they were cultivated by the owners or rented out for other uses.[19] We might take as a case in point

[16] NCR 16a/5 Mayor's Court Book 1540–49, p. 479. On the ingredients for surgical salves, etc., see Gale, 'Enchiridion of Chirurgerie', in *Certaine Workes of Chirurgerie*. On the sixteenth-century Portuguese spice market at Antwerp, from which surgical staples were likely to have been imported to Norwich, see Atkin and Evans, EAA 100, p. 246.

[17] NRO, DCN 70/11 Original Wills 1529–69, fol. 52r.

[18] For example, Robert Erlam, apothecary (1332), owned several properties, including seven cottages with a garden and dovecote in the parish of St Mary Coslany: NRO, NCR 3–4 Private Deeds, box 4. Similarly, amongst many other properties, John Gosselyn, barber (1421), owned of a messuage with buildings and a garden in the parish of St Gregory: NCR 3–4 Private Deeds, box 1. Roger Taylor, *medicus*, leased a messuage with a garden from the Hospital of St Giles, as did John Porter after him: NRO, NCR 24a Box of Accounts 1415–60 (1434–39); on Porter, see the main text above. Harry Coket, barber (1497), owned one garden and one yard in the parish of St Martin at Bale: NRO, NCC will register Multon, fols. 62v–63r. Many others held property described as 'land' or 'grounds': on this, see Fay, 'Health and Disease', table 3.

[19] S. Kelly, 'The Economic Topography and Structure of Norwich *c*. 1300', in *Men of Property: An Analysis of the Norwich Enrolled Deeds 1285–1311*, ed. U. Priestly (Norwich, 1983), pp. 12–21 (p. 30); Rutledge, 'Economic Life', pp. 166, 171, table 2.

a large stretch of land adjacent to Ber Street in the south-east of the city, situated amid a concentration of properties owned by apothecaries (map 7). Superficially, this appears to have been a prime site for an extensive garden for medical ingredients. However, the plot was in fact leased out to textile workers who used it to set up frames for drying and stretching newly manufactured cloth.[20] Thus, whilst property deeds can help us to pinpoint the location of gardens and to suggest something about the purchasing power and wealth of medical practitioners and provisioners, they do not enlighten us about medical horticulture *per se*. In what remains of this section, therefore, we will explore domestic horticulture as a whole, paying particular attention to the houses and property of individuals who – though they could lay no claim to having undergone a formal medical training – nonetheless appear to have been interested not only in gardening and garden produce, but also in healing.

Domestic horticulture in Norwich

The size of plots under cultivation varied considerably across the city.[21] Gardens in the outskirts measuring 3,000–4,000 square feet were sufficient to grow vegetables, herbs and a small amount of fruit.[22] Much larger tracts were also available, like the acre of land owned and rented out by the city from 1346 in the north-western parish of St Augustine.[23] More gardens were to be found amongst the fourteenth-century tenements, cottages and shops on Botolph Street. Such sizeable plots dwarfed those situated behind the crowded street frontage and shops recorded in areas such as Smithy Row (Hosiergate); they were presumably used for a mixture of small-scale commercial and domestic

[20] NRO, MC 146/52 684x5, map 104. On other tenter grounds like this, see Campbell, 'Norwich', p. 11. The spicers, or apothecaries, were quite active investors in property: Rutledge, 'Economic Life', table 2, p. 172.

[21] See e.g. NRO, MC 146/52 684x5 42 (Roger Pictor; John son of Theobald); MC 146/52 684x5 47 (Cecily de Newbrigg); MC 146/52 684x5 130 (Thomas Bavent).

[22] Atkin and Evans, EAA 100, pp. 102–3 and fig. 15 (18: Ranulf de Plumpstede); MC 146/52 684x5 26 (parish of St Mary Coslany). For similar plots in medieval Winchester where citizens grew herbs, vegetables, grapes and other fruit, see D. Keene, 'The Medieval Urban Environment in Documentary Records', *Archives* 16 (1983), 137–44 (140).

[23] *RCN*, II, 366 (1346).

activities (map 7).[24] Silvia Thrupp found similar distinctions in the sizes of various kinds of gardens in London which she has identified as belonging to particular socio-economic groups. Those owned by craftsmen measured approximately twenty feet in length. The larger properties of merchants, on the other hand, were cultivated for fruit and vegetables, and as places for recreation (whether attached to their own properties, or corporately owned via a guild or company).[25] In Norwich in the later sixteenth century, a survey of burgage plots that paid landgable rent (a fixed ground-rent) to the civic corporation provides a reliable guide to the basic distribution of domestic horticultural space towards the end of our period. Higher concentrations were recorded in the peripheral sub-wards of North and South Conesford (where approximately eleven to twelve per cent of properties were described as gardens, closes or grounds), and in West Wymer and Colegate (where the figure was closer to fourteen per cent); whilst the proportion of gardens to other types of space was particularly high in St Giles (accounting for almost twenty percent of the land surveyed, map 2). Given the proximity of the plots in St Giles to the market, it seems plausible that these were used as market gardens.[26]

Garden space was not only widespread but was also apparently highly prized. Several Norwich residents took the opportunity (following the city government's acquisition of the Blackfriars site in the late 1530s) to rent plots of the dissolved friary's garden.[27] In the accounting year ending in September 1544 such lets supplied a healthy injection of cash into the civic coffers, with some important citizens, like alderman Quash, paying as much as £4 a year for a portion of land.[28] The

[24] For example see MC 146/52 684x5 88 (Arnold le Latoner). This property contained a garden behind a two-storey shop. Other undeveloped plots behind tenements on the same frontage were described as 'land'.

[25] S. L. Thrupp, *The Merchant Class of Medieval London, 1300–1500* (Chicago, 1948), pp. 130–1, 136.

[26] I have calculated the distribution of undeveloped land, viz. plots identified as 'gardens', 'grounds', or 'closes' (enclosed plots), from *Landgable*, ed. Rodgers and Wallace, pp. 29–139. Across the city as a whole, about six per cent of properties mentioned in the survey were undeveloped: Rutledge, 'Introduction', in ibid., p. 9, and see p. 21 on the 'widespread coverage' of housing represented by the landgable (probably over eighty per cent of the housing stock of Norwich is accounted for in the text).

[27] NCR 18a/6 CA 1537–47, fol. 57r; *LP*, XV, 410 (72).

[28] Just under £10 was raised from the rents in that year alone: NCR 17b Mayor's Book (Book of Oaths), p. 152. William March meanwhile paid 26*s*. 8*d*. a year

corporation additionally took an active role in improving gardens in its possession. The chamberlain John Florens paid out 5s. during the year 1534/35 as part of a general campaign to tidy up empty properties and public spaces.[29] This outlay comprised wages for:

> 2 gardeners mendyng and wedyng the garden by 13 dayes at dyvers tymes [at Master Percy's tenement] and makyng clene the yerds and garden and ayenst Saynt Olaves gilde.[30]

The care taken at the tenement equates to a visit by the gardeners every two weeks during the growing season. Percy (no lesser personage than the earl of Northumberland's brother) had left the city property worth £100, and the ruling elite clearly felt obliged to maintain his gift.[31]

If private landowners lacked the time, energy or inclination to tend their own garden to a similar standard, the well-heeled could always enrol the services of a professional gardener.[32] Individual members of the civic government, however, seem to have enjoyed taking part in the activity themselves. The horticultural accomplishments of the prominent citizen Thomas Godsalve were particularly noteworthy. In 1534, Godsalve sent 'a mound with pears of my own grafting' to his son's patron – a certain Thomas Cromwell, the king's principal secretary and chief minister.[33] Grafting fruit trees was *the* defining skill of the accomplished Tudor gardener, and information on the subject was available to the interested reader in both manuscript and (after *c.* 1520) print form.[34] The library of alderman Augustine Steward, on the other hand, included a text which discussed various further horticultural skills, including sowing, preparing the ground and propagation.

for an osier (willow) yard, which he presumably exploited as a commercial venture. The precinct of the Austin friary (King Street) also became a garden after the dissolution: Kirkpatrick, *Streets and Lanes*, p. 8.

[29] For more on this, see chapters 5 and 6 below.

[30] NCR 18a/6 CA 1537–47, fol. 99r.

[31] NCR 17b Mayor's Book (Book of Oaths), p. 151.

[32] Rutledge, 'Economic Life', p. 168.

[33] *LP*, VII, 462 (1189); cf. D. M. Palliser, 'Civic Mentality and the Environment in Tudor York', *Northern History* 18 (1982), 78–115 (p. 89), for evidence of York city corporation requiring its tenants to diligently graft and set civic-owned fruit trees (1541). For more on the link between Godsalve and Cromwell – who intervened to ensure that Godsalve's son, John, was returned as an MP for Norwich in 1539 alongside Augustine Steward – see *House of Commons*, ed. Bindoff, I, 152.

[34] B. Henrey, *British Botanical and Horticultural Literature before 1800* 3 vols. (Oxford, 1975), I, 55; Keiser, *Manual*, pp. 3689–90, 3903–4.

The manuscript comprised sections of Palladius's *Opus agriculturae*, a horticultural calendar.[35] Following a different tradition, Bodleian Library manuscript Rawlinson C 816 (at one time in the possession of Thomas Butts), witnesses the compiler's interest in picking the most profitable time of the year to grow healing and other plants; he copied simple rules from printed prognostications regarding propitious times (according to the position of the moon in the signs of the zodiac) to sow, plant and grass into his personal medical notebook.[36]

The type of plants grown and consumed in Norwich can be inferred from samples of soil taken from anaerobic sediments in Norwich cess-pits. The residents ingested quantities of figs, apples and grapes as well as smaller quantities of walnuts.[37] Cherries, celery and parsnips were also eaten, as were beans, peas, leeks, onions, brassica and garlic.[38] The benefits of fruit were discussed in dietary handbooks and tracts on the regimen. Uncooked apples, figs and pears were seen as potentially harmful if they were eaten by somebody with the wrong type of humoral complexion, but also might be given as luxury presents.[39] Meanwhile, apple blossoms and aromatic pears were commended for 'their swete smell', which reportedly 'comforte[d] the spirites'.[40] Even so, orchards had to be properly cared for if their health benefits were to be maintained. Physicians were keen to point out that they should be well tended and tidy, that they should not be over-stocked or screened from fresh breezes, and that fallen apples should be cleared away, lest they putrefied and gave off poisonous, disease-inducing vapours.[41] In warmer times, grapes were produced at Norwich cathedral priory,[42]

35 Beeching and Rhodes James, 'Library of the Cathedral Church', p. 102 on Lambeth Palace Library MS 425(4). Cf. J. Harvey, *Medieval Gardens* (London, 1981), p. 22.

36 See, fol. 85r (pencil foliation), where the compiler quotes from Leonard Digges, *A Prognostication of Right Good Effect* (London: Thomas Gemini, 1555), sig. E2r–v. On Butts, see above, p. 53, and on the tradition of the election of times, see above, p. 46, n. 52.

37 Atkin, Carter and Evans, EAA 26, p. 68.

38 Ayers, EAA 37, pp. 120–2; 'Gardeners' Accounts', ed. Noble, e.g. pp. 32–9.

39 For fruit as presents, see NCR 18a/7 CA 1541–49, fols. 71r, 220v.

40 Harvey, *Medieval Gardens*, p. 6.

41 Boorde, *Dyetary of Helth*, sig. B4v. For Norwich orchards, see e.g. MC 146/52 684x5 19 (parish of St Saviour); MC 146/52 684x5 27 (parish of St Saviour); MC 146/52 684x5 42 (John son of Theobald); MC 146/52 684x5 76 (parish of Michael at Plea).

42 Gilchrist, *Norwich Cathedral Close*, p. 62.

though figs were imported. One John Cropp (d. *c.* 1598), a surgeon and Walloon immigrant who arrived in Norwich in the later sixteenth century, supplemented his income in this line of business.[43] A market existed for ornamental plants too. Roses and lilies were purchased for cultivation around houses and as cut flowers for chambers owing to their therapeutic smell and cheering beauty.[44]

Archaeology supplies further evidence of the residents' enthusiasm for gardening; a variety of horticultural tools have been recovered from several excavations across Norwich. Those owned by residents at the early sixteenth-century site of Pottergate (149N, map 7), for example, were of a size appropriate for clearing plots, moving manure, breaking up ground, pruning and planting out.[45] Other finds recovered from the site help to put these horticultural tools in their proper context. A fragment of a late medieval specimen urinal (fig. 16),[46] a pilgrim badge,[47] a pendant displaying the five wounds of Christ,[48] a book clasp,[49] fragments of painted window glass (one of which incorporated a merchant's mark),[50] and a writing implement or *stylus* were also recovered.[51] The value of this assemblage is greater than the sum of its parts; it gives us insight into the priorities of residents of this street. Unusually, we also have an uncommon degree of confidence concerning their date and provenance,[52] as these objects were lost in the great Norwich fire in 1507.[53] The objects' original owners were clearly literate, pious and rather well off, and engaged both with spiritual

[43] Pelling, *CL*, p. 226; Pelling and Webster, 'MP', p. 224. Andrew Boorde attributed to Avicenna the belief that 'fygges ... nowrysshe more than any other fruyte': their virtues apparently included cleansing of the breast and lungs, opening obstructions in the liver and spleen and increasing 'the sede of generacyon'. Unfortunately, by provoking sweat, they reputedly had the side-effect of engendering lice: Boorde, *Dyetary of Helth*, sig. K2r–v.

[44] 'Gardeners' Accounts', ed. Noble, pp. 44, 79; Henrey, *Horticultural Literature*, p. 73.

[45] Atkin, Carter and Evans, EAA 26, p. 56; Margeson, EAA 58, pp. 194–5, nos. 1527 (pitchfork), 1512 (spade iron), 1518, 1519 (billhooks), 1523, 1524, 1525 (sickles), 1528 (larger pitchfork, associated with post-fire silting and collapse).

[46] Atkin, Carter and Evans, EAA 26, pp. 58, 62 no. 57 (SF149N/1059), p. 83.

[47] Ibid., pp. 56–7 no. 4 (SF149N/1259).

[48] Ibid., pp. 56–7 no. 3 (SF 149N/710).

[49] Ibid., p. 58 no. 28 (SF149N/2121).

[50] Margeson, EAA 58, p. 172 no. 1332.

[51] Atkin, Carter and Evans, EAA 26, pp. 58–9 no. 23.

[52] Margeson, EAA 58, p. 172 no. 1332.

[53] They were subsequently dispersed across the site when it was tidied up.

medicine (souvenirs like the pilgrim badge and the five-wounds pendant might be purchased on trips made for the sake of health), as well as with humoral theory (represented by the broken specimen urinal).[54]

This last object, the much satirized symbol of the Galenic physician, suggests that an individual who lived at Pottergate (or at least generated rubbish that was dumped there) had a grasp of diagnostic practice. Purportedly, urine inspection was a precise technique for gauging the state of an individual's health, and the practitioner needed to have a grasp of humoral theory, including the relationship between the elements, the seasons and human complexions, in order to understand the significance of the colour and odour of urine samples.[55] The therapeutic possibilities following diagnosis by this means were laid out in vernacular texts for a technically inclined but not necessarily academic readership. For example, *The Seynge of Urynes* (printed in 1525 from medieval manuscript sources) suggested herbal recipes for a variety of diseases.[56] Many of its ingredients could be sourced from urban gardens and household cupboards: sage, hart's tongue, parsley, tansy, mustard, honey and saxifrage were recommended for adding to pottage, to cooked fruit or to an alcoholic base for their medicinal properties, whilst a trip to the spicery (apothecary's row in the market) might provide the necessary supplements of sugar, treacle, gromwell, hart's heart bone, ginger, scammony, figs and pepper. Access to a

[54] On pilgrimage in the region, see C. Rawcliffe, 'Curing Bodies and Healing Souls: Pilgrimage and the Sick in Medieval East Anglia', in *Pilgrimage: The English Experience from Becket to Bunyan*, ed. C. Morris and P. Roberts (Cambridge, 2002), pp. 108–40 (esp. p. 136, fig. 26); on pilgrimage by women hoping to conceive male children, see Hill, *Women and Religion*, pp. 24–5; and see *Paston Letters and Papers*, ed. Davis, I, 218, where Margaret Paston tells her sick husband: '[m]y moder hat be-hestyd a-nodyr ymmage of wax of [th]e weytte of yow to Oyur Lady of Walsyngham ... and I have be-hestyd to gon on pylgreymmays to Walsyngham and to Sent Levenardys for yow'. Walsingham lies about 30 miles north-west of Norwich.

[55] Anon., *The Seynge of Urynes* (London: [J. Rastell for] Richard Banckes, 1525), sigs. B3v, B4v–C1r, D4v–E1r. On the elements, seasons and complexions, see sig. D3v.

[56] Anon., *The Seynge of Urynes*, sigs. A2r–B3v, and D4r (for a more complex remedy for dropsy). On the medieval sources, see M. T. Tavormina, 'The Twenty-Jordan Series: An Illustrated Middle English Uroscopy Text', *ANQ: A Quarterly Journal of Short Articles, Notes and Reviews* 18 (2005), 43–67. On local translations into English of uroscopy texts, see above, p. 54 (William Buckenham).

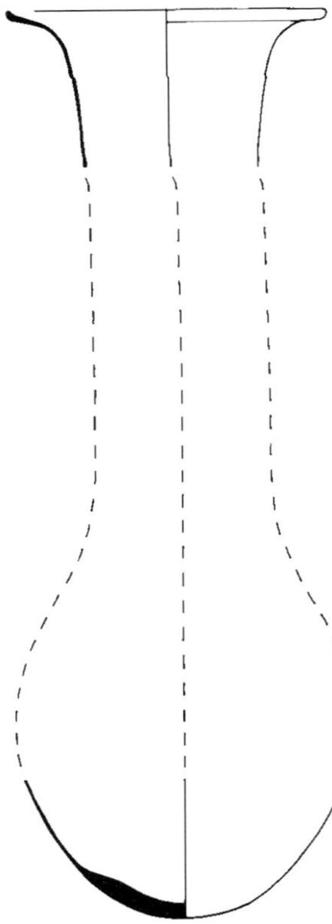

Figure 16: Example of a urine inspection vessel excavated from a property on medieval Nether Westwick (St Benedict's Street), Norwich (site 153N).

practitioner able to let blood might also be required, depending on the diagnosis.[57]

More horticultural tools dating to the late fifteenth or sixteenth century have been recovered alongside another late medieval urinal fragment from Alms Lane in the Colegate district of the city (site 302N,

[57] Anon., *The Seynge of Urynes*, sigs. H2v–3v. This was produced as a companion volume to an extremely popular herbal published at the same press by Richard Banckes, on which see Henrey, *Horticultural Literature*, pp. 12–14; F. R. Johnson, '*A Newe Herball of Macer* and Banckes's *Herbal*: Notes on Robert Wyer and the Printing of Cheap Handbooks of Science in the Sixteenth Century', *Bulletin of the History of Medicine* 15 (1944), 246–60.

map 7).[58] As at Pottergate, there is no documentary evidence that any medical practitioner lived or worked in a tenement at site 302N, which was originally given over both to the brewing and iron-working industries before it was redeveloped for general domestic use.[59] However, we know the livelihood of one owner-occupier at the turn of the sixteenth century, and the evidence is intriguing. Thomas Hendry, a grocer, lived in the most north-westerly of the excavated tenements.[60] Grocers – who sold foodstuffs wholesale – occasionally branched out into offering medical advice and acted, in this respect, much like apothecaries.[61] In fact, the businesses of both sets of merchants united the closely interrelated spheres of therapeutics and diet, diet being generally credited as the principal therapeutic instrument.[62] It was not unknown for grocers also to trade as barbers, and a small number might therefore have been able to perform phlebotomy.[63] Was Hendry one of those inquisitive healers who from time to time aggravated academically trained specialists by assuming the tools and techniques of the physician's trade? We cannot be sure.

The close links between horticulture, food and health were, however, prominently displayed in another source pertaining to Hendry's occupation: the Norwich grocers' Whitsun pageants. Evidence of the staging of this annual event survives from a mid-eighteenth-century copy of the minute book and accounts of the sixteenth-century Grocers' Company. Two versions of the play were transcribed by the guild: one was written in 1533, the other in 1565.[64] The grocers' re-enactment of the fall of man was set in the garden of Paradise – supposedly *the* event

58 Atkin, Carter and Evans, EAA 26, pp. 211–12. The urinal fragment, of late medieval design, was found intruding into an archaeological feature dating from between 1275 and 1400.

59 Atkin, Carter and Evans, EAA 26, pp. 144, 149–63.

60 Ibid., p. 235.

61 See in Pelling, *CL*, pp. 55, 220 and 222 (for the career of Henry Holden).

62 On the powers of foods to alter bodily states, see Albala, *Eating Right in the Renaissance*, pp. 99–104.

63 Pelling, *CL*, pp. 222–3, 227, 241.

64 J. Dutka, 'The Lost Dramatic Cycle of Norwich and the Grocers' Play of the Fall of Man', *Review of English Studies* 35 (1984), 1–13 (p. 6). The company was jointly responsible for staging the pageant with the chandlers, an association that would have seemed appropriate to local audiences: chandlers sold wax for (amongst other uses) the making of plasters and medicinal salves, as well as embalming ointments: R. Fitch, 'Norwich Pageants: The Grocers' Play', *NA* 5 (1859), 8–31 (p. 9); Pelling, *CL*, p. 55.

that first introduced infirmity, pain and mortality into the human condition.[65] In both surviving texts, the surroundings are described as 'a garden of pleasure'. Like the 'paradise' gardens maintained by St Giles's hospital and the Norwich Benedictines, the grocers' version of Eden provided an opportunity for health-promoting light work,[66] and was planted to stimulate 'recreation', 'contemplation', 'delectation' and 'solace'. There were extended opportunities in the texts for word-play on such medico-spiritual themes. Following the commonly accepted principles of the *regimen sanitatis*, the pageants make numerous references to the interrelatedness of emotional well-being, the avoidance of despair and dolour, and corporeal health. In both, Adam takes a tour of the garden, an activity recommended by physicians for exercise and the stimulation of the senses. Conversely, after eating the apple, he laments his 'fowle' presumption which cast him 'fro pleasur to payn', and the lack of any 'remedye' for labour and travail.[67] In the later version of the play, the personification of Myserye revels in the notion that mankind must now 'taste and byte/ Of hardenes and of colde and eke of infirmitie',[68] whilst the serpent's deception is styled in terms used elsewhere to describe disease-inducing vapours; his temptation acts on Eve like 'a darkned myste'.[69] The list of stage properties and receipts which accompanies the two texts shows how Eden's food stores were recreated on the Norwich pageant wagon (a useful platform on which to advertise the grocers' stock-in-trade). The

[65] On the attempts by the medieval and early modern founders of botanical gardens to emulate Eden's ideal, temperate climate and sweet air, see J. Prest, *The Garden of Eden: The Botanic Garden and the Re-creation of Paradise* (Yale, 1981); cf. G. Darley 'John Evelyn's Norwich Garden', *Garden History* 34 (2006), 249–53 (p. 250), on the 'spring' garden of the duke of Norfolk (1663–64).

[66] In one version of the pageant, God commands Adam to 'use thys place in vertuse occupacion', in the other to 'cherish tre and plante/ To dresse and kepe the grounde, and eate what frute hym lyste': 'The Norwich Grocers' Play [Text A]', in *Non-Cycle Plays*, ed. Davis, p. 9, line 46, and 'The Norwich Grocers' Play [Text B]', p. 12, line 20. On digging and weeding as appropriate and healthy light work that might distract men and women from more spiritually perilous pastimes (such as games, gossip or drink), see the foundation statutes of the hospital of St Mary, Great Yarmouth, Norfolk (1386), quoted in Rawcliffe, *Urban Bodies*, p. 98. On work and health more generally, see Part III below.

[67] 'The Norwich Grocers' Play [Text A]', p. 10, lines 83–4; 'The Norwich Grocers' Play [Text B], p. 17, line 121.

[68] 'The Norwich Grocers' Play [Text B]', p. 16, lines 115–16.

[69] Ibid., p. 12, line 24. On the harmfulness of 'myste' see Lydgate 'Doctrine for Pestilence', in *Minor Poems*, II, 702, lines 8, 16 (cf. above, p. 38).

following expenses were approved at a preparatory meeting convened at Blackfriars' in May 1534: apples and figs at the cost of 4*d*., oranges at the cost of 10*d*., three pounds of dates costing 1*s*., and one stone in weight of almonds. These were used to ornament the pageant's Tree of Knowledge.[70] Additionally, the pageant's committee purchased various perfumes,[71] bundles of flowers or posies, nutmeg, cloves and mace, which together synthesized the sweet air and aromas of Paradise during the performance.[72]

Placing insalubrity: uncultivable plots and dumping grounds

Pursuing the associations between well-being and garden space through the documentary and physical record brings us closer to understanding the vernacular health culture of pre-modern Norwich. The evidence, of various kinds, returns us to themes that we encountered from a theoretical, top-down perspective in earlier parts of this book: the importance of sweet air, of exercise and rest, and of the quality and cleanliness of spaces. Not all of Norwich's open spaces were maintained to the highest, most wholesome standard, however. In the final part of this chapter, we will look at plots put to altogether more prosaic uses.

Until its boundaries became fixed in the fourteenth century by the completion of the circuit of the walls, Norwich comprised a set of sprawling and scattered concentrations of habitation.[73] As we saw in the introduction, the area eventually enclosed was large, partly to accommodate these nuclei, and partly to simplify the construction of

70 Fitch, 'Norwich Pageants', p. 24; N. Davis, 'Introduction', in *Non-Cycle Plays and Fragments*, ed. Davis, p. xxxii.

71 The perfumes were burnt inside a large, gilded fumatory. The total spent on perfumes alone increased steadily over the years that the play was staged, amounting to 2*s*. for 6oz in 1557 (when prunes and raisins were also added to the cornucopia of fruit). Depending upon the occasion, the fumatory was either carried by one of the performers or attached to the wagon's set: Fitch, 'Norwich Pageants', pp. 9, 24, 28, 30; Davis, 'Introduction', pp. xxxii, xxxv. Perfumes were also burnt in the griffin during the grocers' annual dinner, held on Corpus Christi day: Fitch, 'Norwich Pageants', p. 28.

72 Fitch, 'Norwich Pageants', p. 29; Davis, 'Introduction', pp. xxxiv–xxxv. On the grocers' thriving import market in the last part of the sixteenth century, see Pound, 'Social and Trade Structure', pp. 61–2.

73 On Richard Spynk's gift to the city, which facilitated the completion of large stretches of the walls, see *RCN*, II, 216–25.

the fortifications themselves; with a circuit of almost two-and-a-half miles to cover, awkward angles and watercourses were best avoided wherever possible. The area thus enclosed included plenty of open space, apt for horticultural use. Some interstitial places – between the main clusters of development and major axial roads – proved unattractive for long-term settlement. As was the case with St Margaret's Fyebridge, distance from central services and markets was one factor that deterred development. Ecclesiastical landholdings also prevented colonization, with the Benedictine cathedral priory, the four orders of friars, the hospital of St Giles, and various smaller institutions all retaining significant tracts (in addition to their own sizeable precincts) within the city walls.[74] Thus, in the early fourteenth century, when other areas of the city were being densely built up, open stretches – including an expanse of agricultural land known as the Gildencroft and further empty plots to the east – were to be found in the northern outskirts.[75] There were also fields in the south and east around Great Newgate and in the parish of St Catherine, and much of the area adjacent to the Butter Hills and to Ber Street (where the city's noxious lime-works were concentrated) was also open (map 7).[76] Marginal and out-of-sight plots were liable to be used for storing or disposing of some of the vast quantities of waste generated by the population. At the close of the sixteenth century, for example, one lime-kiln yard near Ber Street was officially decommissioned, enclosed and given over as a laystall to which compost (well-rotted manure or organic matter), muck (fresher manure and straw) and rubbish (refuse) were permitted to be bought in small quantities at a time.[77] In earlier centuries, a not dissimilar use was made of former quarries that had been exploited for

[74] On these themes, see Ayers, 'Urban Landscape', pp. 19–24; Campbell, 'Norwich', pp. 10–11; E. Rutledge, 'Immigration and Population Growth in Early Fourteenth-Century Norwich: Evidence from the Tithing Roll', *Urban History Yearbook* 15 (1988), 15–30 (pp. 17, 22–3).

[75] Campbell, 'Norwich', p. 11; Rutledge, 'Economic Life', p. 160.

[76] For St Catherine's Croft, see Kirkpatrick, *Streets and Lanes*, p. 14; for Great Newgate, see Campbell, 'Norwich', p. 11, and Rutledge, 'Immigration and Population Growth', p. 18. On the lime-kilns as a source of water and air pollution, see Rawcliffe, 'Health and Safety at Work in Late Medieval East Anglia', in *Medieval East Anglia*, ed. C. Harper-Bill (Woodbridge, 2005), pp. 130–51 (p. 145), and Rutledge, 'An Urban Environment', p. 92. On smoke (of both harmful and beneficial kinds), see Bartholomaeus Anglicus, *De proprietatibus rerum*, trans. Trevisa, fol. 151r–v (book 10, chapter 6).

[77] Kirkpatrick, *Streets and Lanes*, p. 11.

the excavation of iron pan, sand, clay, gravel or other building materials in peripheral plots inside the city defences. Once abandoned, these pits and hollows were used as convenient places to dump garbage and cess, and as places into which old middens were cleared and levelled.[78]

Areas along the river margins, which were uncultivable owing to the poor quality of the land, were similarly employed. To be sure, stretches of river marsh supplied valuable summer pasture (in Conesford, the area sandwiched between the southern sweep of the Wensum and the precincts of the cathedral was used in this way, map 7), but this was not appropriate in more central stretches.[79] Land adjacent to Calke's mills[80] in the north-west of the city proved hard to utilize.[81] Another tract situated nearby between the defences in Coslany and the river, had been described as a 'low and ill-conditioned place' in 1343.[82] Perhaps inevitably, a survey by the civic authorities in the early sixteenth century discovered large quantities of manure were stowed in 'muck yards' along the riverside backlands.[83]

The land employed for more or less officially sanctioned waste disposal was likely to have been viewed as a necessity by the men and women of Norwich, though they may have been reluctant to live too close to the most heavily used areas. Disposal practices were not, however, indiscriminate; even in out-of-the-way locations, concentrations of manure and refuse were intended to be well managed. In 1374/75, John de Gissing was reprimanded by the city authorities for heaping up an island in the river (known as the bitmay) with one hundred cartloads of muck, material that he had removed as part of a private collection service. Apparently, the waste was contaminating the river.[84] Almost two hundred years later, the same plot seems to have been used for a similar purpose, but safeguards were now in place to prevent the river from becoming polluted. The city lease book recorded that the individual renting the island from the civic corporation had to

[78] Atkin and Evans, EAA 100, pp. 11–12 (waste accretion), 159 (midden clearance); Atkin, Carter and Evans, EAA 26, pp. 94–5, 143, 149, 240.

[79] Ayers, *NAFC*, p. 104; Atkin and Evans, EAA 100, pp. 7, 66.

[80] These were probably situated just downstream of the New Mills, in the parish of St Martin at Oak.

[81] The civic assembly instigated proceedings to cleanse the area: Kirkpatrick, *Streets and Lanes*, pp. 73–4.

[82] *RCN*, II, 216–17: 'une place basse et malvoise a faire'.

[83] NRO, NCR 16c/2 Assembly Minute Book 1510–50, fol. 2r–v.

[84] *LJ*, ed. Hudson, p. 65.

ensure that his enterprise did not damage the river 'with eny maner of fylth, rubysshe, coulder[85] or meanour', but that he would 'at all tymes at hys onely costes and chardges keepe the river cleane with dydalles [hand tools used for cleaning watercourses]', leaving the water in a clear state at the end of the rental term.[86]

The procedures by which waste was transferred from households and densely occupied areas to common dumping grounds can be inferred from archaeological evidence. Initially, in Norwich domestic contexts, rubbish and manure tended to be buried permanently in the backyards of tenements. But from about the late fourteenth century, waste of all kinds was deposited away from houses in special off-site locations, or was stored in temporary containers or middens ready for removal.[87] For property owners, engaging with corporate waste-removal strategies offered obvious advantages; in this way, the burden of energy expenditure, as well as financial costs, could be shared. Additionally, rubbish and waste had a value of their own, particularly in large quantities. By Cuningham's time, valuable tracts along the river margins and the valley of the Great Cockey had been consolidated with dumps of waste materials and with silt dredged from the river.[88] Human waste was also removed from properties in much the same way as rubbish. During the late fifteenth century, the tenements at Pottergate had en-suite accommodation on the first floor which connected to external lean-to cellars via a chute. The contents of these cellars were dug out periodically and removed, and were either reburied elsewhere, or collected for use as agricultural fertiliser.[89]

Waste that was not confined to its proper place was a different matter altogether; this was not considered tolerable. It is to an investigation of these substances – and attempts by the residents to control them – that we turn in the third and final section of this book. Here, our focus will be trained upon the allocation of responsibility and accountability regarding environmental cleanliness in the pre-modern city; allocations that were made to both the individual residents (and

[85] On 'coulder', see below, p. 154, n. 66.

[86] NRO, NCR 22g/1 City Lease Book A, fol. 62v.

[87] Atkin and Evans, EAA 100, pp. 31, 105, 184.

[88] Ayers, *NAFC*, p. 100; B. Ayers, 'The Infrastructure of Norwich from the 12th to the 17th Centuries', *Lübecker Kolloquium zur Stadtarchäologie im Hanseraum IV: Die Infrastruktur*, ed. M. Gläser (Lübeck, 2004), pp. 31–40 (p. 34).

[89] Atkin, Carter and Evans, EAA 26, pp. 10 fig. 2, 12–13, 15, 21, 70; and (on cleaning out cess and reburying it) see below, p. 170, n. 17.

especially householders) and the officers of city government acting collectively. In introducing us to the themes of the final part of this book, one prominent citizen whom we met in this chapter (alderman Augustine Steward) will act as our initial guide.

Part III

Governing the City and the Self

> But what of Roome? Sythe yow have browghte (whos vertewes doethe excell),
> A man in whom what Grace hathe wrowghte unnethe mye tounge can tell [I can scarcely say].
>
> Suche one whome Nature so did frame to seeke the peoples heallthe,
> Goodwill and Wisdoome tawhte the same to awgmeant the common wealthe.[1]
>
> Mayoral pageant by Mr Boucke, schoolmaster, 1556

In Norwich during the month of June 1556, a pageant was performed in honour of the mayor, Augustine Steward (then in his third stint in the office), which listed the virtues with which all civic leaders ought to be endowed. The pageant's author, a local grammar school master named Boucke, explained that Norwich surpassed ancient Rome in certain qualitative aspects, not least in the calibre of its governors. In electing Steward, Boucke went on to explain, the citizens had chosen a man destined to improve standards of human welfare. Steward's remit thus conceived included keeping the city fabric 'in coomlye order' and providing support for the genuinely sick and incapacitated ('impotennte') poor.[2] Although the extent of the personal praise heaped upon Steward is surprising to modern readers accustomed to treating the motives of politicians with no small measure of scepticism, Boucke's wider concerns – about physical order, the righteous poor and the

[1] NCR 17b Mayor's Book (Book of Oaths), p. 139, printed in *Records of Early English Drama: Norwich*, ed. Galloway, p. 38.
[2] NCR 17b Mayor's Book (Book of Oaths), p. 140.

general good – were not original. He was drawing on an already old set of medico-political ideas which promoted the notion that decorum and cleanliness were necessary prerequisites for well-being: medieval ideas which had been reframed and aired in the works of reformers and in the activities of parliamentarians of the preceding generation. According to this philosophy, disease, illness and urban decay apparently interacted with, and dangerously aggravated, one another.[3] A scheme proposed in parliament in 1535, for example, provided constructive solutions to the perceived evils of industrial collapse, the dilapidation of the urban fabric and the seeming arrival of swarms of unruly, disease-ridden paupers. The poor, it was suggested, could be employed in waged work upon various civic projects, including the 'makyng of the comen high waies and ... skowryng and clensyng of watercourses through the realme'. Such provisions, it was hoped, would not only bolster trade, but would also bring about better standards in health, not least owing to the 'holsome' bodily effects of labour on those thus employed. Furthermore, the labourers were to be given free, specialist medical help as necessary, and a reasonable wage.[4] In this way, the streets and waterways of cities would not only be made clean of dangerous, putrefying materials, but would also be delivered of mendicant frauds who 'pretende knowlege and conyng in physik, surgery, phiysnamye, palmestrie, destenyes, or other craftie sciences wherby the poore rude and innocent people [are] disceived'.[5]

Steward, if forced to justify the tone of the mayoral pageant, could reasonably claim that he and other aldermen had steered Norwich in the general direction outlined by his fellow members of parliament:[6] firstly, he was mayor at the time of the city's purchase of the hospital of St Giles (the 'Great Hospital'), an institution for the succour and rehabilitation of the 'impotent' poor;[7] secondly, he claimed personal

[3] P. Slack, *From Reformation to Improvement: Public Welfare in Early Modern England* (Oxford, 1998), pp. 6–23, esp. 8–9, 17. See also Pelling, *CL*, pp. 63–5, 79–102.

[4] See extracts printed in G. R. Elton, 'An Early-Tudor Poor Law', *Economic History Review*, 2nd. s. 6 (1953), 55–67 (pp. 58–9) from BL Royal MS 18 C VI. On health, exercise and labour, see Rawcliffe, 'Health and Safety at Work', pp. 130–32 and *passim*.

[5] Elton, 'Poor Law', p. 62. For a characterization of the damages caused by false physicians and prognosticators to credulous and innocent householders, see Copland, *Hye Way to the Spyttell Hous*, sigs. C1r–2v.

[6] Steward was returned as MP for Norwich in 1539 and 1547: *House of Commons*, ed. Bindoff, III, 383–5.

[7] Rawcliffe, *MFTS*, p. 219; NCR 16a/5 Mayor's Court Book 1540–49, p. 376.

responsibility for improving dilapidated tenement plots and buildings in Norwich, and he highlighted the problems caused by the dumping of noxious waste in them; and thirdly, he had on occasion presided at the mayor's court[8] over checks on the qualifications of individuals practising medicine. We will meet Steward acting in each role from time to time in the following two chapters.[9]

His ability to mandate improvements in at least some of these areas was apparently endorsed by none other than John Caius, the future president of the college of physicians in London. The name of the mayor featured prominently in the preface of Caius's *Boke or Counseill Against the Disease Commonly Called the Sweate* (1552) which was written immediately after a particularly disastrous outbreak of the disease.[10] To be sure, Caius carefully demarcated the areas of health policy that a civic leader like Steward might reasonably take responsibility for, and separated them from medicine proper.[11] But he recognized that there were basic principles of urban hygiene that non-university-educated laymen needed to have at their command during times of emergency, and it was these that he set out in his *Counseill*.[12] He noted that he was specifically encouraged in this endeavour by men who had read and enjoyed certain of his earlier translations – a group that included

[8] A court convened at the guildhall where minor offences were tried.

[9] For the wider context, see the discussion on developments in forms of mayoral (and bureaucratic) authority, and the manipulation of built space, in R. Tittler, *Architecture and Power: The Town Hall and the English Urban Community c. 1500–1640* (Oxford, 1991), chapter 5; and, for the material culture of the ruling elite in Norwich – including a metre-long gold, rock crystal and gemstone civic mace, gifted to the corporation by Augustine Steward in 1550 for use in processions by the mayor and aldermen – see M. Thøfner, 'Catholics, Protestants and Strangers', in *The Art of Faith: 3,500 Years of Art and Belief in Norfolk*, ed. A. Moore and M. Thøfner (London, 2010), pp. 34–43.

[10] Caius, *Counseill Against the … Sweate*, fol. 4r.

[11] Ibid., fol. 2v. A properly qualified physician would be needed to 'geve … particular counseil', and to prescribe changes to a person's regimen according to the characteristics of 'place, persone, [and] cause': ibid., fol. 8r.

[12] Ibid., fols. 7v–8r. The physician expected his reader to be cognisant of many terms and ideas pertaining to the functioning of the humours and the nature of human complexions. He also assumed that he would have a basic grasp of anatomy which extended to understanding the primacy of the three principal organs (the heart, brain and liver) and their relation to the bodily 'spirits'; that is, to the physical agents which apparently prompted the body to perform its functions.

Steward.[13] The second section of his pamphlet included a potted history of disease in history's greatest cities – Rome, Troy and Athens – and hammered home two familiar points: the first being Galen's warning against dwelling next to 'merishe, and muddy groundes, puddles or donghilles, sinkes or canales, easing places or carions, deadde ditches or rotten groundes'; the second, a summary of the ills of dietary excesses.[14]

In the next and final chapters of this book, we will address each of these themes in turn. We begin by looking at the long history of urban hygiene through the lens of corporate and individual activities to improve the state of the environment. In chapter 5, we see how ideas about cleanliness similar to those espoused by Caius were used in Norwich to inform practical action in the sphere of clearing 'donghills', 'carions', 'sinkes' and 'canales' from the thirteenth to the sixteenth centuries. In chapter 6, we will discover how the principle of moderation and self-rule (which lay at the heart of the concept of the preventative regimen) was interpreted by Norwich's governing elite when drafting policies for the 'common benefit'. Complementing this, we will look at measures to supervise medical practice, provide for the impotent poor and keep the city fabric in good order: themes explored in Steward's 1556 pageant. Throughout both chapters, we will probe concepts of individual and corporate culpability for harm done either to the city's natural and man-made infrastructure, or to personal well-being. Our source material yet again covers a range of evidence not normally read in conjunction: the financial and administrative accounts of the city authorities, churchwardens' accounts, medical literature, and the verbal denouncements made by residents when reporting cases of careless or polluting behaviour by their neighbours, as well as wills and taxation records. Having already encountered some of the factors governing waste disposal practices in the urban environment, we begin with the punitive legal proceedings taken against individuals who committed environmental infractions, before moving on to consider the corporation's regulatory attempts to improve standards of cleanliness in the city's waterways and streets.

13 Caius, *Counseill Against the … Sweate*, fol. 8r–v. Whilst a student at Cambridge, Caius translated and condensed Erasmus's *De vera theologia* for his 'very friend', Augustine Steward, then aged 39 (some 19 years older than Caius): ibid., fols. 3v–4r.

14 Caius, *Counseill Against the … Sweate*, fol. 15v.

5

Cleaning Up: Reforming the Urban Environment 1300–1570

Norwich's residents from all backgrounds had a duty to preserve the condition of communal spaces. In the following sections of this chapter, we will look first at the legal frameworks, customary obligations and mandates by which residents and governors attempted to enforce observance of this duty from the close of the thirteenth century onwards, before narrowing our focus to examine civic attitudes to waste in the period 1530–70 (that is, in the immediate wake of the publication of the reformed version of *Airs, Waters, Places*). Over this period of about 250 years, we will observe particular constants: the supposed importance of the purity of water and air to human health; the responsibilities of householders and property owners to the civic environment; the relative importance of particular types of urban space or plots (of central or peripheral tracts, visible or hidden ones). The mechanisms for removing waste (hand tools, human and animal muscle power, transportation by cart and boat) were also common across time periods, scaled up or down according to (perceived) need. The story is, however, also one of change and evolution; from the 1530s if not earlier, the ruling aldermanic class assumed the role of guardians of cleanliness (albeit largely for their own benefit), and they were duly held accountable by the residents for their performance.

Reports and regulations: legislating for cleanliness

The earliest extant records of public health from Norwich comprise a series of documents recording fines imposed upon residents in courts held within each of the city's wards and their sub-wards (or 'leets') (map 2). These were assemblies where neighbours were able to present people in their community who committed a range of offences, including actively polluting the local surroundings.[1] In the words of one historian, such courts were 'the bedrock of civic administration in England and were the lowest and most immediate ... units through which a town could be governed'.[2] The first Norwich leet courts for which evidence survives were convened in 1287.[3] A royal prohibition against allowing debris to accumulate in Norwich's waterways had recently come into force, and this led to a series of prosecutions regarding drainage and waste disposal. Complaints ranged from problems relating to the smallest gutters to very serious cases of pollution in the river Wensum.[4] For example, John le Redepriest was accused by the residents of St Peter Mancroft of allowing his sewer to run into a watercourse;[5] meanwhile, the anchorite of All Saints Westlegate, Timberhill, was presented by the jurors of the Ber Street sub-leet for blocking the flow of the Great Cockey (map 8);[6] and one Alan de Freton was reported because he threw dung (*fimum*) and ashes into the Wensum.[7] In the following year, irresponsible waste disposal was again in the forefront of the jurors' minds and cases were reported that involved the dumping of putrid or stinking matter.[8] For example, Roger Benjamin was fined 2*s*. for positioning a muck-heap in the street and hiding offal inside it, thus causing the air to become 'badly infected'.[9] The

[1] Records from the leet courts and sheriffs' tourns survive sporadically from the late thirteenth to the seventeenth centuries. The origins of the leet courts lay in frank-pledge, a system administered by small numbers of adult men grouped into neighbourhood tithings. Tithing members, amongst other duties, monitored and reported on one another's behaviour under the oversight of the civic executive: Rees Jones, 'Household, Work and the Problem of Mobile Labour', pp. 140–1; *LJ*, ed. Hudson, pp. xviii–xxii, xxvi–xxxix; Rutledge, 'Immigration and Population Growth', pp. 15, 18–20.

[2] Rees Jones, 'Household, Work and the Problem of Mobile Labour', p. 136.

[3] They followed a period of serious civil unrest in Norwich: J. Campbell, 'Norwich before 1300', in *MN*, ed. Rawcliffe and Wilson, pp. 29–48 (pp. 34–5).

[4] *LJ*, ed. Hudson, pp. 3, 6, 7 (muck-heaps), 8, 9 (new watercourses), 11 (new gutter/muck-heap), 12 (common ditch).

[5] Ibid., p. 9.

[6] Ibid., p. 6.

[7] Ibid., p. 3.

[8] Ibid., pp. 23–4 (muck-heaps, watercourses), 26–7, 30 (muck-heaps).

[9] Ibid., p. 23. The following report was made: 'De Rogero Beniamin pro quodam fimario posito in via regali in quo sepellivit viscera animalium per quod aer pessime corrumpitur, 2*s*.'. A handful of similar cases were ultimately proven to be spurious or prompted by malicious opportunism: ibid., pp. 26–7.

activities of the leet courts in Norwich mirrored current metropolitan practice: in London, by order of the mayor, offenders who dumped rubbish in the streets faced fines of 4*d*. for each infraction, whilst those failing to safeguard the cleanliness of the watercourses from effluent or rotting matter could expect a hefty penalty of 40*s*.[10]

In 1352, royal letters patent authorized Norwich's bailiffs to force every able-bodied individual under sixty years of age to clean the city by removing dung and filth, and also to pave the streets in order to make future cleaning operations easier. The mandate was issued following a dramatic contraction in the size of the population during the Black Death, and in response to the community's apparent failure to raise a large enough workforce for this task under its own authority. In addition, the letters patent referred to the large number of work-shy inhabitants of the city – already the subject of the Ordinance of Labourers – who might be usefully put to work as part of a cleansing programme.[11] In February 1378, the actions of the ruling elite were again supported by a royal mandate which commissioned the bailiffs to improve the state of the river (then reportedly clogged with weeds) and to view and repair the city's defensive ditches, which were also filled with refuse and manure.[12] Whilst the civic authorities customarily oversaw standards in certain common areas at this time (for example the toll-house site, later occupied by the guildhall, and market were both cleansed on a regular basis under the supervision of a common sergeant), the city defences required more significant resources than could be found by the municipality acting alone.[13]

Nevertheless, shortly afterwards, existing systems of waste removal seem to have broken down. On 21 March 1380, the city assembly disciplined residents and private muck carriers who had heaped up waste ready for removal in the market and other areas but had failed

[10] *Letter-Books*, ed. Sharpe, A, 183, 212.

[11] *Calendar of the Patent Rolls Preserved in the Public Record Office, Edward III*, 16 vols. (London, 1891–1916), IX, 283–4.

[12] *Calendar of the Patent Rolls Preserved in the Public Record Office, Richard II, 1377–81*, 6 vols. (London, 1895–1909), I, 121. News of plague in the north of England at this time may have been the incentive for this move. The ditches which skirted the castle and the city's fortifications were again cleaned in 1385: Blomefield, *Norfolk*, III, 112. Norwich's sanitary measures from this date onwards are also considered in Jørgensen, 'All Good Rule', pp. 307–11, and Rawcliffe, *Urban Bodies*, pp. 217–22, and *passim*.

[13] *RCN*, II, 44, 53.

to arrange for its collection and carriage to suitable places for disposal. Civic officers attempted to coerce the inhabitants into remedying the problem using the powers acquired by royal mandate earlier in the century; an order went out giving them three months to clear up concentrations of waste wherever they were located. To ensure that the residents did not shirk their responsibilities, they were threatened with punitive fines if they did not comply. After the designated period had elapsed, the assembly envisaged, remiss householders would face an immediate penalty of 40*d.*, and the same sum would be extracted for each subsequent day that the waste was suffered to remain in situ. After the initial clean-up, residents would risk further, very stringent fines if any future collections were not removed from the streets within four days.[14]

Subsequently, following subsequent widespread plague epidemics, a parliamentary statute was proclaimed in Norwich and in all other English towns that codified the obligations of city dwellers with regard to the cleanliness of the water supply. The statute condemned the dumping in ditches, rivers or any other body of water of 'dung and other filth' – especially the 'issues and entrails' of butchered animals, but also other putrid substances. It reminded residents that such materials caused the air to become 'greatly corrupt[ed] and infect[ed]' with the result that inhabitants and visitors alike were on a daily basis falling ill with 'many maladies and other intolerable diseases'.[15] It further required the individuals responsible for 'annoying' (or damaging) rivers and watercourses to cleanse them again. The next set of surviving leet court records for Norwich reflect the statute's concerns. In 1391, a gardener was charged with blocking up the Great Cockey in the Westlegate area (modern Red Lion Street), presumably with organic matter. Complaints were also made against three dyers who

[14] Ibid., II, 84.

[15] *SR*, II, 59–60: 'Item pur ce qe tantz des fymes et autres ordures des issues et entrailles sibien des bestes tuez come des autres corruptions sont gettez et mys en fosses, ryvers et autres ewes et auxint plusours autres lieux dedeinz entour et pres diverses citees burgh et villes du roialme et les suburbes dicelles, qe laire illoeqes est grandment corrupt et enfect, et plusours maladies et autres diseases nient suffrables aveignent de jour en autre sibien a les inhabitantz et conversantz es dites citees burghs villes et suburbes come as autres illoeqes repairantz et passantz a tresgrant anusance damage et peril des inhabitantz conversantz repairantz et passantz susditz' (1388). Civic authorities were given the power to compel residents to remove any such matter with the threat of a very large fine (£20).

allowed industrial waste – ashes, pigments (*paste*) and clay (*fimus*) – to clog up waterways and contaminate highways, whilst one property owner, following work on his house, was reported for permitting a reeder to dump thatching material and other builder's waste in the river.[16] Meanwhile, Thomas, a barber from Conesford, was charged with frequently throwing into the highway putrid or tainted blood (*sanguis corruptus*), doubtless accumulated through his practice of phlebotomy.[17] Even more brazen in his actions was William Gerard, who was accused by residents of St Michael Coslany (Colegate) of dumping the body of a dead horse near the boundary of the parish churchyard. The rotting carcass not only caused nausea to passers-by, but, crucially, also the 'corruption' – that is, the unwholesome spoiling or contamination – of the locality.[18] Around this date or shortly thereafter, the jurors of Norwich, like their counterparts in the equivalent courts of London, probably had a fixed series of routine questions to put to witnesses concerning the accumulation of stagnant waste in the neighbourhood.[19]

At a time when outbreaks of epidemic disease occurred in East Anglia perhaps as often as once in each decade,[20] residents were inclined to vote with their feet in response to excessive levels of pollution. In the fourteenth century, for example, sections of the foreshore of the Wensum in the Westwick area of Norwich were reclaimed to form a costly domestic and industrial complex. Some of the wealthy residents of this quarter were dyers who – like their counterparts in the leet courts – pragmatically used the river to wash away by-products

16 *LJ*, ed. Hudson, pp. 70–1, 73, 75.

17 Ibid., p. 70. Another barber, Adam de Hindringham, resident in the Castle Fee, was presented in 1374–75 for 'foully encumbering' the highway with muck all year round, 'on account of which the said road is always deep and disgusting through its blockage': ibid., p. 68 ('unde dicta via semper est profunda et turpis in incumbracionem').

18 Ibid., p. 75. Gerard was fined 12*d*. for his infraction, which was reported in the following terms: 'Willelmus Gerard habuit unum equum per longum tempus iacentem in Regia via … in magnam abhominacionem et corrupcionem' ('William Gerard had a horse lying for a long time in the highway … causing great disgust and corruption'). On the disposal of horses in the castle ditches, see Shepherd Popescu, EAA 132, II, 1006.

19 John Carpenter, *Liber albus*, pp. 287–92; Rees Jones, 'Household, Work and the Problem of Mobile Labour', p. 135.

20 That is, in 1361, 1368–69 and possibly also in 1375, 1383 and 1391: Blomefield, *Norfolk*, III, 95–6, 113; Dunn, 'After the Black Death', pp. 38–9.

(map 7, site 159N).[21] Indeed, all along the city's river banks and water-courses, fullers (cloth processors), metal workers and tanners emptied waste into the Wensum.[22] Where the concentration of industries was fairly light on the foreshore, this seems not to have caused too many problems. However, the colonized area at Westwick was prone to flood. The richer inhabitants slowly abandoned the quarter; perhaps the combination of standing water and industrial effluent created a situation that seemed both dangerous and undesirable.[23]

The seriousness of the potential knock-on effects of excessive effluent in this city of 'running water and ponds'[24] ought not to be underestimated. Across the urban landscape, a large network of both natural and man-made water channels emptied into the Wensum (map 8). The whole drainage system was vulnerable to abuse, but the river became the focus of the most concerted remedial attention. A build-up of nitrogen in the water system caused by industrial waste and human cess led to it becoming clogged with vegetation.[25] The authorities responded by implementing repeated reed cutting operations from the late fourteenth century onwards. In 1366, for example, the civic assembly ordered that a levy should be raised in each of the four wards to fund improvements to the river.[26] In the following spring, the corporation paid John de Gnateshale (who was later returned as a member of parliament for Norwich) and William Staloun to supervise a cleansing programme. They were each paid 6*s.* 8*d.* per week.[27] Subsequently, the authorities bought in professional advice from further afield. The treasurer's account for 1398/99 records the expenses of one man who

21 Atkin and Evans, EAA 100, p. 133.

22 Rutledge, 'Economic Life', pp. 162 (map 9), 165. On riparian industry in North Conesford, see Ayers, EAA 37, pp. 154, 169; Atkin and Evans, EAA 100, pp. 9, 29.

23 Atkin and Evans, EAA 100, pp. 117, 133, 152. On industrial water pollution by the cloth industry as a perceived cause of plague in the later sixteenth century, see below, p. 190.

24 Rutledge, 'An Urban Environment', p. 83.

25 On the probable use of the river to dispose of rubbish and cess in North Conesford, see also Atkin and Evans, EAA 100, p. 44; Ayers, EAA 37, p. 157. The civic assembly's survey of 1503 indicated that several individuals illegally used the river as an outflow from domestic privies: see above, p. 133, n. 83.

26 *RCN*, I, 265. On reed cutting in 1479, see RCN, II, 102. On the frequency of reed cutting on an annual basis (as administered by the city's chamberlain in the 1530s), see NCR 18a/5 CA 1531–37, fols. 33v, 60r, 81v, 97r, 127v, 148v, and 18a/6 CA 1537–47, fols. 10r, 25r, 41r.

27 *RCN*, I, 267.

travelled from Bishop's (King's) Lynn, where relatively sophisticated water control measures were already in place, 'to examine the defects of the common river'.[28] His fee matched that paid to Gnateshale and Staloun, and he presumably acted in much the same capacity as they had done.[29] A further consultation took place in 1401/02 when a specialist from Colchester, one Blaumester, gave advice concerning the smooth operation of the new civic water mills, to be situated upstream.[30] His findings led the corporation to employ a group of labourers to work on clearing the river for a period of no fewer than thirty-five weeks. The costs incurred over the following few years were not insignificant. Over and above the wages of a supervisor for the labourers (of 16*d.* per week), the consultant himself was paid 20*s.* plus expenses, and the commonalty also purchased various scythes and sickles. A few years later, the civic treasurer purchased a cart, horses and harnesses for 'the community'.[31] The cart and cart horses (which were presumably used to remove material dredged from the Wensum, as well as from the streets) alone cost almost £14.[32]

Besides hiring workers, the civic executive again conscripted and taxed householders to assist in the removal of reeds and in dredging. In the summer of 1422 the corporation's assembly stipulated that everybody living adjacent to the river between Calke's mills and Thorpe (one-and-a- half miles downstream of the city defences) should contribute either money or labour to the value of 4*d.*, whenever it was demanded, to help the effort. The city authorities provided the necessary boats and other implements, and constables were installed in every ward to instruct the residents when the work should be carried

28 *RCN*, II, 52; Rawcliffe, *Urban Bodies*, pp. 181–3. At Lynn, a conduit had piped fresh water to the market since the mid-century. *The Making of King's Lynn: A Documentary Survey*, ed. D. M. Owen, Records of Social and Economic History, new series 9 (London, 1984), pp. 16, 214–15. See also V. Parker, *The Making of Kings Lynn: Secular Buildings from the 11th to the 17th Century*. King's Lynn Archaeological Survey 1 (London, 1971), pp. 26–7 (canals and ditches).

29 In the 1570s, the city was still paying two men to clear the river of weeds, but their wages had increased to £8 per annum each: 'River and Street Accounts', ed. Fay, e.g., p. 153 (Wygot).

30 *RCN*, II, 53–4.

31 *RCN*, II, 54–5. The animals were worked hard. The treasurer's expenses included payment for ninety-three horse shoes, twelve appointments with the farrier, and 6½*d.* for horse medicine.

32 *RCN*, II, 55. The sum was balanced by a receipt 'for carting' of £13 4*s.* 6*d.*, which was probably raised by taxing the population.

out.[33] From time to time, and perhaps in recognition of the burden such projects placed on the residents in straitened times, members of the ruling civic elite made donations at their death towards continuing work in the river. Thus the mayor, John Gilbert, gave the city a bequest of £50 to this purpose in the later fifteenth century, supplementing £10 left by the Conesford alderman Ralph Segryme in 1456;[34] a century later, Thomas Howard, 4th duke of Norfolk (who had a residence on the riverside), promised an annuity of 20*s*.[35]

The corporation also instituted new controls in order to diminish the risk of spillage and contamination. Great quantities of waste were apparently being removed from the city by barge, and were either dumped downstream of the city boundary at South Conesford, or spread on fields.[36] From the late fourteenth century, only one individual at a time was allowed to perform this role, and he had to swear an oath to the assembly that he would neither pollute the river nor (in order to maintained a chain of accountability) allow any other man to perform the task.[37] The citizen thus named and approved by the corporation was able to rent a 'common muck boat' from the city's main financial officer, the chamberlain.[38] The muck boat operator was licensed to take payments from householders to remove their waste. In remuneration for his initial outlay on the lease, he also received a rebate of 20*s*. if he agreed to take on responsibility for cleaning out on a regular basis a stream known as Holley's cockey (possibly the

33 *RCN*, I, 277–8.

34 *RCN*, II, 92; C. Rawcliffe, 'Sickness and Health', in *MN*, ed. Rawcliffe and Wilson, pp. 301–26 (pp. 312–13).

35 'River and Street Accounts', ed. Fay, p. 113. For the duke's residence, see above, map 4.

36 *RCN*, II, 91 (on the dumping of waste beyond the city boundary).

37 *RCN*, II, cxxix, 84, 85, 91. The scale of potential penalties for individuals infringing the new order indicates the seriousness with which the issue was viewed: individuals would face a fine of 20*s*. for their first offence, 40*s*. for their second and 60*s*. for a third. Citizens might also lose the liberty of the city or (if an incomer) be forced to leave.

38 By the 1530s, the rent due was 40*s*., rising to 42*s*. in the accounting year 1535/36 when a new muck boat was purchased: NCR 18a/5 CA 1531–37, e.g. fols. 8v, 141r, 150v.

Dalymond Dyke: see map 8).[39] The cost of repairs to the muck boat, meanwhile, was covered by the chamberlain.[40]

Yet another citywide levy for dredging and harvesting reeds was raised in 1517. The authorities ordered the collection of the impressive sum of £40 from the citizens to clean the river, whilst a further £12 was allocated to cover the purchase of a common tumbrel (a horse-drawn cart) and to pay the wages of a 'canelraker', a man permanently employed to clean the streets and carry away muck on a weekly basis.[41] In the summer of the following year, two more carts were purchased to continue the work. Each of the city's sub-wards was obliged to raise a fixed sum (which depended on the size of the district's population) to cover the cost. Meanwhile, householders were required to clear the street in front of their properties, piling up the waste ahead of a collection on a weekly basis (whilst ensuring that the heaps were laid away from the central gutter so that the waste was not washed into the drainage network).[42] The initiative was again underwritten with private funds. In 1518, for example, Elizabeth Thursby, a resident of St Andrew's parish, left a sum of £10 in her will, amongst an extraordinary list of other charitable gifts, to guarantee that the service could continue in her neighbourhood.[43] The long-term, citywide future of the scheme was secured by alderman Robert Jannys one year later. He gave three tenements situated near the market to the corporation, stipulating that the income from the rents should be ring-fenced for the collection and carting away of the 'filthye mater comyng of the makyng clene, foweng [feying: clearing] and swepyng of the ... stretes'.[44]

A further opportunity to reflect on the effectiveness of sanitation in the city came in 1531. At that time, a centralized and permanent royal commission of sewers was proposed in parliament to remedy 'the daily great damages and losses' to the commonwealth which arose

39 NCR 18a/5 CA 1531–37, e.g. fol. 29v. On John Holley, see Hawes, *Index to Norwich City Officers*, p. 84; *Landgable*, ed. Rodgers and Wallace, p. 112.

40 NCR 18a/5 CA 1531–37, fols. 61v, 63r, 131r, 150v. In 1566, a muck boat was described in a lease as a vessel with a freight of 2½ tons: NCR 22g/1 City Lease Book A, fol. 40v.

41 *RCN*, II, 109–10. Additionally, householders were prohibited from casting refuse from their houses into the streets. Later, cockey-cleaners were expected to pay for their own cart and horses: 'River and Street Accounts', ed. Fay, p. 176.

42 *RCN*, II, 110.

43 NRO, NCC will register Gylys, fol. 97r.

44 NCR 16d/2 Assembly Proceedings 1491–1553, fol. 102r.

from the 'misuse' and 'ill-maintenance' of ditches, streams and gutters, as well as bridges, causeways and other related structures throughout the land. Edward Rede, current mayor and MP for Norwich, may have heard a bill on the subject read in the Commons.[45] At any rate, not long after, the corporation commissioned Sir Nicholas Hare, gentleman, to execute a survey of the sewers (watercourses) within the bounds of Norwich.[46] Further cleansing programmes duly followed. In 1533/34, for example, the chamberlain paid an additional £9 5*s*. 8*d*. 'to and for the feyeng [clearing] of the rever' (about six per cent of his total expenditure for the year);[47] this was over and above his regular annual outlay of £2 or £3 on reed cutting activities.[48]

The corporation's efforts to keep water flowing in the city had a particular and very visible impact on the infrastructure. Repeated attempts to improve and control drainage meant that the cockeys – many of which were natural streams that originally meandered along their own route to the river – became increasingly constrained or fossilized in the city landscape. The Great Cockey, for example, was in places lined with stone, brick, tile and timber, which made it easier to clean. One section at Cuttlerrow (map 8) was fenced off to protect it from passing traffic.[49] Earlier, a section of this stream to the south had been redirected and then culverted to a more convenient course, along the back of property developments.[50] Parts of other cockeys were also paved over, to prevent waste from washing in, or paved alongside, to stop the ground adjacent to them from becoming churned up.[51] Access to water was also in places limited by gates and locked doors to discourage residents from dumping waste; for example, sections of the cockeys in the parish of St Edmund (either the Spital or Dalymond dykes) and at the Blackfriars' were protected in this way.[52] Grates

[45] Elton, *Reform and Renewal*, pp. 121–2.
[46] NCR 18a/5 CA 1531–37, fol. 11r.
[47] Ibid., fol. 83v.
[48] Ibid., *passim*.
[49] Ibid., fols. 58v–59r, 100v; NCR 18a/6 CA 1537–47, fol. 9v; on the Great Cockey, see Kirkpatrick, *Streets and Lanes*, pp. 43–4.
[50] Shepherd Popescu, EAA 132, II, 548.
[51] NCR 18a/5 CA 1531–37, fols. 81r (St Lawrence's), 98v (Whitefriars', by Bettes', Conesford), 144r (Salters').
[52] NCR 18a/6 CA 1537–47, fol. 60r (St Edmund's, where the gate weighed sixteen pounds, and was almost certainly made of iron); 'River and Street Accounts', ed. Fay, p. 175 (Blackfriars').

positioned inside the cockeys also preserved the free flow of water by helping to trap refuse and organic matter.[53]

As part of the careful auditing process which governed all civic expenditure, the financial officers of sixteenth-century Norwich chose to keep detailed records of their city cleaning activities. They enable us to ascertain – to the cartload – exactly how much waste was removed from the city's watercourses, and how this process was organized. In the 1530s, up to eight named labourers at one time were responsible for clearing or 'keeping' the various cockeys throughout the year. Each man was paid for the volume of material he dug out, which he would heap up ready for removal by a different contractor.[54] By the 1570s, this body of labourers had been replaced by a single cockey-cleaner who was paid a salary of about £8 per year; and, at this stage, the cockey-cleaner was also responsible for safely disposing of the waste he gathered up.[55] The watercourses receiving most attention were those in the core, built-up, central areas, whilst other, more peripheral waterways were overhauled less regularly. For example, owing to its central location, the Cuttlerrow portion of the Great Cockey both required and received particular oversight. The chamberlains' accounts for just one year – 1534 to 1535 – record that fourteen cartloads of muck were taken out of it on four different occasions. In comparison, areas downstream produced minimal quantities of refuse. In spite of the fact that St Crouch's cockey was the last stretch of the Great Cockey on the corporation's land before it reached the river, it generated only two loads of material in the same period.[56] The system of filtering and clearing waste out of the cockeys before it reached the river seems to have worked. The same individuals were also responsible for routinely cleansing the city's cisterns, which had a range of uses (see map

[53] See, for example, the grate and paving at the cockey next to a dwelling owned by a dyer named Bettes, which was renovated in 1534–35: NCR 18a/5 CA 1531–37, fol. 98v; see also ibid., fol. 29r, 80r–v, 97v, 132r, 144r; 18a/6 CA 1537–47, fol. 9r. A similar system existed in the late thirteenth century in London along the Walbrook: Keene, 'Issues of Water', p. 168.

[54] NCR 18a/5 CA 1531–37, fols. 29r–v, 59r–v, 80r, 97v, 124v, 143v–144r; 18a/6 CA 1537–47, fols. 9r–v, 22r–v, 41r.

[55] 'River and Street Accounts', ed. Fay, pp. 153 (Johnson), 174, 176 (Ebbottes).

[56] NCR 18a/5 CA 1531–37, fols. 97v–98v. Compare also the forty loads extracted from the upstream section of the Great Cockey in the parish of St Stephen known as Salter's cockey, in the same period: ibid. On the identity of Salter's cockey, see ibid., fol. 10r.

8):[57] some acted as filters for the river or cockey water passing through them; others were storage tanks; and some were cesspits.[58] Several of the city's staithes, quays and bridges each also had their own cistern. In total, six were regularly cleaned out by the city authorities, and all produced large amounts of muck which yet again had to be removed at no small cost to the civic treasury.[59] Routine maintenance also had to be budgeted for. In 1546/47, the stone-built cistern in the parish of St Swithin, Westwick, needed extensive repair work. The renovations, which also involved cutting out silt and debris from the river, led to such a large quantity of material being excavated that the resulting spoil heaps impeded traffic. A mason called John Erne was paid to repair the cistern and to stop up certain 'jakes' (latrines) that had hitherto emptied into it.[60]

Profits and waste in Norwich from 1530

The civic authorities had compelling incentives to continue to reform and systematize the mechanisms for waste removal. In the polemical humanist literature of the second quarter of the sixteenth century, deteriorating cityscapes were submitted as evidence of serious deficiencies in the prevailing moral and political order. For example, the Oxford humanist Thomas Starkey (d. 1538), benefiting from his early academic studies with Thomas Linacre (founder of London's college of physicians) and inspired by his experiences in Padua, argued that a lack of beauty in a town – manifest in begging people, wasted grounds

[57] They were located at St Benedict's (i.e. Westwick) gate, in the parish of St Swithin, by the New Mills, at the Blackfriars, at Fyebridge quay, and in the parish of St Martin at Palace. See NCR 18a/5 CA 1531–37, e.g. fols. 10r, 27r–v, 29v–30r, 59r–v, 80r–81r, 97v, 125r, 126v, 144v; 18a/6 CA 1537–47, fols. 9v, 22r–v, 47r.

[58] Pelling, 'Health and Sanitation to 1750', pp. 130–1. For a possible, archaeologically excavated example of a cistern, see J. G. Hurst and J. Golson, 'Excavations at St Benedict's Gates, Norwich, 1951 and 1953', *NA* 31 (1957), 1–112 (p. 47), and (in comparison) on a small barrel cistern for water storage, see Ayers, EAA 37, pp. 51–3.

[59] As an example of the frequency of such operations, the cistern at the church of St Martin at Palace was cleaned six times during the 1530s: NCR 18a/5 CA 1531–37, fols. 30r, 59r–v, 97v, 125r; 18a/6 CA 1537–47, fols. 9r, 47r. The capacity of the cistern at St Benedict's gates, meanwhile, was substantial: in 1544–45, over one hundred loads of 'muck' were extracted from it: NCR 18a/7 CA 1541–49, fol. 161v.

[60] NCR 18a/7 CA 1541–49, fol. 271r.

and empty or ruined houses – indicated a failure in policy and in governance.[61] To guard against such situations, he suggested that each large city or town should appoint special officers who would be responsible for maintaining the physical appearance and cleanliness of the locality. These guardians would, he hoped, 'cause grete helth' and ensure that 'the prestylens [pestilence]' would not be so prevalent in future.[62] The magistrates of Norwich did not then read Starkey's work (it remained unpublished at the time of his death). But in practice they identified the same perceived set of problems; and they viewed themselves as guardians of beauty, order and health in their city.

In the mid-1530s the eyes of the authorities in Norwich were urgently drawn to a particular set of run-down plots scattered throughout the domestic and commercial properties in central areas. They complained that not only had many of the properties damaged in the devastating fire in 1507 still not been rebuilt – lying instead 'as desolate and vacant groundes' – but (more dangerously) unscrupulous people were using these places to dump noxious waste. Several vacant plots, 'nighe adjoyninge to the highe stretes', were apparently 'replenished with moche unclennes and filthe', causing great harm to the inhabitants and passers-by.[63] In 1534, in collaboration with the governors of Lynn, the corporation of Norwich petitioned for an act of parliament to enable it to compel citizens to renovate void ground and fire-damaged houses on pain of forfeiture.[64] This was more than empty rhetoric used to justify a land grab.[65] A few months before the bill for acquiring burnt-out plots was considered in parliament, the civic assembly – acting under the guidance of alderman Augustine Steward – passed a local ordinance which forbade the dumping of 'vile things' on 'brent [burnt-out] grounde', in the castle's defensive

[61] Thomas Starkey, *A Dialogue Between Pole and Lupset*, ed. T. F. Mayer, Camden Society fourth series 37 (London, 1989), pp. 48–9, 58–9, 117–19.

[62] Ibid., p. 117.

[63] 'An acte for reedifieng of voyde groundes in the citie of Norwich', 26 Henry VIII c.8, in *SR*, III, 504–5. On this, see R. Tittler, 'For the "Re-edification of Townes": The Rebuilding Statutes of Henry VIII', *Albion* 22 (1990), 591–605.

[64] On Lynn, see 'An acte for the reedifienge of voyde groundes within the towne of Lynne', 26 Henry VIII c.9, in *SR*, III, 505–6.

[65] The ordinance suggests that the muck identified in the parliamentary statute existed as a real substance, not simply as a calculated rhetorical flourish. This is notwithstanding the fact that allegations concerning accumulations of 'dung and filth' had been used in the fifteenth century as a means to justify enclosures of public thoroughfares: Rutledge, 'An Urban Environment', p. 83.

ditches or in Cockey Lane (map 9, inset i), on pain of a respectably sized fine of 2*s*. and referral to the justices of the peace for further punishment.[66]

When the bill had passed into law, the Norwich authorities had a structured and publicly accountable schedule for reform.[67] The legislation gave the owners of vacant lands or dilapidated tenements a period of two years in which either to rebuild, or to enclose the boundary of the plot 'with walls of mortar and stone'. If they failed to meet this obligation, the corporation was free to seize the property for its own use without incurring any fees or charges. The mayor or his agents then had a further two-year period in which to make improvements, at which point the land (if it remained unimproved) would revert back to its first owner.[68] The provisions of the act were proclaimed on thirteen Norwich properties in January 1535/36, and the two-year period allowed for redeveloping and/or enclosing was begun. Several vacant sites situated around Tombland, as well as in central areas close to the market – namely, in Cuttlerrow (modern London Street) and Sporrerrow (modern White Lion Street) – were duly seized (map 9, insets ii and iii).[69] The following summer, a number of MPs from other

[66] NCR 16d/2 Assembly Proceedings 1491–1553, fol. 156v (4 September 1534). The ordinance referred to 'caulder muck'. 'Colder' in contemporary documents can refer to stone rubble or chippings (and, indeed, Norwich labourers were paid for 'coldryng' or breaking up stone to make a surface for metalling roads: NCR 18a/7 CA 1541–49, fols. 167r–9r), but in Norfolk and Suffolk dialect, colder or caulder also signifies things that are worthless, including rubbish or chaff: *Middle English Dictionary*, ed. H. Kurath and S. M. Kuhn (Ann Arbor, 1952–2001), C, 385. Given the association here with 'vile' things and 'muck', it seems likely that senses relating to rubbish or (putrid/noxious) waste were intended. See also Dyer, *Decline and Growth*, p. 36, on the visibility of waste as the issue of concern.

[67] On previous acrimonious litigation between members of the elite and the commonalty, and the suspicion that property owners were exploiting renovation plans for their own advantage (which may have compelled the move to secure endorsement from parliament), see Wood, 'Kett's Rebellion', pp. 292–3, 407 n. 28 (on TNA, STAC 2/2/225–7).

[68] To safeguard against setting an unfortunate precedent which excluded other interested parties, parliament annexed a schedule to the act requiring that unrenovated land should not, in fact, pass immediately to the corporation, but firstly to the lord of the fee (the feudal lord from whom the land was held). Only if the latter also failed to 're-edify' the ground within a year could the city lay its claim: *SR*, III, 505.

[69] *RCN*, II, 167. Plots in the parishes of St Giles's and St Gregory's were also taken into the commonalty's hands. In April 1537, the chamberlains were authorized

English towns and cities followed the lead set by Norwich and Lynn, and petitioned for similar rights over the great number of vacant plots in their localities.[70]

A few members of the governing elite benefited personally from these developments. Alderman Augustine Steward, for example, used the momentum generated by the 1536 seizures to drive through a scheme to acquire land for himself. Steward had good reason to be familiar with the recent proceedings; he was the city's auditor at the drawing up of the initial petition in 1534. His kinsmen, Reginald Lytleprowe and Edward Rede, presented it to parliament, and by the time of its ratification, Steward had been elected mayor.[71] Using language that echoed both the civic ordinance and the act of parliament, he persuaded the corporation to part with a handful of 'void' plots in Tombland at knock-down prices, arguing that many people had 'soore accombred and replenysshed' the empty dwellings 'with muk and such other vile mater to the grette noysaunce of all the Kynges liege people passing by the same'.[72] The corporation agreed to his terms and Steward secured the second plot for the nominal fee of 4*d.* in yearly assize rent.[73] Other leading citizens followed suit. Robert Ferrour, alderman of East Wymer and erstwhile mayor, and Thomas Bathcom, a former councillor for Mancroft, acquired Tombland wastes through the same mechanism. The rents that they paid to the city in return for their gains were tiny. Bathcom, for instance, paid just 20*d.* per annum for each of his four tenements, despite the fact that they had been previously leased for 20*s.*; Ferrour, meanwhile, paid only 2*d.*[74]

to take possession of any of these properties that were still suffering from neglect: *RCN*, II, 122.

70 'An acte for reedyfyeng diverse towns in the realm', 27 Henry VIII, c.1, *SR*, III, 531–2. See also: 'An acte concerning decay of houses and inclosures', 27 Henry VIII, c.22, *SR*, III, 553–4; 'An acte concernyng the assuraunce of a voyde plotte ... in Chepe in London', 27 Henry VIII, c.49, *SR*, III, 619–20; 'For reedifieng of towns', 32 Henry VIII, c.18, *SR*, III, 768; 'For reedification of townes westward', 32 Henry VIII, c.19, *SR*, III, 769.

71 *House of Commons*, ed. Bindoff, I, 152 and III, 185, 383; Hawes, *Index to Norwich City Officers, passim.*

72 *RCN*, II, 122.

73 *RCN*, II, 123. Assize rent was a fixed, annual sum levied by the chamberlain for encroachments onto vacant ground: Rutledge, 'Introduction', in *Landgable*, ed. Rodgers and Wallace, p. 12.

74 *RCN*, II, 123.

The aldermen were clearly making opportunistic acquisitions. The legal instrument gained through parliament did not suffice to eliminate the problem of empty grounds in Norwich. For example, during the late 1560s and early 1570s, vacant properties were still in existence by Tombland, where Steward had expanded his property portfolio.[75] Nonetheless, the aldermen named above do appear to have honoured their agreements with the city to rebuild. In a survey of 1568–70, none of the plots recorded as being previously in the hands of these men or their successors were described as 'void',[76] and Steward had passed on the new buildings he commissioned to his heirs.[77] In the next chapter, we will see how the city corporation tried to stimulate rebuilding and the value it attached (in terms of salubriousness) to quality architecture. For the time being it is enough to note the avowed motives of the aldermanic elite. Their concerns about filth and the threat of disease were clearly pitched at the right register; combating a threat to health was accepted as a compelling justification for their actions.

The reforms may, however, have had a secondary – and unintentionally deleterious – impact on the landscape. With certain ad hoc dumping grounds cordoned off or redeveloped, the question of where to put waste safely remained open. A few years after Steward issued his ordinance to prevent the dumping of 'muck' on burnt-out Norwich plots, the authorities were struggling to organize the removal of significant quantities from various central and outlying locations. A sense of the scale of the problem can be readily ascertained, as the city officers again opted to quantify the amounts of muck involved: in 1541/42, sixteen or seventeen cartloads were removed from a heap in the street near the Three Bells inn 'whyche hade lyen ther 2 or 3 years byfore'; similar amounts were also taken from and around the market.[78] The situation seems to have been aggravated by serious rain storms which blocked drainage systems.[79] In the following year, a deposit of fifteen loads was hampering ingress at St Benedict's (Westwick) gate. This accumulation had reportedly also 'lyen of long tyme' under the walls.[80] Reports made in the leet courts in late spring 1541

[75] *Landgable*, ed. Rodgers and Wallace, p. 98. These were, however, probably enclosed.

[76] Ibid., pp. 97–100.

[77] On rebuilding by Steward, see NCR 18a/6 CA 1537–47, fol. 205v.

[78] NCR 18a/7 CA 1541–49, fol. 20r.

[79] Ibid., fols. [19br], 20r.

[80] Ibid., fol. 59r; 'River and Street Accounts', ed. Fay, p. 108.

highlight a range of related problems: nineteen individuals were denounced for keeping noxious drains and for allowing 'corrupt' water to issue thence into the streets; two others for damaging the river with muck. A haulier named Keteringham (who was often employed by the city to remove cockey-waste) was reported for leaving a further sixteen cartloads of muck in the high street, whilst two individuals were presented for not cleansing cisterns on their land.[81] The remedies instituted by the city included a redoubled cleansing effort, alongside modifications and repairs to the infrastructure of the cockeys: paving, linings, frames, grates, fencing and arches were installed; gullies and breaches stopped up.[82]

As part of a related effort to address sanitary standards, the city government set about improving conditions in the highways and streets (not least because well-maintained street surfaces were easier to clean and thus less waste was in danger of washing into gutters and watercourses).[83] Under fifteenth-century orders and by-laws, Norwich residents were required to remove refuse from the streets bordering their property on a regular basis, and to resurface them as often as was needed.[84] The city fathers took active steps to ease the financial burden on those who were least able to pay. For example, in 1542/43, they covered the costs of paving around the house of an impoverished woman, one Hemmyng, living in the vicinity of the old Augustinian Friary. The outlay for this charitable act and for other paved surfaces was offset by the sale of the bells from the church of St Faith (St Vedast), which was organized by the North Conesford alderman Thomas Codd.[85] Occasionally, payments were also made from the city's hamper (a fund of civic profits administered by the mayor and senior civic officials) to subsidize improvements, such as those made to the paving around the White Horse inn in 1548.[86]

During the 1530s and 1540s, the Norwich city government directly funded two further, major campaigns to ameliorate the quality of

[81] NCR 5d/1 Sheriffs' Tourn, May 1541, Wymer. On Keteringham, see NCR 18a/5 CA 1531–37, fol. 98r and *passim*.

[82] NCR 18a/7 CA 1541–49, fols. 19v–[19bv].

[83] On this concern, see NCR 16d/2 Assembly Proceedings 1491–1553, fol. 102.

[84] *RCN*, II, 96–8; on the wider context, see D. Jørgensen, 'Cooperative Sanitation: Managing Streets and Gutters in Late Medieval England and Scandinavia', *Technology and Culture* 49 (2008), 547–67 (pp. 551–7).

[85] NCR 18a/7 CA 1541–49, fol. 64r.

[86] NCR 16a/5 Mayor's Court Book 1540–49, p. 530.

paving on property owned by the corporation itself. In the accounting year 1531/32, for example, the city's chamberlain paid for the resurfacing of public areas in Fyebridge in the north of the city, at the market at the centre and at the entry to Ber Street gate to the south. Both stone and gravel were laid.[87] A few years later, during the dissolution of the religious houses, quantities of stone and tile were purchased by the chamberlains from the dismantled Greyfriars and from the Blackfriars (which was being redeveloped as a civic venue).[88] Between 1542 and 1545, this material was used to lay new surfaces in various locations across the city which received the heaviest footfall or traffic. Such areas included the perimeter of the church of St Peter Mancroft; around certain of the city's tenements; in those parts of the market left out in earlier campaigns (including Cobblerrow); at the watering spot for horses at Heigham ('Hells') gate (an especially important precaution owing to the mixture of heavily churned mud and manure which might otherwise accumulate); at the New Mills (where the movement of carts posed similar problems); at St Stephen's gate; in Tombland; and in streets around the former Augustinian friary and Blackfriars' hall.[89] Meanwhile, the corporation honoured its own responsibilities as a property owner and landlord, especially when during the city's economic recession in the 1540s, it was unable to find tenants for a number of its rental holdings. To ensure the maintenance of appearances, the chamberlains paid for the areas surrounding certain unoccupied, city-owned tenements to be swept.[90]

Wealthy individuals petitioned for, and helped to pay for, similar initiatives. In 1534/35, a group of parishioners undertook to lay a paved surface at St Augustine's gate (members of the group raised enough between them to purchase fifty 'thak [i.e. brick] tyles'). A more substantial campaign was implemented by Augustine Steward at

[87] NCR 18a/5 CA 1531–37, fol. 63r.

[88] NCR 18a/6 CA 1537–47, fols. 109v–10r; 16a/5 Mayor's Court Book 1540–49, p. 553. Norfolk having no natural supplies of stone except flint, the opportunity to acquire a substantial amount of new material was too good to miss. On the acquisition of the Blackfriars' (in which alderman Steward played a key role), see *House of Commons*, ed. Bindoff, III, 384.

[89] NCR 18a/7 CA 1541–49, fols. 60v–4r (1542–43), 110r–11v (1543–44), 162r–3r (1544–45): substantial improvements were also made in the parish of St John Timberhill, at Swinemarket Hill, by the castle ditches, to plots and a watering place in St Martin at Oak, and at the Common Inn.

[90] NCR 18a/7 CA 1541–49, fol. 60r.

Tombland in 1535/36, which cost over £5 to accomplish.[91] Assistance was similarly provided by Sir John Godsalve, the king's lieutenant at the castle, who in September 1548 offered to donate stone and sand to the poor people whose houses adjoined the streets around the castle ditches so that they could meet their obligations with regard to street resurfacing. He used this gesture as a form of leverage with the then mayor – Edmund Wood – as well as with Augustine Steward and other aldermen to tackle a related problem. Certain people were again dumping 'donge' and 'fylthe' into the broad defensive ditches surrounding the castle.[92] Godsalve's bid to enhance the appearance and thus the dignity of this royal institution was not immediately realized (in the event, Kett's rebellion derailed medium-term efforts to improve the situation), but in late May 1551 the mayor and aldermen paid for the removal of 114 loads of 'muck' from the ditches (map 9).[93]

Both manpower and additional resources were needed to maintain hard-won standards. In a will proved in 1548, the alderman and mayor Edmund Wood left a total of £66 13*s*. 4*d*. (100 marks) which, he hoped, would contribute in perpetuity towards 'the provision of a commen carte to be mayntened for ever within the citie of Norwiche to carry away the filthe of the streates'. The bequest came with a supplement of £20 for dredging the river.[94] Wood's generous gifts were in fact used to fund a new system of city cleaning; in the same year that Caius published his tract on the perils of poor sanitation, the civic assembly complained that, due to lack of money and other provisions, and despite 'dyvers good and godly actes and ordynaunces ... [the] streetes remayne fowle and fylthye and also the ... ryver decayethe and fyllethe moore and moore'.[95] As a remedy, it established a body of twelve river and streets 'surveyors' who were given specific authority to ensure the free flow of water and enforce higher standards of cleanliness in public

91 NCR 18a/5 CA 1531–37, fols. 91v, 132v.
92 NCR 16a/5 Mayor's Court Book 1540–49, p. 514; Shepherd Popescu, EAA 132, II, 544–5. In fact, the residents of Norwich had dumped waste in this location from time to time since the mid-twelfth century: Shepherd Popescu, EAA 132, I, 457, 539. For waste dumping here in 1534, see above, p. 153–4.
93 NCR 18d Clavor's Book 1 [Hamper] 1550–1601, fol. 53r.
94 London, The National Archives, PROB 11/32/288, Will of Edmund Wood, Alderman of Norwich, Norfolk (1548), fol. 145v.
95 *RCN*, II, 127.

areas of the city.[96] The status with which the committee was invested is apparent from its expensive new account book purchased at the end of 1556 (fig. 17).[97] In it, as well as the accounts themselves, the names of the officers appointed were recorded, along with their particular duties.[98] Of this number, two were nominated for each of the four wards: one to survey and report on the defects of the cockeys and streets, and one to collect quarterly levies from the wealthier citizens. Additionally, a surveyor oversaw the work of 'watermen' who were responsible for cutting and cleansing the river. The primary duty of the latter was to maintain discipline amongst the workmen and to ensure that they did not 'tract time' (or take longer than necessary), but he also identified which parts of the river were in greatest need of attention.[99] The first entries in the account book record the receipt of £14 8*s*. 9*d*. from the collectors in the wards.[100] This was enough to pay the wages of the men who cleared and disposed of muck, reeds and other waste, whilst securing a considerable reserve fund for future activities or emergencies.[101] The surveyors also received a substantial annuity of £14 direct from the chamberlain, most of which was money ring-fenced from the city's income from the rent of the civic water-powered corn mills (the New Mills).[102] The subsequent expansion of the surveyors' activities can be determined by a simple rule of thumb: in the 1530s, the average routine expenditure on the river and cockeys combined (under the auspices of the chamberlain) cost about £6 to £8 per annum. By the time of the new account book, the figure was averaging about £30 per annum, rising closer to £40 per annum in 1570 (a rate of increase that outstripped even the exponential rise in inflation during the 1540s, and steadier price increases thereafter).[103]

96 The structure, authority and income of the committee are outlined in *RCN*, II, 127–31.

97 The folio-sized volume itself cost 18*d*.: 'River and Street Accounts', ed. Fay, p. 126.

98 The committee was comprised mainly of members of the city's common council, led by two aldermen.

99 'River and Street Accounts', ed. Fay, p. 123.

100 Ibid., pp. 124–6.

101 On the levies, including a surviving assessment for 1561, see 'River and Street Accounts', ed. Fay, p. 114.

102 Ibid., p. 113.

103 NCR 18a/5 CA 1531–37, fols. 10r, 31r, 34r, 59v, 60v, 81r–v, 97r, 98v, 125r, 127v, 145r, 148v; NCR 18a/6 CA 1537–47, fols. 9v, 10r, 22r, 25v; 'River and Street Accounts', ed. Fay, pp. 129, 136, 143, 147, 151, 156, 164, 168. For a guide to inflation, see S. Rappaport, *Worlds Within Worlds: Structures of Life in Sixteenth-Century*

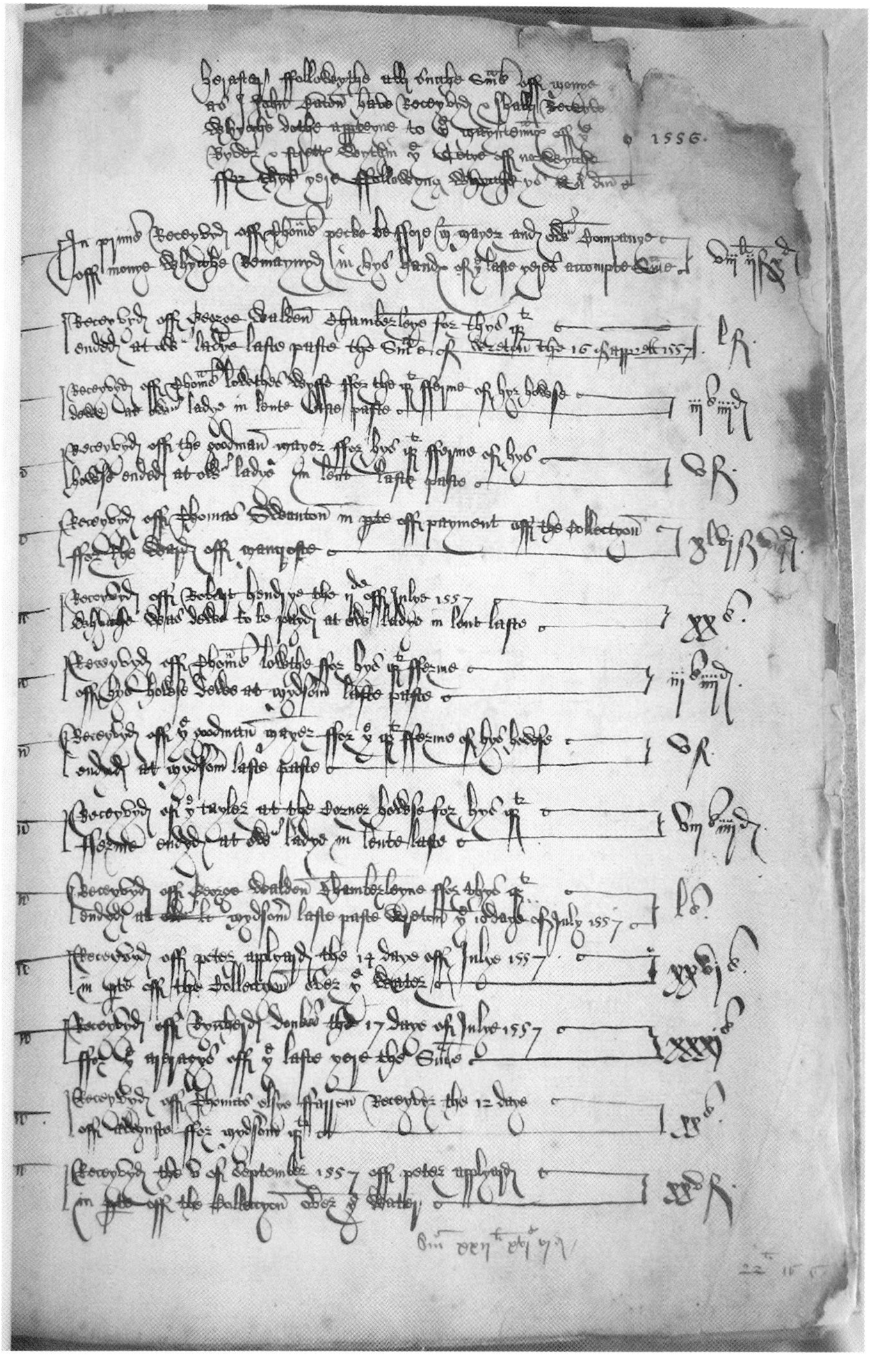

Figure 17: Account book of the Norwich river and streets surveyors, 1557.

At the same time, the corporation looked for ways to transfer onerous financial commitments back to the citizens. Requirements relating to sanitation and drainage were therefore sometimes written into corporation leases. For example, in 1552, the tenant of one particular property (a piece of riverside ground) was required to construct an underground drain leading from the street to the river, and to keep the drain clear of 'fylth, rubbysshe [and] cowlder', as well as regularly to cleanse and maintain the street in front of the property boundary.[104] In the 1560s, the mayor and aldermen similarly placed an additional responsibility on the lessee of the muck boat to effect repairs to a dilapidated cistern adjacent to the old common staithe in Conesford (map 8).[105] (This plot came as part of the lease, and was, therefore, probably used to store muck ahead of it being loaded and removed by boat.) But the corporation was careful that the arrangement should prove both sustainable and realistic; the stone required for the repairs was to

London (Cambridge, 1989), p. 155. The committee's very visible annual activities for clearing and maintaining the watercourses at times may have seemed to suggest that greater responsibility belonged to corporate rather than private agents in the battle to improve hygienic standards. One group of hopeful seventeenth-century residents appears to have been under the impression that the corporation's responsibility for the state of drainage extended to repairing cockeys that ran under private houses and grounds. A legal query was raised to determine the question, but the position of the corporation remained unambiguous, as the following transcript demonstrates: 'Case: The corporation of Norwich have from time to time made divers laws, orders and constitutions about clearing the river and emptying the cysterns and cockeys and to oblige the inhabitants to sweep the streets and carry away the dirt as often as needfull which would otherwise be carryed on any sudden shower into the common river. The corporation at their own expence have repaired and cleansed the cockeys, traps and cysterns and so much of the common shores or sewers as run through the streets and publick places within the said city but never repaired or cleaned the common shores or sewers running under the houses or grounds of private owners.' The text went on to explain that a common sewer running between the cockey in St Andrew's and the river under the houses and tenements of John Custance, mayor, and others, was blocked, and caused the properties to become flooded during heavy rainfall. The question remained as to how the householders (who, significantly, included the city's leading official) might be compelled to effect repairs at their own expense. NCR 10f Liability of Householder to Repair Common Sewers [1726 or 1750].

104 NCR 22g/1 City Lease Book A 1537–1664, fol. 61r.

105 The area around the staithe had apparently been seriously polluted: see below, p. 172.

be supplied by the chamberlain, who also retained responsibility for cleaning out the cistern.[106]

Unfortunately for their neighbours, individual aldermen were not always as diligent as they might have been in maintaining standards in their own properties and the adjacent streets. Any oversight was liable to upset residents who might legitimately complain (in light of the manoeuvres of Augustine Steward and others) that expensive refurbishment campaigns seemed mostly to benefit wealthy property owners. Perhaps, therefore, it was with some relish that the community presented to the leet courts two senior aldermen for failing in their duties. William Rogers, it was reported in late February 1550/51, had failed to repair the pavement in front of one of his tenements (an offence all the more aggravating owing to the suggestion that Rogers was in this respect at least a negligent landlord).[107] He was required to pay an on the spot fine of 3*s*. 4*d*., and would have had to find a further 20*s*. had he allowed the problem to persist to midsummer.[108] Master Myngey was similarly reprimanded in the autumn of 1554 by the residents of Conesford and Ber Street for 'not sufficiently repayre[ing] the strete' for which he was responsible. Myngey's fine was 2*s*.[109] Individual civic officers were also vociferously criticized for failing to address certain health risks. Thus in 1551, the chamberlains were reported by residents at the sheriffs' Lenten leet court for damaging the 'King's highway at the cokkeye within the precinct of [the parish of St Gregory] to the great nuisance of the people and lieges of the lord King, that is to say, at the cockeyes in the parishes of Saints Gregory, Lawrence and Seynte Croyse [St Crouch]',[110] and 'for not lokyng to the corrupt lane callyd saynt Bartylmewes Lane [in the sub-leet of Ber Street]'.[111] The

[106] NCR 22g/1 City Lease Book A 1537–1664, fol. 40r (1566).

[107] Roger's wife, Katherine, later made a bequest to the river and street surveyors for improvements in the river (1556): 'River and Street Accounts', ed. Fay, p. 113.

[108] NCR 5c/3 Leet, 26 February 1550/1 [ward not legible].

[109] NCR 5d/5, Sheriffs' Tourn, October 1554, Conesford, Ber Street and Trowse.

[110] 'Et quod camerarii predicti nocent regiam viam apud le cokkeye infra presinctum huius lete ad graunde nocumentum populi et leges [i.e. *lieges*] domini regis, videlicet, apud lez cockeyes in parochiis sanctorum Gregorii, Laurentii et Seynte Croyse': NCR 5c/3 Leet, 26 February 1550/51, St Gregory, reproduced in *RCN*, I, 386–7 (English translation); *LJ*, ed. Hudson, p. 86 (Latin transcription).

[111] NCR 5c/3 Leet, March 1550/51, Ber Street; *RCN*, I, 387; *LJ*, ed. Hudson, p. 88. The chamberlains were also presented for several other offences, including: laying muck outside Westwick gates and at the cockey in the parish of St

chamberlains were fined 4*s.* and 5*s.* respectively on these occasions. In 1569, mayor Nicholas Norgate (whom we met in chapter 1 as the author of a recipe to cure colic), left in his will a plot of land outside Magdalen gate for the commonalty to use as a public muck-heap.[112] Perhaps his gift was intended as much to salvage the reputation of his fellow brethren, as for its obvious sanitary benefits. Ordinary householders were not, however, exempt from censure either; in October 1554, following outbreaks of epidemic disease in the city, several individuals were reported to the authorities in the ward Over-the-Water for 'castyng owt … thir fylthy and corrupt washe [liquid refuse] into the stretes into the infeccion of the Kyng and Quenes lege people'.[113]

The duties of the residents of all classes were reiterated in no uncertain terms in a civic by-law passed on 21 September 1559 some months after the publication of Cuningham's *Cosmographical Glasse.* The by-law required every owner of a house or grounds adjoining a paved public street to repair or resurface that street in stone within a period of three months, or risk a punitive fine. As a direct response to a devastating outbreak of infectious fever during the previous year, the by-law stressed the sanitary benefits of easy-to-clean streets.[114] The ordinance lamented that standards had lapsed recently, as residents had become increasingly lax in discharging their duties to pave and clean:

Swithin (NCR 5d/1 Sheriffs' Tourn, May 1541, Wymer, see map 8); for failing to keep two cockeys clean near the houses of Nicholas Manne and Thomas Elys, respectively, so that they became 'noysom aswell to the Kynges leage peple as also to the Kynges ryver' (NCR 5c/3 Leet, 26 February 1550/51 [ward not legible]); for not making clean the cockey in St Swithin's and that 'withowt Seint Benettes [Benedict's] gattes' (NCR 5c/3 Leet, April 1551, Wymer); for problems at the cockey at the New Mills, for 'annoying' an (unnamed) stream, for failing to refurbish the head of 'the drayne att whight fryers brygge', and for 'the comen drayne of the systerne att the comen stathe' (NCR 5d/4 Sheriffs' Tourn, no date [1550x51], Conesford); and for a corrupt cockey in an unknown location (NCR 5c/3 Leet, 1550x51, East Wymer). Notably, in early July 1550, the civic assembly had passed a general order for the 'reformation of gutters' (or 'water drains') which required the breaking up of noisome cases: NCR 16d/2 Assembly Proceedings 1491–1553, fol. 218r.

112 The National Archives, PROB 11/51/41, Will of Nicholas Norgate, Alderman of Norwich, Norfolk (3 Feb 1569), fol. 39a. On Norgate's recipe, see above, p. 53.

113 NCR 5d/5, Sheriffs' Tourn, October 1554, Beyond the Water.

114 *RCN*, II, 133–4. For national legislation in a similar period on the same topic, see the following statutes for highways: *SR*, IV.1, 284–5 (2&3 Philip and Mary c.8, 1555); 441–3 (5 Elizabeth I c.13, 1562–63); 620–1 (18 Elizabeth I c.10, 1575–76).

> Whereas tyme oute of mynde there hathe bene a comely and decent order used within this cittye for the pavyng of the stretes ... whiche thing hath not only bene a great ease and helthefull commodyte to the inhabitauntes ... but also a goodly bewtefying, and an occasyon that dyverse havyng accesse to the same cittye from farre and strange places have moche commended and praysed the same, and the majestrates in the foresight for the mayntenaunce thereof ... [N]ow of late tyme thorough the great gredynes and obstynacy growne into dyverse mens hartes (whiche neyther regarde the comodyte of helth, ther owne eses and ther naybors, nor yet the bewtefying of the cittee) ... [so that they] suffer the paving of the strete ageynst ... [dilapidated] howses or grounde to decaye and be broken to the great discommodyte and annoyaunce of the neybours and travaylors thorough or by the same, and to the disworshipp of souche as be majestrates at this present.[115]

The significance of the by-law for historians lies not only in the association between proper paving and health (the risks would have been self-evident to onlookers), but also in the light that it sheds upon the delegation of responsibilities. Magistrates, it makes plain, are duty bound to guide, have foresight and make provisions. It was the duty of residents, on the other hand, to behave and govern themselves and their dependants with due care for their own and their neighbours' welfare. Thus the guardianship of the city's 'beauty and health' was apportioned. Towards the end of our period, the corporation's power to command greater resources did indeed enable it to act in a way that was increasingly strategic and policy driven, and to make use of a wider range of technologies. In 1575/76, for example, the surveyors of rivers and streets began a programme of excavating flint for paving and building material; these flints were grouped into batches according to size, and were sold to residents so that they could meet their obligations with regard to street paving and renovation.[116] The new endeavour made use of a larger workforce and required expensive up front purchases (for example, the building of a crane which cost more than £11). Because the activities of the committee were in part financed through ward-based collections, the move was effectively publicly funded; by spreading the costs over a wider proportion of the

[115] *RCN*, II, 133.

[116] See 'River and Street Accounts', ed. Fay, pp. 115–16, 181, 184, 187, 189–90, 193–4, 197. On the stone mines, see M. Atkin, 'The Chalk Tunnels of Norwich', *NA* 38 (1983), 313–20.

population and devising a mechanism to ensure perpetual income, the corporation was becoming less dependent upon large-scale but unpredictable philanthropic gifts to drive its improvement plans.

In this chapter, we have seen a range of ways by which the governors of Norwich imagined that they might achieve better standards of cleanliness. Capital expenditure, administered through central departments and financed through compulsory levies and gifts, was one means; the authorities also placed the residents under both moral and legal pressure to assist in maintaining standards on a day-to-day level; and they made legal pronouncements in concert with central government. The long series of exceptionally detailed records from the archive of Norwich corporation is of particular significance to the medical historian: in the case of financial accounts, for example, we have an almost unmatched opportunity to gauge not only professed, rhetorical or proscriptive statements about the significance of air and water cleanliness, but also attested *activity* for their improvement. In the final chapter of this book we will continue to use the archive to look at broader campaigns to improve sanitary and health standards in the city in the mid-sixteenth century. In the evolving political and social circumstances of the time, the language of decay and disease attained a particular cultural currency, and produced a fruitful moralistic vocabulary (borrowed equally from medical sources and from political jargon) by which to condemn individuals who failed to take precautions to preserve their own (or others') health.

6

Housing, Self-Management and Healing in the Tudor City

The concern elicited amongst the governors of Norwich over the state of the watercourses and streets was matched by an equal concern for the state of the city's housing stock and other buildings.[1] Thomas Starkey summed up the relative shortcomings of English towns compared to those on the Continent. No one, he suggested, could 'be so blynd or obstynate to deny the grete dekey, fautys and mysordurys ... of our commyn wele ... when he lokyth apon our cytes, castellys and towyns, of late days ruynate and fallen downe'.[2] Norwich merchants who sat on the city's ruling council, and who traded in northern Europe, had first-hand experience of these differences; in comparison, Continental cities appeared 'so gudly, so wel byldyd and so clene kept'.[3] According to the particular logic of mid-Tudor reformism, derelict or deteriorating properties had a direct impact on the moral and physical well-being of the residents. Negligent landlords who failed to maintain wind- and water-tight housing to a proper standard were accounted foolhardy not only for squandering and devaluing their assets (and thus jeopardizing the security of a city's economy), but also for displacing an apparently endless stream of impoverished and ailing tenants who, with no other options open to them, were forced to refer themselves

[1] For the wider context, see P. Clark, 'Improvement, Policy and Tudor Towns', in *Authority and Consent in Tudor England*, ed. G. W. Bernard and S. J. Gunn (Aldershot, 2002), pp. 233–47.

[2] Starkey, *Dialogue Between Pole and Lupset*, p. 47. His remedy was to fund the rebuilding of such 'commyn ornamentys as ... magnyfycent and gudly housys [and] ... other commyn places' by taxing people according to their ability to pay: ibid., p. 117.

[3] Ibid., p. 62.

to the mechanisms of charitable assistance.[4] The gravity of this situation would have seemed self-evident. Since the publication in 1535 of William Marshall's tract entitled *The Forme and Maner of Subvention or Helping for Pore People* (a translation of regulations for poor relief implemented at Ypres), as well as the passing of the national legislation it inspired, a close relationship between begging and the transmission of disfiguring diseases – especially the pox – was firmly established in the civic consciousness.[5] For these reasons, Norwich councillors felt compelled to scrutinize the state of the city's domestic and commercial buildings with a critical eye.

Rebuilding the domestic housing stock

The extent of the problem of dereliction in Norwich in the mid-sixteenth century is hinted at in a series of land tax (landgable) records, financial accounts and property deeds. Concentrations of empty plots could be found in the sub-wards of Colegate and Fyebridge, and the situation remained particularly bad in the sub-ward of St Giles, which – in addition to its many gardens – included the fire-wasted rows of Pottergate that Cuningham erased from his plan.[6] There were yet more dilapidated properties in Tombland, as well as close to the hospital of St Giles.[7] Property in St Michael at Plea was apparently 'decayed by casuall fyer' in the 1530s,[8] and in the Castle Fee (an area of the castle's baileys under civic jurisdiction) there were several empty and burnt-out

[4] Copland, *Hye Way to the Spyttell Hous*, sigs. C3v–[4]r. In the text, the proctor of the eponymous hospital condemns 'Landlordes that do no reparacyons/ But leve theyr landes in desolacyons/ Theyr housyng unkept wynd and water tyght/ Letyng the pryncypals rot down ryght/ And suffreth theyr tenauntes to renne away/ The way to our hous we can them not denay'.

[5] On the medico-moral advice to magistrates about this time regarding poverty, transience, disease and sexual behaviour, see Slack, 'Mirrors of Health', pp. 271–2.

[6] About fourteen per cent of all properties in St Giles's sub-ward were labelled 'void' (empty), whilst the figure was closer to six per cent in Colegate and Fyebridge, and four per cent or less in all the other sub-wards: calculated from *Landgable*, ed. Rodgers and Wallace, pp. 29–139. On the other hand, and in contrast to the distribution of gardens, there were very few 'void' properties recorded amongst the tenement rows in South Conesford, or in Mid Wymer.

[7] For fire-damage at the Great Hospital's holdings at Holme Street, burnt in 1549, see 'Account Rolls of the Great Hospital', ed. Phillips, p. 20; for Tombland, see above, p. 78.

[8] NCR 18a/5 CA 1531–37, fol. 6r.

plots, including (probably) one of those seized by the corporation in 1536 (map 9).[9] The amount of empty housing in Norwich naturally also fluctuated in proportion to the size of the resident population and to the strength of the economy. Indeed, whilst the total population of Norwich seems superficially to have remained static between 1520 and the late 1550s – standing at about 11,000 people – cycles of famine in the 1520s and early 1530s, together with epidemics and food shortages between the mid-1540s and 1560, caused sharp peaks in mortality. Even when numbers were at their highest, though, the city was so large that the supply of land and property significantly exceeded demand.[10] The corporation was seriously alarmed that, in the prevailing market, private landlords were renting to large numbers of impoverished immigrants whose only means of subsistence was to beg.[11]

In order to combat the problem of landlords who failed to vet the financial position of tenants, as well as to augment its own income, the corporation sponsored various rebuilding schemes. For example, it refurbished the roofs and fittings in thirteen houses belonging to the city in Conesford, and a few further properties elsewhere. Pains were taken to make the houses waterproof and wind-tight: repairs to doors, windows and chimneys were frequent.[12] Further negotiations enabled the corporation to acquire another row of ten dilapidated houses closer to the city centre, in the Castle Fee, which had been in the possession of John Underwood (d. 1541), suffragan of Norwich and titular bishop of Chalcedon (map 9, inset T).[13] In 1536, the suffragan agreed to lease

[9] For the Castle Fee, see M. Tillyard with E. Shepherd Popescu and N. Ives, *Norwich Castle: Excavation and Historical Survey Part IV: People and Property in the Documentary Record*, EAA 23 (Dereham, 2009), pp. 18, 25. In 1531, the chamberlain of the city asked to be excused the sum of 4*s.* 6¼*d.* that had customarily been received from certain tenements in the Castle Fee. It was not, ultimately, collected, because some of the properties had been 'brent by soden fyer', while others stood 'spere [spare, unoccupied]': NCR 18a/5 CA 1531–37, fols. 12v–13r; and see NCR 16d/2 Assembly Proceedings 1491–1553, fol. 165v. On the 1536 seizure, see above, p. 154.

[10] On the population, see Appendix II. The same area had housed a population of nearer 25,000 in the 1330s, and was home to 37,000 towards the end of the eighteenth century: see Rutledge 'Immigration and Population Growth', pp. 16, 27.

[11] *RCN*, II, cii, 125 (1546). For the wider context, see ibid., pp. 132–3 (1557), 172–5 (1544, 1548, 1551), and below.

[12] For example, see NCR 18a/5 CA 1531–37, fols. 31r–2v, 56r–v, 59v, 77r. In one case, the corporation paid 2*s.* for six feet of glass for a single window (fol. 32v).

[13] Underwood had acquired these properties in a piecemeal fashion from 1513 onwards: Tillyard et al., *People and Property*, pp. 31–3.

most of his holdings to the city for a peppercorn rent.[14] Alderman Steward, avowedly driven by his 'goode will for the maynetenaunce of the citie', played a significant part in securing the properties for the corporation. He redeemed two long-term leases in the row at his own personal cost of £6 18*s*. 4*d*. Steward reported that his attempt was to encourage Underwood to rebuild other plots, but, in effect, Steward was buying him out.[15]

The corporation moved on to tackle yet another eyesore on the main Tombland frontage, not far from the 'suffragan's tenements'. In the accounting year 1543/44, it secured a four-hundred-year lease of the dilapidated church of St Mary the Less (map 9, inset S). The chamberlain set about replacing the church glass and erecting substantial flint walls around the churchyard.[16] A house situated on the same plot, meanwhile, was completely overhauled. One of the first jobs contracted (as was often the case when property was transferred) was to clean out the cesspit in the cellar.[17] The chamberlain took care to ensure that the contents were dug out and disposed of at night when the streets were empty (at least theoretically) and no one was at risk of harm from any vapours escaping and infecting the air; indeed, as there were outbreaks of plague in the city at this time, he would have appeared grossly negligent if he had permitted the labourers to move the stinking waste during the day.[18] Considerable work was also required on the tenement's main structure. The roof, chimneys and hearths, the cesspit and wooden components of the privy itself, the house's window frames, floorboards and ironwork were all replaced. The resulting rubble and debris were carted away, and the street adjacent to the property was diligently swept. The finished accommodation included bay windows

[14] *Records of Early English Drama: Norwich*, ed. Galloway, p. lxxxv.

[15] *RCN*, II, 122–3. Following renovation work, the chamberlains were able to raise their rents from 18*s*. 10*d*. in the accounting year 1539/40 to £6 19*s*. in 1551, when the refurbishments were finally complete: NCR 18a/6 CA 1537–47, fol. 35v; NCR 18a/8 CA 1551–67, fol. 5v.

[16] NCR 18a/7 CA 1541–49, fols. 116v–17r.

[17] For clearing cesspits after property transfers, and at properties owned by the commonalty, see NCR 18a/5 CA 1531–37, fol. 59v (on cleaning and closing up a 'draught' or privy); NCR 18a/8 CA 1551–67, fol. 17v (on a jakes at the suffragan's tenements); NCR 18a/7 CA 1541–49, fol. 105r (on clearing a jakes at night in Cobblerrow, the material from which was reburied under the marketplace: see map 9, inset H). And see below, n. 25.

[18] NCR 18a/7 CA 1541–49, fol. 168r. The waste was buried in a pit made in Tombland for the purpose.

overlooking the house's own garden.[19] The total cost of the project was recouped within six years, and the civic administration was quick to pass on any further charges to the tenants.[20] By 1551, the corporation's chamberlain was collecting rents worth just under £20 per annum from all of its tenements – including those in Conesford, the suffragan's and that at St Mary's – a decent return on the £56 11*s.* 8¼*d.* in total it had spent on refurbishments up to September 1550.

As was also the case with repairs to the waterways and streets, the improvement plans of the elite for the city's housing stock benefited from timely injections of cash and enthusiasm from individual members of the aldermanic class (although private contributions were not in this case administered through the civic treasury).[21] Thus, in 1569, Sir Peter Rede, the son of the alderman and mayor Edward Rede, gave four of his tenements to the parish church of St Peter Mancroft. Significantly, the tenements were located in St Lawrence's parish, an area that had been affected by the 1507 fires, and the plots may well have been some of those that had been burnt out (map 9).[22] Rede stipulated that the churchwardens – as the administrators of his gift – should keep each one in good repair. Any profits were to be distributed amongst the city's poor and used to maintain a fund for the ringing of St Peter's bells to help traders in the market to judge the time.[23] The churchwardens duly kept careful accounts of the repairs that they implemented (which initially related to the tenements' windows, roofs, floorboards, fences and drains,[24] as well as the cleaning out of a well and a 'house of office', that is, its privy and cesspit).[25] An extraordinary sixty-seven

[19] Ibid. fols. 167v–9r.

[20] After the early 1550s, the city retained responsibility for maintaining the churchyard only: NCR 17b City Revenues and Letter Book, fol. 9r.

[21] On the veritable renaissance of Norwich mercantile housing between *c.* 1520 and 1560, along with domestic rebuilding by a broader section of urban society in response to the 1507 fires, see C. King, 'House and Society in an English Provincial City: The Archaeology of Urban Households in Norwich, 1300–1700' (unpublished PhD thesis, University of Reading, 2006), pp. 200–14, 245–6, 262.

[22] For the location and nature of the tenements, see *Landgable*, ed. Rodgers and Wallace, p. 80.

[23] Rede's gift was a continuation of charitable provisions made by his father, but restructured to replace doctrinally suspect references to purgatory and good works with acceptable Protestant alternatives: NCR 20f/17 Book of Charity Founders Wills 1549–1791, fol. 5r; The National Archives, PROB 11/30/434, Will of Edwarde Rede, Alderman of Norwich, Norfolk (28 May 1545), fol. 209r–v.

[24] NRO, PD 26/110, Account Book of Rents 1569–1641, fols. 1–7.

[25] Ibid., fol. 3v.

loads of 'yarthe [earth] and other moucke' were also carted away from the yards, which perhaps suggests that the area had either been used as a dumping ground, or perhaps had not been cleared after the 1507 fires.[26] The concerns of Rede and the churchwardens thus closely mirrored those of the corporation with regard to its own tenements, and there can be little doubt that this scheme was inspired by the same ideas about clean, dignified housing, city space and the 'common weal' that were evident in the city government's renovation plans.

A further factor compelling the city authorities' pursuit of dignity and beauty in the urban fabric was the perceived relationship between physical decay and opportunities to indulge in damaging human behaviour. A combination of the derelict nooks and crannies of urban space, material pollution and the congregation of beggars indulging 'in idleness and sloth', with no 'order of lyvynge', was viewed as providing just the right circumstances for subversion of the social order.[27] Such a fear was voiced explicitly in the city assembly in February 1538 when a citizen and councillor, the grocer William Moraunt, petitioned for improvements in the area around the old Common Staithe (St Clement's staithe). It was, he claimed,

> noyfully [noxiously] kepte and a deformyte to the strete adjoyning, and a like place for ill-disposed pepille entendyng to done mischef to stond in to awayte ther praye in the nyght.[28]

Later, the Norwich magistracy had an extended opportunity to reflect upon the abuses 'ill-disposed pepille' might wreck on the landscape. In August 1549, Kett's rebels engaged in running battles with royal forces in the streets of Norwich.[29] The destruction caused to domestic buildings by arson attacks in South Conesford was widespread throughout

[26] Ibid., fol. 3v.

[27] On the urban haunts of the poor, including streets, churches, and doorways, see Marshall, *The Forme and Maner of Subvention*, sig. A2r. Similarly, according to the Norwich Mayor's Book of the Poor (1571), the indigent were to be found in 'churche porshes, mens sellers, doores, barnes, haye chambers and other back corners': *RCN*, II, 345.

[28] Kirkpatrick, *Streets and Lanes*, p. 87.

[29] Wood, *The 1549 Rebellions*, pp. 65–6. At the outbreak of rebellion, the civic authorities put themselves in a perilous position; having initially misread the situation, they were slow to condemn the participants. In the wake of its suppression, and in addition to the physical sanitizing and reordering they were required to undertake, they thus also had some ground to recover in the eyes of the central government: Wood, 'Kett's Rebellion', pp. 291, 294–7.

the parishes of St Peter Southgate, St Edward, St Etheldreda and St Clement Conesford, with property in St Etheldreda's and St Edward's in particular being especially badly hit (map 9).[30] Decisive action by the earl of Warwick put an end to the uprising, and the officers of the corporation set about implementing emergency repairs across the city. The chamberlain made immediate payments for restoring the gates, cleansing the streets, lanes, ditches and staithes, for extinguishing a fire in Conesford and, he complained, '100 leke thynges not possybyll to be wryten'. Great expense was incurred in repairing the guildhall and prisons. A phalanx of labourers was employed for 'makyng clene the market place' where rebels had been hanged, as well as the guildhall and the new Common Hall (Blackfriars), which had been 'wonderfully sore noyed with horsemucke'. At the market alone, these men worked for eighty-five labouring days and removed 272 loads of detritus.[31]

Moderation in all things: regulating idleness and gluttony

We have seen that the authorities in Norwich were on occasion prone to draw deterministic conclusions about the relationship between the quality of space and human behaviour: disgusting, ill-used or poorly maintained spaces seemingly provided opportunities for damaging or toxic activities. Additionally, there existed a prevailing expectation that citizens would choose to behave well, and to show solicitude to the environment and to each other: to handle noxious materials responsibly. The city's ruling oligarchy, meanwhile, created for itself a mandate to coerce residents into better standards of behaviour. In the next section, we will investigate the city fathers' attempts to combat failures in self-governance amongst the residents – especially the poor – through legal means, applying concepts derived from national medico-political discourse.

The renaissance in Greek medical theory during the 1520s and 1530s reminded readers that lifestyle greatly influenced health; as Hippocrates

[30] The collector of landgable rent could only record occasional receipts for buildings in these areas: NCR 18d, Landgable 1 1541–49, fol. 3r; Rutledge, 'Introduction', in *Landgable*, ed. Rodgers and Wallace, p. 4. (St Clement's was subsumed into St Julian's parish in 1482, although the landgable accountants marked the former boundary).

[31] NCR 18a/7 CA 1541–49, fol. 305r–v.

decreed, 'labores, cibaria, pocula, somnus, venus, mediocria sunto'.[32] This dictum had an obvious corollary: disease was determined by one's ability to self-rule; health was an individual matter. To be sure, the lives of a very small number of 'impotent sick' remained, theoretically, a corporate concern; the fate of the very aged or very seriously incapacitated was genuinely 'in other men's hands'.[33] Their shamefaced but piteous circumstances left them 'arayed with honger, thirste, rayne, colde, sores, stynkynge sycknesses, sadnesse [and] hevynesse', circumstances that might be reversed through the provision of prudent civil policies (including, perhaps, a brief stay for rehabilitation in a 'common' hospital).[34] Conversely, the illnesses of an apparent army of fraudulent beggars – who, in the absence of great age or incapacity, still chose not to work for a living – were inexcusably brought about by their own dissolute living.[35] Accordingly, the 'counterfeit' poor who appeared lazy, gluttonous and drunk, whilst revelling in 'other vyces not to be named', were deemed responsible for their own physical suffering; they paid no heed to the golden rule of temperance.[36] Norwich's civic policy was intended to keep both groups – the sturdy and the incapacitated poor – under firm control.[37]

Aspects of the 1531 poor law were swiftly implemented in the city; official beggars were marked out as licensed and approved. The infirm poor were still suffered to 'beg after the olde custome', but only if they possessed a copy of a seal-print which confirmed their

[32] 'Labour, food, drink, sleep, sex: these in moderation!': Hippocrates, *Epidemics*, VI.vi.2; cf. Hippocrates of Cos, *Hippocratis octoginta volumina* (Rome: ex aedibus Francisci Minitii Calvi, 1525), p. 444. Referring to 'diet' in the dual sense, not only with regard to eating and drinking, but also as a mode of living, the author of 'The Pageant of Knowledge' made a similar point a century before: 'among all there ys nothyng more mete / To helthe of man then temperat [moderate] diete': Lydgate, *Minor Poems*, II, 728. On themes of (self-)governance and food, see Albala, *Eating Right in the Renaissance*, pp. 206–8, 217–24.

[33] Marshall, *The Forme and Manor of Subvention*, sig. B6r.

[34] Ibid., sigs. A8v, D8v. On the local importance of William Marshall's analysis, see Rawcliffe, 'Sickness and Health', p. 306; Rawcliffe, *MFTS*, p. 217; Pelling, *CL*, p. 81.

[35] Marshall, *The Forme and Maner of Subvention*, sig. B5v.

[36] For a discussion of the prominence of debates concerning temperance versus gluttony in contemporary *regimina* see Wear, *Knowledge and Practice*, pp. 178–84.

[37] On the broader context (and for Europe-wide developments), see S. Cavallo, *Charity and Power in Early Modern Italy: Benefactors and their Motives in Turin, 1541–1789* (Cambridge, 1995), pp. 23–86, esp. pp. 23–9.

status as 'impotent persons'.[38] In 1532/33, the corporation paid for two painted staffs to distinguish the 'master beggars'. These individuals (who were probably required to monitor and report on 'vagabonds') received a wage so long as their deportment seemed to merit it, but their behaviour was also closely regimented.[39] For example, one Purdy, a master beggar in 1548, was placed in the stocks and had his staff removed following complaints about his conduct.[40] In February 1542, the authorities attempted to make the 'legitimate' poor more visible; the chamberlain purchased forty tin badges, which were given as distinguishing markers to incapacitated beggars (a tiny fraction of the numbers – we might guess – that were in need given rampant price rises).[41] Those not identified as genuinely incapacitated risked physical punishment. In 1538/39, the chamberlain paid out 6*d.* for 'whippyng of certain vacabundes about the market and for writines sette over ther hedes', a penalty allowed by the statute.[42] Individuals who failed to comply with the orders were also pursued in the mayor's court. Thus, on St Valentine's day 1543, Master Leche, Edward Rede and Nicholas Stywhat, in their capacity as JPs, exhorted William Fax, husbandman, to 'giff hym self to labour and labour effectually to his power' and 'leve and eschew idleness'.[43] A few years later, John Chapman of Hull was sent to a Norwich prison because he was found begging, but was not sick.[44]

The severe plague in 1544–45[45] and the subsequent dearth in food supplies apparently heralded an influx of poor immigrants into the city from its rural hinterland.[46] In February 1545, during the mayoralty of Robert Rugge, the authorities commissioned a survey to ascertain the number of beggars then living in the city. The survey also recorded the length of the term each had dwelt in Norwich and the names of their

38 *RCN*, II, 161.

39 NCR 18d Clavors' Book 1 [Hamper] 1550–1601, fol. 55v; *RCN*, II, xcix. On the painting of hand staves for the master beggars, see: NCR 18a/5 CA 1531–37, fols. 62v, 101r, 131v.

40 *RCN*, II, 174. For the location of the pillory, see map 4.

41 NCR 18a/7 CA 1541–49, fol. 70r (and see NCR 18/6 CA 1537–47, fol. 114r–v).

42 NCR 18a/6 CA 1537–47, fol. 25v.

43 NCR 16a/5 Mayor's Court Book 1540–49, p. 134.

44 Ibid., p. 517.

45 Slack, *Impact of Plague*, p. 61.

46 NCR 16a/5 Mayor's Court Book 1540–49, p. 372b (on dearth).

landlords.[47] Not long after, when the dissolution of the religious guilds eliminated a source of charitable giving to sustain the poor, Norwich began a centralized system of public assistance. In November 1548, William Rogers, as mayor, required the aldermen to present him with a list of the names of every resident in their wards, the amount of money raised by every parish for poor relief, and the amount each parishioner paid weekly to the same end.[48] The data gathered facilitated the implementation in May 1549 of an assessment for the poor, which was supplemented by substantial donations. Altogether, a sum of £280 was raised, whilst residents refusing to contribute to the assessment were threatened with imprisonment.[49] Norwich thus seems to have been the first provincial city in England to levy a compulsory poor rate.[50]

Beggars were also employed in appropriate work. One of the master beggars, for example, was required to keep horses away from the city's magnificent, arcaded market cross (presumably, so that they did not foul the area).[51] A concern with finding minor occupations anticipated statutory provision,[52] and was a policy repeated by the corporation in later years. In one case, the chamberlain employed a poor man to sweep the streets in front of its Conesford tenements, thus in one stroke solving (in a short-term and limited fashion) two of the city's perceived problems: poverty and dirtiness.[53] A sizeable rebate of the city's fee farm,[54] granted under the provisions of a parliamentary statute in 1548, sought to stimulate further programmes of this sort, by helping urban administrations nationwide in 'settinge poore people on woorke' on various projects for the benefit of the commonwealth. The ruling elite in Norwich grasped this opportunity with both hands.[55] Between the late 1540s and 1567, the chamberlains used the fee farm rebate to effect repairs to the city walls and to employ a small army of

47 *RCN*, II, cii, 172. The policy was extended in the following year during Augustine Steward's mayoralty: ibid., p. 125.

48 NCR 16a/5 Mayor's Court Book 1540–49, p. 532; *RCN*, II, 174–5.

49 *RCN*, II, c, 126.

50 Pelling, *CL*, p. 81; Rawcliffe, *MFTS*, p. 232.

51 NCR 18a/5 CA 1531–37, fol. 62v. See also NCR 18a/5 CA 1531–37, fol. 28r (for a beggar paid to knock down walls in the Free Chamber at the guildhall, 1531–32), and 18a/7 CA 1541–49, fol. 309r (for poor men clearing stones at the city walls that were damaged in Kett's rebellion).

52 Elton, 'Poor Law', p. 64 (on 27 Henry VIII c.25).

53 NCR 18a/6 CA 1537–47, fol. 140r.

54 A fixed annual amount owed to the Crown for the land held by the corporation.

55 *SR*, IV, 43–4 (2 and 3 Ed. VI, c.5); NCR 18a/7 CA 1541–49, fol. 343r.

labourers, spending more than £200 in the process.[56] The city's repair campaigns thus went some way to sponsoring productive (albeit poorly esteemed) work, compensating for the lost opportunities for building and labouring brought about by the closure of the religious houses.[57]

The medico-moral rationale for the city's actions was confirmed by the physician John Caius.[58] In his tract which outlined the precautions a person might take to preserve his body from the sweating sickness, Caius made a case for sweeping reform of provisions for the poor. Recognizing that 'miserable persons' were now relieved at public expense, Caius continued by advocating the Ciceronian distinction that 'compassion should be shewed upon them, whome necessitie compelled to do or make a faute: and no compassion upon them, in whome a faulte made necessitie'. Thus, those obliged to beg through age, impotency or sickness should not be penalised, whereas those 'whyche might laboure and serve and wil not for idlenes ... [are] not to be pitied, but rather to be punished'.[59] He prefixed his thoughts with the statement that, although on occasion he encouraged 'solace' (rest) for medical reasons, he wished 'no man to be idle, but [rather] to be occupied in some honest kinde of thing necessary in a common welth'.[60] Making plain the close association between labour and health in medical theory, he argued that public humiliation might reasonably galvanize the work-shy into action:

[56] NCR 18a/8 CA 1551–67, fols. 17r, 34v, 55r, 71r, 96v, 117r, 127r, 148r, 174v, 201v, 202r, 223v, 226v, 243v, 273v–4v, 276v, 298v–9r, 334r, 357v, 358v. Between 1550 and 1560, £145 was paid out, comprising as much as six per cent of the corporation's total expenditure over the same period. Further remedial work was required by 1567, when £140 was earmarked for this purpose: Pound, *Tudor and Stuart Norwich*, p. 105. References to the refurbished walls later prominently featured in a pageant staged in honour of a visit by Elizabeth I to the city in 1578: *Records of Early English Drama: Norwich*, ed. Galloway, pp. 253–4.

[57] For the concern of Norwich's governors that skilled builders were leaving the city, see NCR 16d/2 Assembly Proceedings 1491–1553, fol. 227v. See also D. Woodward, *Men at Work: Labourers and Building Craftsmen in the Towns of Northern England, 1450–1750* (Cambridge, 1995), pp. 1–2, 17, for the mid-century collapse in demand for building work, and attitudes towards building and labouring.

[58] On Caius's links to Norwich, see above, p. 56–7.

[59] Caius, *Counseill Against the ... Sweate*, fol. 30r.

[60] Ibid., fol. 29r–v.

If the ... profite of honeste labour and exercise, conservation of healthe, preservation from sickenesse, maintenaunce of lyfe, advauncement, safety from shamefull deathes, defence from beggerye, dyspleasures by idlenesse, shamefulle diseases by the same, hatefulle vices and punishemente of the immortalle soule canne not move us to reasonable laboure and excercise, and to be profitable membres of the commune welthe, let at the least shame move us ...[61]

The governing elite again appealed to medical ideas when it set about devising Norwich's more famous measures in the final third of the sixteenth century. A survey of the poor living in the city in 1570 recorded not only the disease status of individuals, but also their 'maners and merits'. The preamble to the Mayor's Book of the Poor argued that indigents reportedly:

cared not for enie exercize of bodie ... to get them clothes or lodgynge ... [and therefore] fell into such absurd diseases of bodie, both they and ther children, that the charge of healing of one cost more then woolde suffise twentie persons.[62]

Such feckless creatures failed to bring up their children to be able to 'serve or doo good in the common welth'. Rather, bloated with food, they 'fell to lust and concupiscence'.[63] For want of adequate clothing, 'though the colde strooke so deepe into them', their 'fleshe was eaton with vermyne and corrupte diseases grewe upon them' and their bodies infected one another.[64] In this sense, the poor posed a 'public

[61] Ibid., fol. 29v. On exercise, see Wear, *Knowledge and Practice*, pp. 160–1. Cf. the earlier prescriptions, made in a similar tone, in John Lydgate and John of Burgundy, *Governall of Helthe*, sig. A4v: 'exercyse is ... tendynge of slothes hete, and wastynge of superfluytes, and saddynge of lymmes, and sleynge of sykenesses, and dryvynge awaye of vyces, medycyne of langores, wynnynge of tyme, and dette of youth, and joye of olde or age, and helpe of helth, enemye of ydelnes and dystroyenge of all evyll'.

[62] *RCN*, II, 344.

[63] NCR 20c Mayor's Book of the Poor 1, no folio number; *RCN*, II, 344.

[64] *RCN*, II, 344–6. On adequate clothing as a defence against injurious air (which, the authors argue, displaced an appreciation of the health benefits of perfuming in the late sixteenth century), see Cavallo and Storey, *Healthy Living*, pp. 105–6. For not dissimilar concerns about cold and about clothing expressed by John Paston III, see *Paston Letters and Papers*, ed. Davis, I, 594 (1475): writing at Norwich, he noted, 'I have be seek ever sythe I cam on thys syd the see, but I trust hastyly to amend, for all my seknesse that I had at Caleys, and sythe I cam over also, cam but of cold; but I was never so well armyd for the werre as I have now armyd me for cold. Wherfor I avyse yow take exampyll by me if it happyn yow

health' issue; that is to say, each failure in self-governance cost the community financially. The mayor, John Aldrich (alderman Steward's kinsman), appealed directly to the principles of Greek medicine when he argued that men and women should, therefore, balance their intake of food, whilst taking appropriate 'exercise' through gainful employment and honest labour.[65]

Closely associated with laziness was the matter of the excessive consumption of food and drink. Serious and repeated food shortages and escalating grain prices forced political commentators to cogitate on the theme. Thomas Starkey argued that, just as man's body achieved a state of healthiness from a judicious balance of provision and consumption, society also required a balance of population and resources.[66] The likely result of any imbalance was clear enough; however, prior to the middle of the century, the civic authorities in Norwich largely managed to forestall outright rebellion by reacting in time to food crises. In 1522, faced with escalating grain prices, the mayor and aldermen bought wheat for Norwich residents using the commonalty's funds.[67] Bad harvests led the authorities to adopt further precautions in the city in February 1532. Stringent measures had to be taken on behalf of the poor to ensure that they could buy grain at a reasonable price in the market, and, in early July, each ward was assessed for its holdings of wheat, malt and barley.[68] Again, in the winter of 1543, the authorities purchased 360 coombs[69] of wheat for 'the ease of the poor inhabitants of the city'.[70]

There was also a concern to monitor the exploitation of food resources at the other end of the social scale. During his second mayoralty, Edward Rede organized a search of Norwich's administrative archives to find evidence to justify a policy for limiting feast-making amongst craft guilds, the enormous cost of which, it was argued, 'sore decayed'

to be seek, as ye wer when I was at Caleys: in eny wyse kepe yow warme. I weene Herry Woodhous nor Jamys Arblaster ware never at onys so many cotys, hose, and botewx [boots] as I doo, or ellys by God we had gone therfor. What we shall yet I can not sey, but I bere me bold on 2 dayes amendyng.'

65 *RCN*, II, 346.

66 Starkey, *Dialogue Between Pole and Lupset*, pp. 31–2.

67 Rawcliffe, 'Sickness and Health', p. 314. On the wider context, see P. Slack, 'Dearth and Social Policy in Early Modern England', *Social History of Medicine* 5 (1992), 1–17.

68 *RCN*, II, xcvii, 116–18, 163.

69 A measure of about 18 stone.

70 NCR 18a/7 CA 1541–49, fols. 122v–3r.

the city. The findings, which referred back to an early civic charter and to legislation passed in 1495, were used to justify an ordinance pronounced by the convocation of aldermen on 7 September 1531. It was noted that private citizens charged with the obligation to finance guild feasts found it impossible to recoup their expenditure, with the result that 'many of them fled and dayly went from the … citie and enhabited them selffe other where for povertie'. Such 'importune charges' had allegedly left 'many houses, habitacions and dwellynges … onlaten [which then] grue to ruyn'.[71] Using words that echoed Thomas Starkey's famous turn of phrase,[72] the ordinance suggested that Norwich thereby 'felle ... to desolacion'. In spite of earlier, unambiguous directives to remedy the problem, many companies, fellowships and brotherhoods 'of ther froward, folysshe myndes, prodigall and pervers disposicions' had sponsored lavish feasts, 'to the grette hynderaunce and enpoverysshing of the comon weall of the same cite'.[73] The economic difficulties were indeed pressing; recession was beginning to bite.[74] Accordingly, the guilds were restricted to organizing only two communal meals a year (to be eaten on the same day) for which they had to produce detailed written accounts.[75]

During his third mayoralty in 1543, Rede took the programme further and issued an edict to limit how much food each citizen might consume at any one sitting. Following the model of earlier sumptuary laws, the mayor himself was limited to six platters, whilst the aldermen, sheriffs and all other inhabitants below the rank of knight had to settle for five dishes only (unless they happened to be eating with the mayor himself, when they might enjoy another).[76] Whilst six platters

[71] *RCN*, II, 111–12.

[72] Or perhaps 'coincided with'. On the difficulties of dating Starkey's work, see Mayer, 'Introduction', in Starkey, *Dialogue Between Pole and Lupset*, pp. vii–xvii (pp. x–xii).

[73] *RCN*, II, 112.

[74] On the decline of the city's cloth exports in the 1530s, see Allison, 'Norfolk Worsted Industry', p. 79.

[75] From 1531, only individuals whose incomes were assessed and found able to bear the costs were to be elected to the position of feast-maker: *RCN*, II, 113.

[76] *RCN*, II, 124. It is possible that Rede (who was conservative in his convictions) was actually fighting a rearguard action: in 1542/43, he hosted the duke of Norfolk at his house, presenting him with a 'purpose pygge [porpoise]'. Perhaps the occasion (which implies a degree of excessive consumption) solicited criticism; it was after all staged at a time of general food shortages: NCR 18a/7 CA 1541–49, fol. 71v.

may seem more than plenty, they were frugal by the standards of contemporary, celebratory dinners.[77] The order not only had the effect of neatly reaffirming precedence within the urban hierarchy, but also diminished the potential for criticism from the lower orders. Rede's policies also reflected a concern voiced in the medical literature, which argued that the rich, just as much as the poor, should be subject to ordinances controlling food intake. Thomas Cromwell's ally, Sir Thomas Elyot, meditated on the theme in his manual *The Castel of Helthe*, stressing the almost apocalyptic consequences of gluttony:

> It maye seme to all men that have reson what abuse is here in this realme in the contynuall gourmandyse and dayely fedynge on sondry meates at one meale, the spirite of gluttony triumphynge amonge us in his gloryouse charyot callyd welfare, dryvynge us afore hym, as his prysoners into his dungeon of surfet where we are turmeded with catarres, fevers, goutes, pleuresies, frettynge of the guttes, and many other sycknesses, and fynally cruelly put to death by them ... For the remedy wherof, howe many tymes have there ben dyvised ordynaunces and actes of counsayle, although perchaunce bodyly helthe was not the chyefe occasyon therof, but rather provision ageynst vayne and sumptuous expenses of the meane people. For the nobilitie was exempted and had libertie to abyde styll in the dongeon yf they wolde ... But whan, where and howe longe were the sayd good devyses put in due execution for all that thereof shuld succede double profite (that is to say, helth of body and increse of substance) by eschewyng of superfluous expenses in sondry dyshes.[78]

Those bold enough to infringe the new Norwich ordinance faced exorbitant fines. In contrast to the 1531 measures, the richest members of Norwich society were no longer exempt from the requirements of moderate living; instead, they were to suffer the greatest punishments for excess. Henceforth, a mayor could expect to pay a considerable 100*s.* for gluttonous indulgences; aldermen and sheriffs 40*s.*; and commoners a relatively lenient 20*s.* (itself perhaps as much as their annual

[77] For evidence of the quantities that might be consumed, see the itemized list of food and drink supplied to the duke of Norfolk at the personal expense of William Mingay, mayor, in 1561: NRO COL 13/53 [seventeenth-century copy].

[78] Elyot, *Castel of Helthe*, fol. 45r–v. On this, see also Slack, 'Mirrors of Health', p. 271.

wage).[79] Rede's reforms seem to be Elyot's advice in action.[80] Should it have needed reiteration, John Caius later provided the Norwich elite with a full exposition of the medical position. Caius examined the common perception that only Englishmen now suffered from the sweat, whereas in former years (and as recently as 1529) other nations had also endured the 'great mortalitie'.[81] The cause, he deduced, was of course the Englishman's notorious tendency toward great excess.[82] People who gorged themselves weakened their bodies, rendering them more vulnerable to the assaults of putrefied air, the primary cause of the sweat. Implicating the rich on the one hand, and the unemployed on the other, he concluded that those who suffered most severely:

> were either men of welthe, ease and welfare or of the poorer sorte such as wer idle persones, good ale drinkers and taverne haunters. For these, by the great welfare of the one sorte, and large drinkyng of thother, heped up in their bodies moche evill matter, [which, owing to] their ease and idlenes coulde not waste and consume it.[83]

As if such a state of affairs was not bad enough, gluttons, according to Caius, immoderately consumed all local resources, 'to the … hinderance of theim which have nede, and great dearth and scarcitie in their common welthes'.[84] As he was writing, Norwich's ruling elite was taking further steps to ensure that staple foods were available to its residents. In 1550, the mayor (anticipating dearth) had raised a loan with which to buy grain. This was sold for reasonable prices to the poor. Just over a year later, in May 1551, the city commissioned bakers to bake grain from the common store into bread, for similar

[79] Based on John Pound's analysis of the 1525 subsidy return. At that date, forty per cent of taxpayers had a yearly income of 20*s.* in wages: Pound, *Tudor and Stuart Norwich*, p. 31.

[80] On wider attitudes to food consumption, feasting and provisioning in Norwich during this period, see McClendon, *The Quiet Reformation*, chapter 3. My argument here is that the regimenal aspects of moderating food consumption were considered as significant by (certain) of the actors involved as 'economic', 'political' and 'theological' considerations. Cf. the municipal measures to control intake, fasting and meat production in London at a later date: Dorey, 'Controlling Corruption', esp. pp. 24–31, 35–41.

[81] Caius, *Counseill Against the … Sweate*, fol. 16v.

[82] Ibid., fols. 16v–17r.

[83] Ibid., fol. [19r–v].

[84] Ibid., fol. 17r.

distribution.[85] Thus, the mayor and aldermen together shared a role suggested to them by Caius, who recommended that for 'oversight of good and helthsome victalles, ther wer appointed certein masters of helth in every citie and toune, as there is in Italie'.[86] Henceforward, by 'saving victualles', the magistrates could hope to increase 'vertue, witte and health' in the populace.[87]

Controlling healing practice and institutional provision for the sick poor

Whilst attempting to control the behaviour of the city's residents regarding cleanliness and healthy living, certain officials in Norwich also sought directly to regulate specific aspects of the healing arts. In mid-July 1539, the aldermen met to determine the fate of George Hill, an apothecary who had recently been committed to prison 'for that he hath used the science off surgerye' despite 'nat beyng expert theryn nor yet admytted therunto according to the lawe'.[88] Reportedly, Hill had attempted to treat several people in the city, and had seriously hurt one woman owing to his lack of skill. The aldermen decided that Hill should leave the city forthwith. Moreover, he was required no longer to 'medle' in surgery unless his competency was lawfully recognized (which is to say, until he was examined and approved by the bishop of Norwich and a board of expert surgeons, and given sealed testimonial letters by them).[89] Thus Norwich's magistrates acted according to statutory provision and followed a precedent long established in London, where, intermittently, private suits in medical matters had been brought to the city courts. Another, similar case was heard in May 1547, when Augustine Steward was back in charge. Steward ordered one Merydieth to present himself to the civic authorities before Pentecost, bringing with him letters 'tesiffeng his experience in the science of

[85] *RCN*, II, ci, 126–7. In this way, the mayor and alderman were able to minimize the profits of middlemen, who inflated prices. See C. Dyer, *Standards of Living in the Later Middle Ages: Social Change in England c. 1200–1520*, 2nd edn (Cambridge, 1998), p. 198.

[86] Caius, *Counseill Against the … Sweate*, fol. [21v].

[87] Ibid., fol. 26v.

[88] *RCN*, II, 168.

[89] *SR*, III, 32 (3 Henry VIII c.11); J. R. Guy, 'The Episcopal Licensing of Physicians, Surgeons and Midwives', *Bulletin of the History of Medicine* 56 (1982), 528–42 (pp. 532–4); *PMR* (1364–81), 236 (1377); *PMR* (1413–37), 127 (1421), 174–5 (1424).

fiscik' from his former employer, Sir Edmond Wyndham.[90] The court also reserved for consideration on the same day the misdemeanours of another, unnamed surgeon, whom it placed under recognisance for good behaviour.[91]

In this way, Norwich's city fathers (whilst acting within their jurisdiction for overseeing standards of commodities or services sold) engaged with a hotly debated topic. Since the preceding century, pressure groups of physicians and surgeons had battled against what they characterized as a mass of ignorant, worldly individuals who took it upon themselves to profess cures and healing techniques despite being neither properly trained nor book-learned.[92] In 1485, the physician Thomas Forestier had complained of the prognostications made by 'carpenters and mylwardes' during an outbreak of the sweating sickness in London, since they were ignorant of the Galenic variables of complexion, age, region, times of the year, climate and the properties of medicines.[93] The act of 3 Henry VIII c.11 (1512) similarly railed against 'common artificers as smythes, wevers and women', who 'boldely and custumably take upon theim grete curis and thyngys of great difficultie',[94] whilst Caius warned his readers against purchasing medicinal distillations from 'unlearned' healers, including 'simple women, carpenters, pewterers, brasiers, sopeballe sellers, pulters, hostellers, painters, [and] apotecaries'.[95] Although Hill obviously fitted the definition, it is unlikely that either Merydieth or the anonymous surgeon would have identified themselves with any of these groups. But they would certainly have been aware of developments at a national level; the identities and authority of healing personnel were in flux. In London, by comparison, attempts were being made to formally reorganize medicine and surgical services (largely in response to widespread alarm concerning the spread of the pox). Thus, in 1540, the companies of surgeons and barbers were unified into one body, and

[90] NCR 16a/5 Mayor's Court Book 1540–49, p. 374.

[91] Ibid.

[92] In 1421, a group of physicians petitioned parliament for a ban on practice except by those who had graduated as a bachelor or doctor of medicine. The petition requested that the sheriffs in each county enquire after any non-graduate or female practitioners: *Rotuli Parliamentorum*, ed. J. Strachey et al., 6 vols. (London, 1767–77), IV, 158.

[93] BL, Add. MS 27582, fol. 70r.

[94] *SR*, III, 31 (3 Henry VIII, c.11).

[95] Caius, *Counseill Against the … Sweate*, fol. 28r.

parliament passed a statute which conferred upon the London college of physicians the authority to inspect the goods of apothecaries.[96] The move was contested by a lobby of what historians call 'irregular' practitioners (who included members of the interest groups condemned by Caius and others). The metropolis nonetheless provided a model of how highly educated, status-hungry practitioners (of both medicine and surgery) might attempt to integrate into an urban community already dominated by craft-based and mercantile institutions with their own strong identities.[97] The market for healing in Norwich seems to have been responding, in its own way, to these wider developments; and, in uncertain times, it was in the interests of Norwich practitioners (especially incomers) to secure endorsements where they could get them. The benefit for the aldermanic elite, on the other hand, accrued from the status evidently attached to striving for 'the peoples heallthe'.

Not long afterwards, a more formal policy of cooperation came into being between approved healers and the governing elite in Norwich. In 1549, John Porter was appointed as a surgeon and barber to the refounded Great Hospital, and was paid by the corporation for his services.[98] Although Porter did not stay long, the new civic post was intended to be a permanent one.[99] The benefits of his contract included 'mete, drynk and lyvery, and fir wode, and ... his oineytements and other such thinges belonging to surgery', in addition to a wage of £7 in cash. As we saw in an earlier chapter, he also had the use of a property with a garden annexed, and was additionally entitled to a supply of wool to provide 'for rolles [bandages] and clouthes'.[100] Porter was a

[96] *SR*, III, 793–6 (32 Henry VIII, c.40 and c.42).

[97] Pelling, 'Appearance and Reality', pp. 83, 96–7, 103. For an evocative portrayal of the tensions generated between the various stakeholders, see Ryrie, *The Sorcerer's Tale*, pp. 43–6.

[98] NCR 16a/5 Mayor's Court Book 1540–49, p. 479; Rawcliffe, *MFTS*, pp. 227–8. The corporation had previously made arrangements with a surgeon to heal battle injuries: in 1545, Peter Freeman, surgeon and barber, had been given a reward of 5*s*. by the city council for 'helyng of Wyllam Warner, late a soldyer for the citie, who came home [from France] very sore hurt': NCR 18a/7 CA 1541–49, fol. 218r. Similarly, Porter was paid for treating a captain injured during Kett's rebellion: NCR 18a/7 CA 1541–49, fol. 313r.

[99] Porter was the first of a series of a few such men who performed medical services on behalf of the city and for the sake of charity: Pelling, *CL*, pp. 88–90.

[100] NCR 16a/5 Mayor's Court Book 1540–49, p. 539; above, p. 121. The wealth that might be accrued through civic service and private practice is apparent from the prosperity of Richard Durrant, bone-setter: he died with over £280 to bequeath, in addition to large debts owed to him: Pound, 'Social and Trade

figure of some local importance, and had been prominent in the affairs of the guild of barbers and barber-surgeons from 1540.[101] Even after his resignation as hospital surgeon, he continued to act as an informer for the corporation in matters of professional standards; thus in 1559, he presented Allen Sendall to the mayor's court for practising surgery without possessing either learning or knowledge.[102] Not long after, the city guilds introduced regulations to promote better standards amongst practitioners; from 1561, the refounded company of barbers and surgeons required its members to attend a lecture once every three weeks.[103]

The generous terms of John Porter's appointment offer a stark contrast to the corporation's treatment of existing 'spital house' staff. In late August 1541, John Crafford, a husbandman and proctor licensed to collect alms for the poor at the small hospital at St Giles's gate (not to be confused with the much larger, civic institution at which Porter worked), and William Rye, a proctor and the keeper of the house at St Stephen's gate, were forced to present themselves at a meeting of the city's aldermen (map 7).[104] Both were charged with abusing the right of the inmates to beg for alms under the king's letters patent. Crafford compelled poor, lame and diseased folk to beg to provide income for the house, with the threat that he would otherwise not support them. In contrast, and contrary to the tenor of the act of 1536 'against sturdy beggars',[105] Rye took in at least one man who could reasonably be expected to work, and he purchased counterfeit licences to beg. Both Crafford and Rye were bound by recognisance. They were

Structure', p. 62. On Durrant's annual wages for healing the poor, see NCR 18d Clavors' Book 1 [Hamper] 1550–1601, fol. 70r.

101 Pelling and Webster, 'MP', p. 213 and see above, p. 58.

102 Pelling and Webster, 'MP', p. 214.

103 *Barber-Surgeons of Norwich*, ed. Williams, pp. 9–10. Some practitioners, however, clearly resented aldermanic interest in physic: in 1562, one Doctor Bylney refused to pay tallage to the guild of barber-surgeons, and was duly threatened with referral to the mayor. Bylney was initially dismissive, stating, 'Mr Mayor have as mouche to do with me as the Pope have to do with me.' When in fact called in front of the mayor, Bylney rapidly capitulated, denied the words and promised to pay his fees to the company: ibid., p. 20.

104 *RCN*, II, 169–70. On the prevailing moral climate, which informed the actions of the ruling elite, see Copland, *Hye Way to the Spyttell Hous*.

105 *SR*, III, 558 (27 Henry VIII c.25).

also ordered to deliver to the mayor before late October all the licences that they had sealed and given out.[106]

The situation did not improve immediately. In a move that preceded the confiscation of the seals of four of the minor spital houses (St Stephen's, St Giles's, St Augustine's and St Benedict's) by the corporation in February 1543,[107] Crafford was again hauled before the mayor. Apparently, he had continued to accept individuals – poor but not diseased – who referred themselves to his care. Under a second recognisance of 100*s*., he was reminded that he was obliged:

> to rule the … spitelhous according to the purpose and intent of the fundacon and the first orderyng [and] bildyng thereof and … not mayntaen ner harbergh within the seid house any vacabunds mighty and sturdy beggers but onlye lazers [that is, those afflicted with an disfiguring disease, including 'lepers'], sike and diseased people.[108]

In future, Crafford was required to report to the justices of the peace any 'sturdy beggars' who sought access to the hospital. The custodian of the spitals of St Augustine and St Benedict's gate were bound over to abide by the same conditions.[109]

Shortly afterwards, the behaviour of the deputy governor of the institution at St Benedict's gate – Stevyn Popelton – was also called into question. A query was raised about Popelton's whereabouts during the days preceding a fair at Cawston (a village some eleven miles north of Norwich); presumably he was suspected of some offence, although the details are not recorded. Popelton produced alibis from a retinue of inmates and proctors, including the poor and sick from St Benedict's spital, St Augustine's spital and Fyebridge spital. These individuals had congregated on separate nights at two private houses, probably with the intention of attending and begging at the fair. Neither the word of Popelton nor that of the proctor of Fyebridge, Edmond Hurst, was considered sufficient to establish Popelton's disputed whereabouts, and he was required to present a more credible witness.[110] The warning shot was not sufficient; the spital house staff either failed to gauge the changing climate, or doggedly persisted with their previous

[106] *RCN*, II, 170.
[107] NCR 16a/5 Mayor's Court Book 1540–49, p. 134.
[108] Ibid., p. 130.
[109] Ibid.
[110] Ibid., p. 132.

modus vivendi. In early March 1548, one recidivist, Robert Adamson – Popelton's former superior as governor of the house at St Benedict's gate and Rye's successor at St Stephen's – was arrested and imprisoned.[111] The event must have prompted yet further investigations, for in the following November all the proctors of St Stephen's, St Giles's, St Augustine's and the Fyebridge spital houses were again required to present themselves to the mayor's court, which was presided over by William Rogers. Each had to confirm how many 'lazers' were currently living at his house. At that time it was:

> ordered and agreed that thei and every of [the proctors] shalbe bounden with sureties that they nor any of them shall not recyve, suffer or maynteyn in ther houses ... any person or persons but such as shalbe admitted by the mayor ... and also to kepe good and honest rules.[112]

The effect was two-fold. Rogers, as mayor, had redefined the role of the houses on humanist lines; at this point, he seems to have envisaged their exclusive use by victims of reputedly infectious diseases. He had also reaffirmed the corporation's prerogative to vet candidates before they entered a house. The treatment of the proctors and redefinition of the role of the spital houses was seemingly a contentious one amongst the aldermen; the clerk finished with the observation that 'many other [related] matter wer debated but not concluded'.[113] But the corporation had manoeuvred the spital houses into a position over which it could assert its control. At the same time, it apparently avoided a backlash from the citizens who, in matters of social and physical hygiene, appeared accepting of the notion that individual civic agents – theoretically acting as a representative of the commonalty as a whole, although in reality members of a privileged, selective and self-appointing elite – might assume judicial powers that in previous generations would have been determined at the micro-community level: that is, between the spital houses and the people of their wards.

[111] Ibid., p. 517.
[112] Ibid., p. 530; *RCN*, II, xcviii–xcix.
[113] NCR 16a/5 Mayor's Court Book 1540–49, p. 530. Over the next seventy-five years or so, successive administrations pushed for further municipal controls or ceded powers to the spital house keepers depending on what was most convenient at the time, although individuals judged unsatisfactory by any particular regime could not expect to stay in post for long: Pelling, 'Healing the Sick Poor', in Pelling, *CL*, pp. 99–100.

EPILOGUE

In the years immediately following the publication of Cuningham's plan (1559), life in Norwich underwent a series of marked developments. Specifically, the city experienced a social revolution. In 1564–65, Dutch and Walloon textile workers were invited by the corporation to settle in Norwich in order to stimulate its flagging textile manufacturing sector. From an initial few hundred, the number of incomers had risen to 4,000 by 1571, an increase of about thirty-five per cent of the size of the population of the time.[1] On occasion, the new arrivals were treated with outright hostility by individual citizens, whilst the attitude of officers in the corporation also seems to have been ambivalent.[2] Thus, when a devastating outbreak of plague hit the city in 1578,[3] the 'Stranger' community received much of the blame for aggravating it through allegedly unhygienic practices: a lack of domestic cleanliness – including the 'corrupte kepinge of ... howses and necessaries [prives]'[4] – was one issue; industrial pollution was another.[5] The assembly recognized that the processes of scouring woollen baize in the river were 'bothe daungerous and very onholsome in eny tyme, but most [of all] in the Somer tyme and in the tyme of syckenes' (thus tacitly recognizing that practices which might be generally tolerated were irresponsible at riskier times of the year). In late March 1579, it placed a ban on the scouring of cloth within the river or waterways in central parts of the city.[6] The mayor of Norwich also wrote a letter

1 Pound, 'Government to 1660', p. 41. The size of the Dutch/Walloon community rose again to *c.* 5,000 people in 1576: ibid.

2 Ibid.

3 Perhaps the greatest mortality crisis to hit Norwich since 1348–50: Slack, *Impact of Plague*, p. 129.

4 *RCN*, II, 335.

5 NCR 16d/3 Assembly Proceedings 1553–83, fol. 276v; *RCN*, II, 336.

6 NCR 16d/3 Assembly Proceedings 1553–83, fol. 276v.

to the Dutch and Walloon congregations demanding that the new arrivals implement much tighter controls on the disposal of effluent. Henceforth, the letter requested, the Strangers must take care to sluice away by-products accruing from the treatment of wool (an important part of their industrial activities), because the fumes would otherwise 'breede in ... bodies dyvers corrupte humours, to the great daunger of their bodies in this infectious time'.[7] The dust and other material produced by combing wool and 'chamber wash' were also identified as agents infecting the air. From then on, chamber wash was not to be conveyed anywhere for disposal during the day, but only at night, and then only 'in a close tubb or elles coveryd with a clothe'; likewise, wool combing was not to take place 'towardes the open strete' but 'inwardly in backehowses', out of harm's way.[8] Other orders – derived from hygienic advice produced by Queen Elizabeth's privy council – followed in early April; they related to the cleansing of domestic accommodation, clothes and bodies, and instructed the Strangers to make use of appropriate prophylactic 'fumes and preservatyves'.[9]

Despite the mayor's readiness to condemn the incomers on hygienic grounds, we have from time to time glimpsed in the pages of this book the invigorating impact that the Stranger community had on local health culture. For example, we noted in passing the importance to Valentyne Bourne of the availability of Dutch and French medical texts; the enterprising side-line of John Cropp, Walloon surgeon, as an importer of figs (considered a laxative and purgative); and the activities of Martin Corembeck on behalf of the college of physicians.[10] The Strangers were simultaneously credited with an almost miraculous capacity to rejuvenate the housing market, renovate tenements and cultivate land: activities, as we have seen, that were closely allied to concepts of salubrity in local health culture. One report from *c.* 1575 stated that, following their arrival, the 'cittie is [again] well inhabited, and decayed houses re-edified and repaired that were in rewyn'.[11]

[7] *RCN*, II, 336.

[8] NCR 16d/3 Assembly Proceedings 1553–83, fol. 276v.

[9] *RCN*, II, 336–7.

[10] See above, pp. 51, 58, 126. On the laxative properties of figs, see, *inter alia*: Thomas Newton, *Approoved Medicines and Cordiall Receiptes with the Natures, Qualities and Operations of Sundry Simples* (London: Thomas Marshe, 1580), fols. 28v–29r.

[11] Pound, 'Government to 1660', pp. 42–3; W. J. C. Moens, *The Walloons and their Church at Norwich*, 2 vols. (London, 1887), II, 262; and see *RCN*, II, 332–3, for the problem of empty or un-let housing acting as an incentive to Norwich's

Themes of diligence, industry and the rejuvenation of civic space, seemingly embodied by the Strangers, were amply celebrated in civic pageants organized to celebrate the arrival in the city of Elizabeth I in 1578.[12] Her appearance occasioned various repairs to, and cleansings of, public spaces and facilities, which developed the policies of the authorities in the period 1530–52. The arrangements for the 'bewtefiyng of the cittie' included a reorganisation of muck storage (especially the removal of a 'great muckehill' by Brazen Doors), along with further refurbishments to (and, in one case, the widening of) the streets and to the bridges. The river was improved (and the privies adjoining it, closed), whilst the market cross was repainted, the old pillory taken away and a new one installed. Industrial polluters (cloth workers, wool and tallow processors) were naturally placed under tight control. Animals grazing the common areas of the city were removed, whilst owners of tenements were required to supply a 'convenient necessary [suitable privy]' for the occupants to ensure that human effluent could not find its way into the streets (or else risk a 5*s.* fine).[13] Subsequently, in 1579, and no doubt in response to the aforementioned epidemic that was then raging, the civic assembly conducted a survey of suitable places where the 'muck and filth' removed from the streets could be laid.[14] Whilst Galenic and Hippocratic principles were clearly at the heart of these measures, and indeed had been integrated into the civic corporation's strategies for health maintenance for most of the period covered here, at the close, beliefs regarding the environmental causes of disease did not go entirely uncontested. The establishment of Puritan groups within Norwich encouraged a providential view of disease which rendered the Hippocratic and Galenic dynamics of environment and lifestyle apparently irrelevant.[15] Fuller exploration

governors to petition the Privy Council, via the duke of Norfolk, for letters patent to allow the Strangers to settle.

12 *Records of Early English Drama: Norwich*, ed. Galloway, pp. 253–5; NCR 16d/3 Assembly Proceedings 1553–83, fols. 279v–80r. The refurbished walls were prominently featured in the enactments staged for the queen (in one instance they were deployed as part of a stage set).

13 NCR 16d/3 Assembly Proceedings 1553–83, fol. 271r; *Records of Early English Drama: Norwich*, ed. Galloway, p. 244. This is the first mention of the possibility of human waste entering the streets of Norwich that I have found: perhaps with the increase in population, disposal of waste was again becoming a serious problem.

14 NCR 16d/3 Assembly Proceedings 1553–83, fol. 283r.

15 On Protestantism amongst Norwich's aldermen from 1558, and the city's subsequent attractiveness to Puritan divines (as well as the survival of conservative

of each of these topics must take place outside the present enquiry; the precise ways in which the Dutch and Walloon settlers complemented and influenced the city's native philosophies of healing and hygiene deserve fuller analysis using, for example, the still largely untapped resources of the Norwich city archives and those of Flemish cities such as Ypres.[16] Our focus has instead concentrated upon the application of notions of topography and hygiene in urban health culture.

In the foregoing pages, we have noted the importance accorded to the purity of air and water in civic attitudes to health; the ghettoization of conjoined cases of poverty and disease; the qualitative judgements made by Norwich residents about the relative salubrity and acceptability of different types of urban plots and grounds; and various corporate and individual attempts to improve the appearance of the built environment for hygienic as well as for economic reasons. Our cast of actors, meanwhile, comprised an extended network of agents, including the disenfranchised and sick poor, but also householders, manufacturers, guildsmen and women, civic officers, professional religious, MPs, cosmographers, academics, and members of the gentry and nobility, as well as a relatively small number of individuals who styled themselves as practitioners of medicine or surgery, or who sold therapeutic commodities. In identifying the relevant groups of stakeholders, it has become apparent that the pervading ethos of sanitary reform did not simply devolve down to civic communities from academic, religious or political circles, but was reciprocal and mutually influential; improvements to the fabric and social cohesion of urban centres coloured and sustained the nature of governmental and medical discourse on the hygiene of towns. Cuningham's interests in the healthiness of places (and of Norwich in particular), which rode upon the crest of a revival of enthusiasm for Hippocratic and Ptolemaic pronouncements on the environmental determinants of human form and

factions), see R. Houlbrooke and M. McClendon 'The Reformation', in *MN*, ed. Rawcliffe and Wilson, pp. 255–76 (pp. 260–76). In 1580, one Norwich mayor argued that segregation controls were irrelevant in the face of plague because the life span of every man was predetermined by God: *Acts of the Privy Council of England*, new series, 46 vols. (London, 1890–1965), XI, 437; Slack, *Impact of Plague*, p. 231.

16 The influence of the policies pursued by city councils in Flanders upon the corporation of Norwich regarding its treatment of the sick and 'sturdy' poor during the late 1560s and 1570s has been noted in Pelling, *CL*, p. 81; Rawcliffe, 'Sickness and Health', p. 306.

behaviour, were likewise developed against a particular backdrop: the observable difference between body shape, disease status and personal status evident in the inhabitants of his native city, and its division into salubrious and waste-ridden parts. Meanwhile, the social value attached to the implementation of urban sanitary improvements (and to the charitable gifts that funded them) provided malleable material from which personal, corporate and civic identities could be forged.

When devising improvement schemes in the sixteenth century, the city government experimented with various models of organization. For initiatives relating to the fabric of the city, magistrates attempted to redeploy a certain amount of corporate and private wealth. The activities of the city chamberlains, for example, were funded through the income generated by renting out the corporation's properties (including the water mills, city gates and the muck boat). Later, the chamberlains delegated powers to the river and street surveyors, a committee predominantly made up of common councillors elected by enfranchised citizens in the wards, working under the direction of two aldermen. This was an exercise in bureaucracy, financed by a combination of public levies paid by wealthier citizens, the existing funding streams exploited by the chamberlains and (very significant) philanthropic donations by individual members of the aldermanic class. Other models were trailed in different areas of health policy. In the case of the city's premier institution for the sick poor (the Great Hospital), day-to-day governance was delegated to a 'master', assisted by aldermen as well as common councillors in particular duties (including signing off the hospital's accounts), and (for healing matters proper) a surgeon.[17] This system in particular proved a difficult one to manage: the autonomy of various masters was periodically called into question.[18] Meanwhile, certain aldermen and mayors styled themselves as guardians of the health of the populace; a role which served to augment their personal status and thus their credibility and legitimacy as governors. Nonetheless, they wisely balanced their own interests with those of other relevant groups. In matters pertaining to the regulation of surgical and medical practice, for example, the mayors and aldermen cooperated with local trade guilds (and acted as an instrument of authorization and authority on their behalf),

[17] 'Account Rolls of the Great Hospital', ed. Phillips, p. 7; Rawcliffe, *MFTS*, p. 228.

[18] On such tensions, see 'Account Rolls of the Great Hospital', ed. Phillips, pp. 7–8; Rawcliffe, *MFTS*, pp. 234–5.

notwithstanding the attempts of the London college of physicians to impress upon Norwich citizens the superiority of its own particular brand of exclusivism and elitism. In the case of the small spital houses, individual mayors exercised a measure of executive authority relating to the admittance of inmates and regulation of the houses. Elsewhere, the elite used its influence in parliament to petition for powers to make improvements and refurbishments to the city fabric, and (at an earlier date) solicited royal mandates in the form of letters patent with which to raise funds or manpower for city cleaning efforts. The association between hygiene, appearances and personal executive power was clearly indicated to the populace when, in 1576/77, five men were paid for drawing water with which to wash the streets at the accession of the new mayor.[19]

At the same time, the emphasis placed upon the responsibility of individual residents did not diminish. Inhabitants presented their neighbours, social superiors and civic officials in the local courts for punishment if they seemed to have polluted the environment. Attitudes to the changeability and the ungovernability of the world at large (the winds, seasons, and other people's behaviour, as well as planetary movements) necessitated that men and women should look to their micro-environment – rooms, houses, gardens, streets – and to precautionary clothing and lifestyle choices in order to preserve their bodies; for similar reasons, waste materials were allocated particular, appropriate spaces within the wider city landscape. Sickness, conversely, was on occasion viewed as the inevitable result of a failure in self-governance. Almost incidentally, we have noted that domestic squalor, stagnant water and filthy streets were not the generally accepted conditions of urban life, despite received opinion on standards of cleanliness in pre-modern towns. Poorly maintained houses and sewers were condemned by medical authorities, city dwellers and civic authorities alike precisely because of the threats to human health that they posed.

Finally, this text constitutes an experiment in an integrated method which explores the material nature of pre-modern health culture: it uses evidence of ceremonies and pageantry, work routines, technologies, built space, artefacts and land use, as much as the content of

[19] 'River and Street Accounts', ed. Fay, p. 179. The mayor was Thomas Layer, who had previously acted as a treasurer for the river and streets committee (ibid., p. 148).

manuscripts, images or printed manuals and textbooks to gauge developments in, and the sharing of, ideas and knowledge. Alone, each form of evidence is partial, but, when read together, the data allows us to detect the wider resonances of medical culture as it was *enacted* within a community. These resonances are hard to access in traditional, exclusively text-based medical histories. Health and topography were intimately intertwined in the pre-modern urban mindset. Our lines of enquiry must evolve accordingly to do justice to this relationship.

APPENDIX I

A NOTE ABOUT PATHOGENS AND RETROSPECTIVE DIAGNOSIS

> Since bones afford not only rectitude and stability, but figure unto the body, it is no impossible Physiognomy to conjecture at fleshy appendencies, and after what shape the muscles and carnous parts might hang in their full consistences. ... Physiognomy outlives ourselves, and ends not in our graves.[1]
>
> Sir Thomas Browne (d. 1682)

The study of the material remains of pre-modern health culture – of 'sewers and skeletons' – has occasionally been treated with ambivalence by medical historians.[2] For their part, osteoarchaeologists and palaeopathologists seek to explain (amongst other things) the functional consequences for an individual of a range of particular congenital and acquired disorders; the socio-economic determinants of health within a population; cultural and social responses to disease; pre-modern surgical and remedial treatments; and the origins and epidemiology of infectious diseases.[3] Historians of medicine, whilst embracing aspects

[1] Sir Thomas Browne, *The Religio Medici and Other Writings* (London, 1906), pp. 121–2.

[2] The point should not be over-emphasized. There is an established tradition of uniting osteoarchaeological data and historiography: for example, see C. Dyer, *Standards of Living in the Later Middle Ages*, p. 192; *Death in Towns: Urban Responses to the Dying and the Dead, 100–1600*, ed. S. Bassett (Leicester, 1992); Rawcliffe, 'Sickness and Health', in *MN*, ed. Rawcliffe and Wilson, pp. 301–26 (p. 304); and see M. Green, 'Integrative Medicine: Incorporating Medicine and Health into the Canon of Medieval European History', *History Compass* 7 (2009), 1218–45 (p. 1221), which advocates the integration of historical, bioarchaeological and palaeomicrobial sources.

[3] A small selection of the many possible examples of the areas of interest mentioned here include (for the medieval period): Lewis, *Urbanisation and Child Health in Medieval and Post-Medieval England* (populations); C. J. Knüsel, 'Orthopaedic Disability: Some Hard Evidence', *Disability and Archaeology*, ed. N.

of the spatial and material culture of pre-modern health care,[4] have on occasion defined their agenda against that of historical epidemiologists and palaeopathologists, largely as a consequence of reacting against anachronistic forms of 'retrospective diagnosis' in their own field. They particularly seek to avoid any suggestion that concepts or diagnoses of diseases transcend time and place, or that they are somehow static, common or innate, or that they are independent of the interpretations offered by the individuals who experience, witness or define them.[5] For example, in a witty and textured article, the historian Peregrine Horden argued that 'in the history of ... pre-nineteenth-century ... public health measures, sewers and skeletons are not quite enough'.[6] Horden admitted that what he calls the 'materialist-biological' account

Finlay, *Archaeological Review from Cambridge*, 15 (1999), 31–53 (impairment); A. Sullivan, 'Reconstructing Relationships Among Mortality, Status and Gender at the Medieval Gilbertine Priory of St Andrew, Fishergate, York', *American Journal of Physical Anthropology* 124 (2004), 330–45; and A. L. Grauer, 'Patterns of Life and Death: The Palaeodemography of Medieval York', in *Health in Past Societies: Biocultural Interpretations of Human Skeletal Remains in Archaeological Contexts*, ed. H. Bush and M. Zevelebil, BAR IS 567 (Oxford, 1991), pp. 67–80 (bio-archaeology). On medical artefacts see, for example: C. J. Knüsel, R. L. Kemp and P. Budd, 'Evidence for Remedial Medical Treatment of a Severe Knee Injury from Fishergate Gilbertine Monastery in the City of York', *Journal of Archaeological Science* 22 (1995), 369–84; and Gilchrist and Sloane, *Requiem*, pp. 103–5.

4 See, for example, *Spaces, Objects and Identities in Early Modern Italian Medicine*, ed. S. Cavallo and D. Gentilcore, *Renaissance Studies* 21 (1998); Cavallo and Storey, *Healthy Living, passim.*

5 For sophisticated investigations of the issues at stake, see A. Cunningham, 'Identifying Disease in the Past: Cutting the Gordian Knot', *Asclepio* 54 (2002), 13–34 (p. 34) reprinted in A. Cunningham, *The Identity of the History of Science and Medicine* (Farnham, 2012), which suggests in all periods 'people died of what their doctor (or their bystander) said they died of [; and] that's that'. See also J. Arrizabalaga, J. Henderson and R. French, *The Great Pox: The French Disease in Renaissance Europe* (New Haven, 1997), pp. 16–19; J. Arrizabalaga, 'Problematizing Retrospective Diagnosis in the History of Disease', *Asclepio* 54 (2002), 51–70; D. Harley, 'Rhetoric and the Social Construction of Sickness and Healing', *Social History of Medicine* 12 (1999), 407–35; P. D. Mitchell, 'Integrating Historical Sources with Paleopathology', in *A Companion to Paleopathology*, ed. A. L. Grauer (Chichester, 2012), pp. 310–23.

6 Horden, 'Ritual and Public Health in the Early Medieval City', p. 18; cf. a companion piece, P. Horden, 'The Millennium Bug: Health and Medicine around the Year 1000', *Social History of Medicine* 13 (2000), 201–19 (pp. 208–11). For a different, though equally positional, view which argues that material findings should not be unthinkingly subjected to the agendas of historians, see D. Austin, 'The "Proper Study" of Medieval Archaeology', in *From the Baltic to the*

can 'capture some of the story' but, he contended, 'it will do that only in the narrow terms of biomedicine and demography'. Religious and moral philosophies and concepts of pollution comprised the principal explanation for disease in the medieval Christian West. These might too easily be eclipsed, Horden implied, by a methodology that utilizes modern concepts of hygiene or pathogens at the expense of such culturally specific categories as space, ritual, symbolism and concerns about communal purity.[7]

In addition to the underlying theoretical concerns, other factors have also discouraged a fuller integration of historical and material evidence. The potential to draw meaningful conclusions about pre-modern health and medical culture from material sources has to some extent been undermined by a persistent deferral of analysis in favour of the accumulation of data.[8] Early attempts to explain the material evidence tended to endorse a strictly teleological view of sanitary and medical developments: in historiographical terms, such analyses were guilty of Whiggishly emphasizing hygienic advances as high points on the journey to modernity.[9] Meanwhile, at the coalface of new research, both the palaeopathological and historical literature has naturally tended to be of a technical and specialist nature, inhibiting the dynamic questioning of the integrated evidence and discouraging interaction between experts in the different fields.

Black Sea: Studies in Medieval Archaeology, ed. D. Austin and L. Alcock (London, 1990), pp. 9–42.

7 The position reflects the historiographical impact of M. Douglas, *Purity and Danger: An Analysis of Concepts of Pollution and Taboo* (London, 1966). See also M. Jenner, 'Early Modern English Conceptions of "Cleanliness" and "Dirt" as Reflected in the Environmental Regulations of London, *c.* 1530–1700' (unpublished DPhil thesis, University of Oxford, 1991).

8 P. V. Addyman, 'The Archaeology of Public Health at York, England', *World Archaeology* 21 (1989), 244–63 (p. 261): Addyman was concerned that the data collected from excavations on subjects such as standards of accommodation, water quality, food supplies, pollution, hygiene and disease was so vast that it would not be synthesized for decades to come. (In the event, the work by Addyman and others on York served to capture the historical imagination, and was promoted through the public outreach work of the city's Archaeological Trust.) As a related issue, data sets have not always been comparable: this problem is tackled directly in C. Roberts and M. Cox, *Health and Disease in Britain From Prehistory to the Present Day* (Stroud, 2003), pp. 26–30, 221–86, and T. Waldron, *Palaeopathology* (Cambridge, 2009).

9 Horden, 'Ritual and Public Health in the Early Medieval City', p. 19.

But all is not lost. Palaeopathologists argue that the old characterizations of the discipline are outdated.[10] They have developed a forward-looking research agenda which draws upon a wide range of anthropological, archaeological and historical methods and themes, and which further opens up enquiries into the identities and experiences of diseased or physically impaired people in the past.[11] Meanwhile, interdisciplinary work on subjects such as the nature, construction and social significance of water supplies and sanitation facilities contributes syntheses from the materialists' perspectives which are attuned to cultural and social circumstances.[12] The challenge now remains fully to integrate these varied forms of evidence. The present book makes such an attempt by viewing together the body, burial context, landscape, and the social and intellectual milieu.[13] In this way, we might be able to circumvent some of the pitfalls identified by Horden and others.

My approach assumes that individuals with certain developmental disorders, or those suffering from particular types of infections, or the victims of serious accidents and physical trauma can be identified

[10] See the critique of my paper 'Text, Space and the Evidence of Human Remains in English Late Medieval and Tudor Disease Culture: Some Problems and Possibilities' in C. Roberts, 'The Bioarchaeology of Leprosy and Tuberculosis: A Comparative Study of Perceptions, Stigma, Diagnosis and Treatment', in *Social Bioarchaeology*, ed. S. C. Agarwal and B. A. Glencross (Oxford, 2011), pp. 252–81 (p. 253).

[11] For an introduction, see several of the papers in *Social Bioarchaeology*, ed. Agarwal and Glencross; see also J. R. Sofaer, *The Body as Material Culture: A Theoretical Osteoarchaeology* (Cambridge, 2006); and M. R. Buzon, 'The Bioarchaeological Approach to Palaeopathology', in *A Companion to Paleopathology*, ed. A. L. Grauer (Chichester, 2012), pp. 58–75.

[12] R. J. Magnusson, *Water Technology in the Middle Ages: Cities, Monasteries and Waterworks after the Roman Empire* (London, 2001); Keene, 'Issues of Water in Medieval London to *c.* 1300'; Jørgensen, 'Cooperative Sanitation: Managing Streets and Gutters in Late Medieval England and Scandinavia'. For an older but still valuable study, see J. Grieg, 'The Investigation of a Medieval Barrel-Latrine from Worcester', *Journal of Archaeological Science* 8 (1981), 265–82.

[13] In this respect, I take inspiration from so-called 'osteobiographies': see, for example, trials in Knüsel, 'Orthopaedic Disability', and R. Gowland, 'The Social Identity of Health in late Roman Britain', in *TRAC 2003: Proceedings of the Thirteenth Annual Theoretical Archaeology Conference*, ed. B. Croxford et al. (Oxford, 2004), pp. 135–46 (pp. 139–44); and see R. Gilchrist, *Medieval Life: Archaeology and the Life Course* (Woodbridge, 2012), esp. chapter 2.

on the basis of lesions and other features in human skeletal remains;[14] although it recognizes that the nature of bone itself (and the limits on our ability to identify all but a relatively small proportion of disease processes in it) places defined limits on the scope of the evidence.[15] It is also sensitive to historiographical concerns about the fundamental incompatibility of concepts of aetiology and diagnosis before and after the development of germ theory.

Let us take leprosy as an example of the issues at stake, as the disease is encountered repeatedly in chapter 3 of this book. The diagnostic criteria of medieval leprosy and modern leprosy are not conterminous. Whilst Hansen's disease (which is still sometimes called 'leprosy' today) has a specific mycobacterial identity, medieval *leprosy* incorporated a wide range of physical and spiritual diseases and symptoms which play no role in a modern diagnosis.[16] A complicating factor in the case of 'leprosy' is that comparison of the modern clinical presentations of osseous changes of Hansen's disease with palaeopathological samples excavated from medieval *leprosaria* seems to suggest that certain pathological characteristics of the modern disease *were* encompassed within the medieval one (even accepting that medieval *lepra* was, conceptually, much broader). But the problems of nomenclature and of specificity are largely surmounted if, rather than emphasizing the bacterial identity of any particular disease condition evident in skeletal remains, the emphasis is instead placed upon the particular collection of manifest *physical changes* displayed in that person's body as inferred from osteological lesions (a method that, as it so happens, was also conceived by Norwich's most famous physician, Thomas Browne, more than four hundred years ago). Figures 18 and 19 indicate one means by which inferences might be drawn using the analysis of osseous anomalies, human anatomy and an appreciation of clinical disease presentations. Figure 18 shows a face from a skull recovered from the medieval leper house of St James and St Mary Magdalene in

14 It can, therefore, be contrasted with the particular epidemiological method used in J. L. Boldsen and L. Mollerup 'Outside St Jørgen: Leprosy in the Medieval Danish City of Odense', *American Journal of Physical Anthropology* 130 (2006), 344–351 (p. 349), in that it retains faith in traditional palaeopathological methods of differential diagnosis using patterns of lesions in an individual skeleton.

15 For a concise and engaging introduction to some of the problems of diagnosing illness from bone, see Walron, *Palaeopathology*, pp. 1–9.

16 On this range, see Rawcliffe, *Leprosy*, pp. 46–54, 86–7 and *passim*.

Chichester, West Sussex.[17] Analysis of the whole skeleton suggests that this person had contracted Hansen's disease, and that he experienced facial changes including the collapse of his nose. Figure 19 shows that the same man had also sustained a compound fracture to the lower shaft of the femur (thigh bone). This healed badly and became infected: the reconstruction shows a discharging abscess from the bone cavity. Meanwhile, the toes show septic changes and destructive remodelling of the underlying skeleton. Extrapolations about a person's appearance may be drawn even without the aid of such skilful visual reconstructions by postulating (using current palaeopathological standards) the potential range of soft-tissue consequences or biomechanical adaptations which may have been associated with the presenting osseous lesions. The focus of the question then becomes: what do we know about the ways in which the manifestly sick, disfigured, or deformed were treated in life – and in death – by the society in which they lived? What does this tell us about pre-modern concepts of health and of corporate hygiene? Thus, the present book discusses skeletal evidence from Norwich of individuals showing similar deformities to those displayed in the reconstructions in order to explore the nexus of ideas surrounding disease, landscape and social status. It is, admittedly, an approach of little value to disease ecologists, but it is a *modus vivendi* for investigators whose primary interests lie in decoding the healing philosophies, practices and attitudes of the past (whether they identify themselves as osteoarchaeologists or as medical historians).

[17] This individual's pathologies are discussed in C. J. Knüsel and S. Göggel, 'A Cripple from the Medieval Hospital of Sts James and Mary Magdalen, Chichester', *International Journal of Osteoarchaeology* 3 (1993), 155–65. See also Magilton, Lee and Boylston, *Lepers Outside the Gate*, pp. 226, 233 and catalogue of skeletons, pp. 55–6 (skeleton 115).

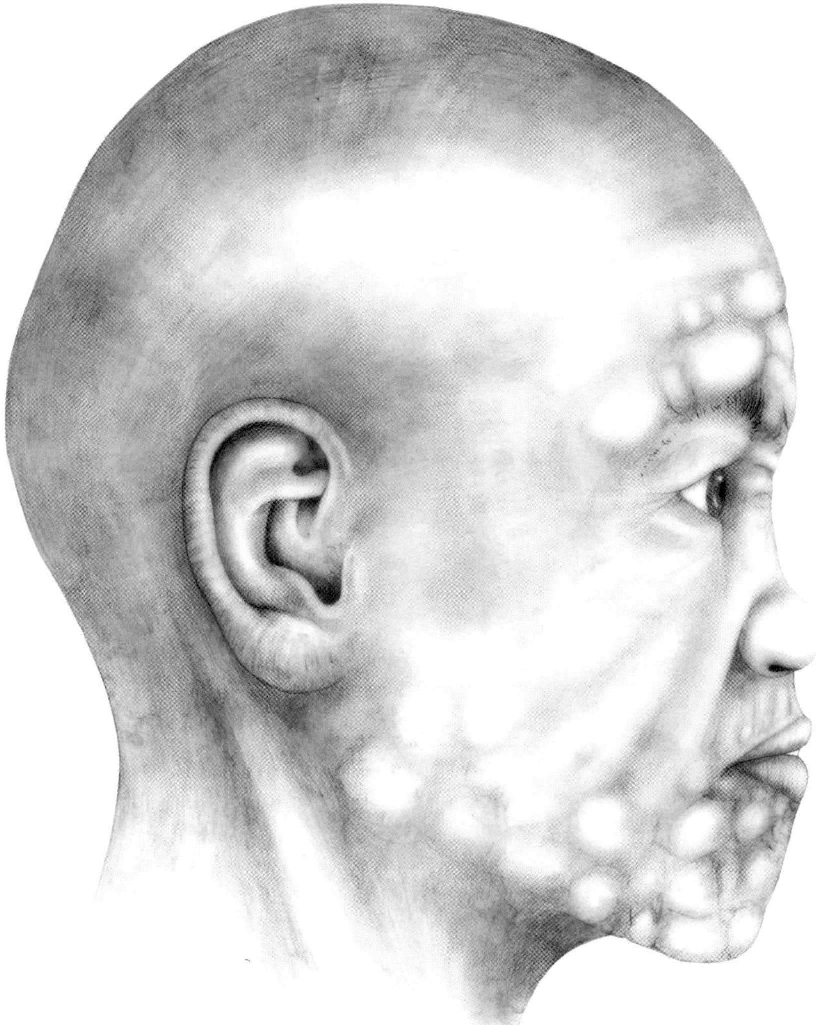

Figure 18: A face, modelled by Caroline Erolin, from a skull recovered from the medieval leper house of St James and St Mary Magdalene in Chichester, West Sussex.

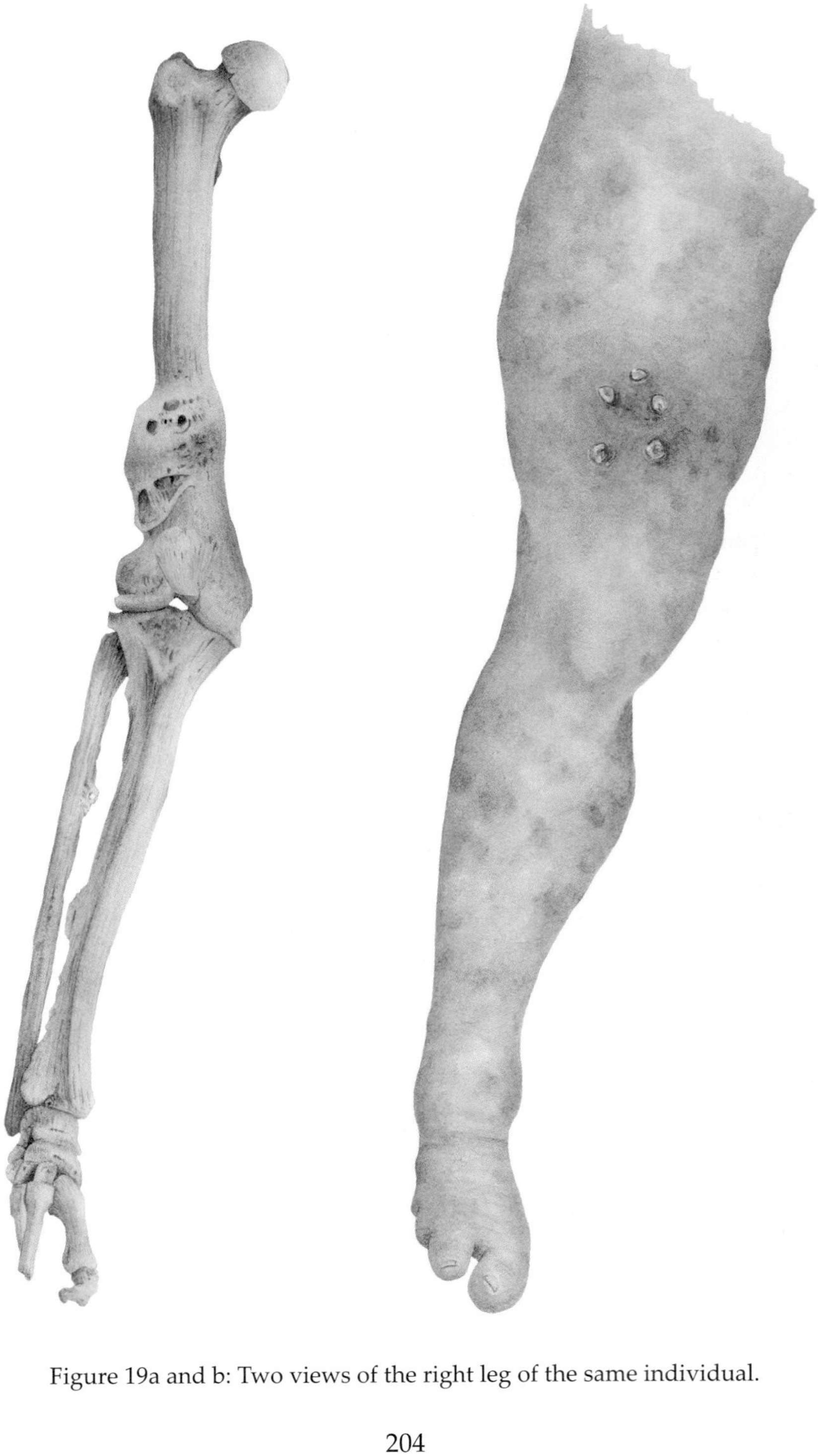

Figure 19a and b: Two views of the right leg of the same individual.

APPENDIX II

A NOTE ABOUT THE POPULATION OF NORWICH, 1100–1600

Norwich's population at the time of the Domesday survey was probably in the region of about 5,000–10,000 souls. By 1311, the figure was closer to 15,000–17,000, rising again (despite famine in the early fourteenth century) to about 25,000 in 1333.[1] Following plague epidemics in 1349–50, 1369 and 1375, the estimated number of residents in 1377 (extrapolated from poll tax returns) was closer to 7,500–8,000, although influxes of rural immigrants helped to make good earlier losses.[2] Levels subsequently stagnated. Countrywide, the population was at its nadir in 1450, recovering only slowly.[3] An estimated minimum population of 8,500 in 1525 has been suggested on the basis of the subsidy of that year.[4] More recently, this figure has been revised upwards to *c.* 11,000–12,000.[5] During the period from the 1530s to 1550s, numbers again fluctuated according to the contrary effects of inward migration and plague or other epidemics, although by the early 1560s, the population probably stood again at the 1525 level.[6] On the subsequent arrival of *c.* 5,000 Dutch and Walloon immigrants from 1565, who were invited to settle in the city by the authorities in order to bolster the flagging textile industry, see the epilogue to the main text.

[1] Rutledge, 'Economic Life', pp. 157–8; Rutledge, 'Immigration and Population Growth', p. 27; Ayers, 'The Urban Landscape', p. 10.

[2] Atkin, Carter and Evans, EAA 26, p. 3 (following Helen Sutermeister's unpublished calculations); Dunn, 'Trade', pp. 213–14.

[3] Dyer, *Decline and Growth*, p. 6.

[4] Pound, *Tudor and Stuart Norwich*, p. 28.

[5] Slack, *Impact of Plague*, p. 128; C. Rawcliffe, *The Hospitals of Medieval Norwich*, pp. 24, 31 n. 37 (following A. King, 'The Merchant Class and Borough Finances of Late Medieval Norwich', unpublished DPhil thesis, Oxford University, 1989).

[6] Pound, 'Government to 1660', pp. 35–6

APPENDIX III

A NOTE ON THE HISTORIOGRAPHY AND ARCHAEOLOGICAL RECORD OF NORWICH

The activities of the city's government produced an extraordinarily full series of manuscript records which are held at the Norfolk Record Office. A selection of the archival material was published in a two-volume work edited by William Hudson and John Tingey at the start of the twentieth century.[1] The city's material and topographical records are equally accessible. Large-scale investigations into the early development of the city began in 1971 with the creation of an interdisciplinary research group known as the Norwich Survey.[2] The Survey was responsible for the archaeological excavation of 31–51 Pottergate (site 149N). Destroyed by a citywide fire in 1507, this row of tenements preserved evidence of the living standards of moderately prosperous Norwich families (see chapters 2 and 4).[3] Helen Sutermeister, a documentary researcher for the Survey, made early inroads into the subject of the health and well-being of Norwich's residents whilst preparing her doctoral thesis (unfinished at her untimely death). Specifically, she addressed the use and development of the city's waterways and cisterns, refuse collection, human remains, sanctions against 'measly' (i.e. leprous) pigs and putrid food, lead-poisoning and the impact of Norwich's housing revolution on living standards.[4] The publication of James Campbell's maps of the medieval city in *The Atlas of Historic Towns* series in 1975 complemented the Survey's work. His legacy is evident in the fact that maps and plans have been situated at the forefront of the subsequent historiography of the city.

[1] Referred to here as *RCN*.

[2] A brief history of the Norwich Survey is given in Atkin and Evans, EAA 100, pp. 1, 235–46, and see A. Carter, 'The Anglo-Saxon Origins of Norwich: The Problems and Approaches', *Anglo-Saxon England* 7 (1978), pp. 175–204 (p. 183).

[3] Atkin, Carter and Evans, EAA 26, pp. 9–85.

[4] Her notes are archived at NRO, MC 146/52 624x4 'Draft: Health etc.', pp. 1–8.

After the cessation of the Norwich Survey, aspects of its research aims were developed by the Norfolk Archaeological Unit (superseded by NAU Archaeology) and by members of the Centre of East Anglian Studies (CEAS) at the University of East Anglia. The subject of 'health and place' has often recurred in publications by both groups. For example, Carole Rawcliffe (CEAS) has examined the social and cultural importance of pollution, exercise through labour, and cleanliness to the medieval ruling elite of Norwich, and has recently published a monograph on the same themes on a national stage for the period 1250–1530.[5] Simultaneously, from evidence of legal documents, the zoning of industry and from tithing rolls, Elizabeth Rutledge has drawn inferences about the damage inflicted by noxious trades upon local air quality and waterways, and about the ease with which infectious diseases may have been transmitted in densely occupied tenements. She has also investigated the nature and layout of the city during the fifteenth century.[6] A two-part collection of essays on Norwich's history and topography consolidates and greatly extends our knowledge of all aspects of life in Norwich,[7] whilst publications on the city's main religious and political establishments – the Benedictine cathedral priory, the Great Hospital, the religious houses and the castle – provide a valuable wider context for the present study.[8] A significant quantity of original source material has been rendered accessible through the efforts of the Norfolk Record Society.[9] Meanwhile, excavations by NAU and NAU Archaeology have revealed evidence of the quality of the urban environment, as well as of medieval industry and domestic

[5] Rawcliffe, 'Health and Safety at Work', pp. 130–51; Rawcliffe, 'Sickness and Health'; Rawcliffe, *Urban Bodies,* and see C. Rawcliffe, *Medicine and Society in Later Medieval England* (Stroud, 1995); Rawcliffe, *MFTS*; Rawcliffe, *Leprosy*.

[6] Rutledge, 'Economic Life', p. 160, map 9 on p. 162, developing and revising Kelly, 'The Economic Topography and Structure of Norwich *c.* 1300', pp. 13–39 (esp. pp. 22–5); Rutledge, 'Landlords and Tenants: Housing and the Rented Property Market in Early Fourteenth-Century Norwich'; Rutledge, 'An Urban Environment: Norwich in the Fifteenth Century'.

[7] *MN*, ed. Rawcliffe and Wilson; *NS1550*, ed. Rawcliffe and Wilson.

[8] Gilchrist, *Norwich Cathedral Close; Norwich Cathedral: Church, City, Diocese 1096–1996*, ed. I. Atherton et al. (London, 1996); Rawcliffe, *MFTS*; Emery, EAA 120; Shepherd Popescu, EAA 132.

[9] *Inter alia,* the records of a landgable (or ground-rent) assessment from 1568–70 published by the NRS is used repeatedly in the present work as a guide to the nature of land use: *Norwich Landgable Assessment 1568–70*, ed. M. Rodgers and M. Wallace, NRS 63 (Norwich, 1999). See also titles edited by John Pound, Claire Noble and Elaine Phillips *op cit.*

arrangements, rubbish and sewage disposal.[10] NAU also excavated the parish cemetery of St Margaret Fyebridge (site 780N), which includes a series of chaotic interments of the city's poor, criminal and sick residents. The findings are used extensively in chapter 3. The analysis presented there would not have been possible without the work of Ann Stirland and Jayne Bown.[11] The revised synthesis of both the material and documentary records by the former county archaeologist for Norfolk, Brian Ayers, provides an incomparable introduction to the city and its physical structures.[12] Finally, the work of the historian Margaret Pelling (which has repeatedly set the agenda for medical historians over the last forty years) includes several treatments of Norwich material. Of most relevance here is a group of articles relating to practitioners, to social policy and poverty, and to water technology.[13]

[10] Ayers, EAA 37; Margeson, EAA 58; Shepherd Popescu EAA 132, I, 479–80, 501, 539; II, 545, 753.

[11] Stirland, EAA 129; Bown and Stirland, 'CAP'.

[12] Ayers, *NAFC*; see also Ayers, 'The Infrastructure of Norwich from the 12th to the 17th Centuries', and other works referenced below.

[13] Pelling and Webster, 'MP'; M. Pelling, 'Healing the Sick Poor: Social Policy and Disability in Norwich, 1550-1640', in Pelling, *CL*, pp. 79–102; Pelling, 'Health and Sanitation to 1750'.

APPENDIX IV: MAP OF NORWICH PARISHES

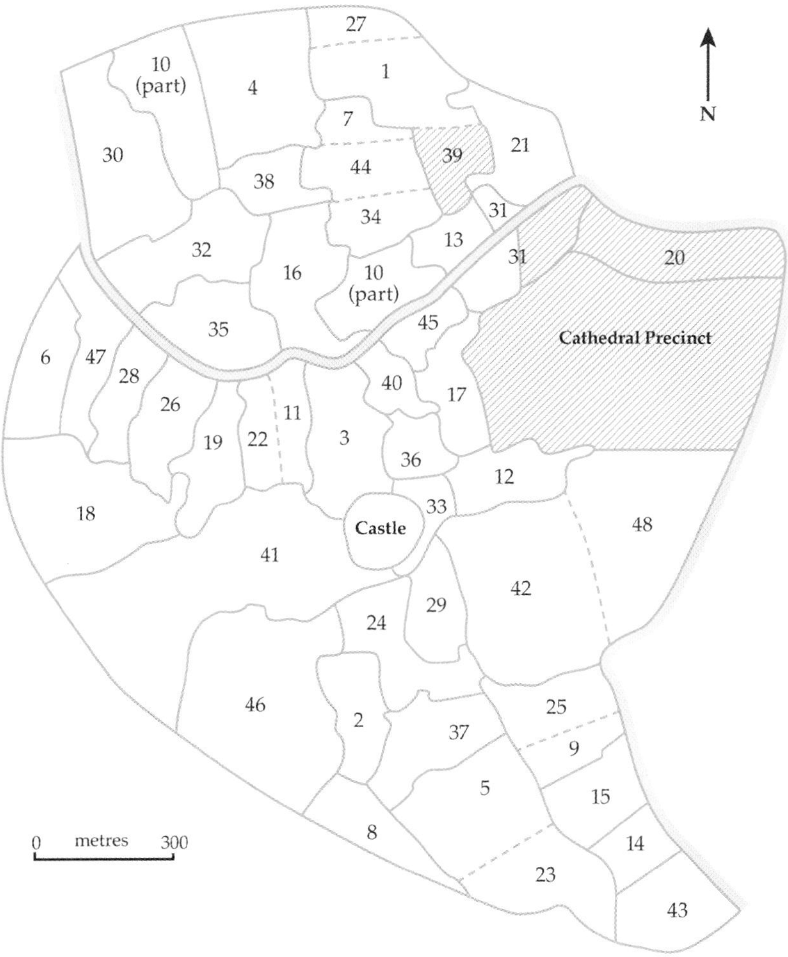

1. All Saints Fyebridge
2. All Saints Timberhill
3. St Andrew
4. St Augustine
5. St Bartholomew
6. St Benedict
7. St Botulph
8. St Catherine
9. St Clement Conesford
10. St Clement Fyebridge
11. St Crouch
12. St Cuthbert
13. St Edmund
14. St Edward
15. St Etheldreda
16. St George Colegate
17. St George Tombland
18. St Giles
19. St Gregory
20. St Helen
21. St James
22. St John Maddermarket
23. St John Sepulchre
24. St John Timberhill
25. St Julian
26. St Lawrence
27. St Margaret Fyebridge
28. St Margaret Westwick
29. St Martin at Bale
30. St Martin at Oak
31. St Martin at Palace
32. St Mary Coslany
33. St Mary the Less
34. St Mary Unbrent
35. St Michael Coslany
36. St Michael at Plea
37. St Michael at Thorn
38. St Olave
39. St Paul
40. St Peter Hungate
41. St Peter Mancroft
42. St Peter Parmentergate
43. St Peter Southgate
44. St Saviour
45. SS Simon and Jude
46. St Stephen
47. St Swithin
48. St Vedast (St Faith)

BIBLIOGRAPHY

Manuscript sources

London, British Library Department of Manuscripts
Add. MS 27582.

London, London Metropolitan Archive, Guildhall Library
MS 9171/18ff.

London, The National Archives
PROB 11/30; 11/32; 11/51.

Norwich, NAU Archaeology
130–2 Magdalean Street Excavation Archive.

Norwich, Norfolk Record Office
COL 13/53.
DCN 70/11 Original Wills 1529–69.
DN/Reg 30 'Tanner's Index' vol. I: Archdeaconry of Norwich and Archdeaconry of Norfolk.
MC 146/52 624x4; 684x5.
NCC will registers Alblaster; Aleyn; Gylys; Jekkys; Multon; Whytefoote.
NCR 3–4 Private Deeds.
NCR 5c/3 Leets before the City Sheriffs.
NCR 5d/1, 4–5, Sheriffs' Tourns, 1541–54.
NCR 10f Portion of a Wall Note *c.* 1550; Draft for the Minutes of an Assembly held 12 August 19 Henry VIII (1527); Liability of Householder to Repair Common Sewers [1726 or 1750].
NCR 16a/5 Mayor's Court Book 1540–49.
NCR 16c/2 Assembly Minute Book 1510–50.
NCR 16d/2 Assembly Proceedings 1491–1553.
NCR 16d/3 Assembly Proceedings 1553–83.
NCR 17b Mayor's Book (Book of Oaths); City Revenues and Letter Book.
NCR 18a/5–8 Chamberlains' Accounts, 1531–37, 1537–47, 1541–49, 1551–67.
NCR 18d Landgable 1 1541–49; Clavors' Book 1 [Hamper] 1550–1601.

NCR 19b River and Streets Accounts 1556–1618.
NCR 20c Mayor's Book of the Poor 1.
NCR 20f/17 Book of Charity Founders Wills 1549–1791.
NCR 22a/4 Agreement Concerning the Supply of Water and Cleaning of the Cockeys (1583).
NCR 22g/1 City Lease Book A 1537–1664.
NCR 24a Archive of the Great Hospital Box of Accounts 1415–60.
NCR 24a Great Hospital Account Rolls 1560–69.
PD 26/110, Account Book of Rents 1569–1641.

Oxford, Bodleian Library
MS Bodley 178.
MS Tanner 397.
MS Tanner 407.
MS Rawlinson C 816.

Printed primary sources

Adams, S. ed., *Household Accounts and Disbursement Books of Robert Dudley, Earl of Leicester, 1558–1561, 1584–86*, Camden 5th series 6 (Cambridge, 1995).
Alberti, Leon Battista, *On the Art of Building in Ten Books*, trans. J. Rykwert, N. Leach and R. Tavernor (Cambridge MA, 1988).
Anon., *Eenen Calendier Historiael* (Norwich: Anthony de Solemne, 1570).
Anon., *The Seynge of Urynes* (London: [J. Rastell for] Richard Banckes, 1525).
Apian, Peter, *Cosmographicus liber* (Landshut: Johann Weissenburger, 1524).
Bartholomaeus Anglicus, *De proprietatibus rerum*, trans. John Trevisa (London: Thomas Berthelet, 1535).
Bartholomaeus Anglicus, *On the Properties of Things: John Trevisa's Translation of Bartholomaeus Anglicus De Proprietatibus Rerum*, ed. M. C. Seymour, 3 vols. (Oxford, 1975–88).
Bartholomaeus Anglicus, *De proprietatibus rerum: Volume I: Introduction générale, Prohemium, et Libri I–IV*, ed. B. Van den Abeele, H. Meyer, M. W. Twomey, B. Roling, R. J. Long, De Diversis Artibus 78, n.s. 41 (Turnhout, 2007).
Bartholomaeus Anglicus, *De proprietatibus rerum: Volume VI: Liber XVII*, ed. I. Ventura, De Diversis Artibus 79, n.s. 42 (Turnhout, 2007).
Boorde, Andrew, *Dyetary of Helth* (London: Robert Wyer, 1542).
Boorde, Andrew, *The Boke for to Learne a Man to be Wyse in Buyldyng of his Howse for the Helth of Body* (London: Robert Wyer, 1550).
Boorde, Andrew, *The Breviary of Healthe* (London: William Powell, 1552).
Brewer, J. S., et al., ed. *Letters and Papers, Foreign and Domestic, Henry VIII*, 21 vols. (London, 1880–91).
Browne, Sir Thomas, *The Religio Medici and Other Writings* (London, 1906).
Bullein, William, *The Governement of Healthe* (London: John Day, 1558).

Bullein, William, *Bullein's Bulwarke of Defence Againste all Sicknes, Sornes and Woundes* (London: John Kyngston, 1562).

Caius, John, *A Boke or Counseill Against the Disease Commonly Called the Sweate or Sweatyng Sicknesse* (London: Richard Grafton, 1552).

Caius, John, *The Works of John Caius, M.D*, ed. E. S. Roberts (Cambridge, 1912).

Calendar of the Patent Rolls Preserved in the Public Record Office, Edward III, 16 vols. (London, 1891–1916).

Calendar of the Patent Rolls Preserved in the Public Record Office, Richard II, 1377–81, 6 vols. (London, 1895–1909).

Calendar of the State Papers Relating to Scotland and Mary, Queen of Scots, 1547–1603: Vol. I. A.D. 1547–1563, ed. J. Bain (Edinburgh, 1898).

Carpenter, John, *Liber albus: The White Book of the City of London*, ed. H. T. Riley (London, 1861).

Chaucer, Geoffrey, *The Love and Complayntes bytwene Mars and Venus* (Westminster: Julian Notary, ?1500).

Copland, Robert, *The Hye Way to the Spyttell Hous* (London: Robert Copland, 1536).

Cuningham [Kenningham], William, *A Newe Almanacke and Prognostication … Made for the Meridian of Norwich and … Serving for All England* (London: John Day, 1557 for 1558).

Cuningham, William, *The Cosmographical Glasse: Conteinyng the Pleasant Principles of Cosmographie, Geographie, Hydrographie or Navigation. Compiled by William Cuningham Doctor in Physicke* (London: John Day, 1559).

Cuningham, William, *A New Almanach and Prognostication … Faithfully Calculated for the Longitude of London and Pole Articke of the Same* (London: Rowland Hall, 1563 for 1564).

Cuningham, William, *A New Almanach and Prognostication … Diligentlye Calculated for the Longytud of London and Pole Articke of the Same* (London: Richard Serll for William Jones, 1565 for 1566).

Davis, N., ed., *Non-Cycle Plays and Fragments Edited on the Basis of the Edition of Osborn Waterhouse*, EETS ES Supplementary Text 1 (London, 1970).

Davis, N., ed., *Paston Letters and Papers of the Fifteenth Century*, 3 vols., EETS SS 20–2 (Oxford, 2004–05).

Dee, John, 'Preface' to Euclid, *Elements of Geometrie*, trans. H. Billingsley (London, 1570).

Digges, Leonard, *A Prognostication of Right Good Effect* (London: Thomas Gemini, 1555).

Dormer Harris, M., ed., *The Coventry Leet Book 1420–1555*, 4 vols., EETS OS 134–5, 138, 146 (London, 1907–13).

Elyot, Thomas, *The Castel of Helthe* (London: Thomas Berthelet, 1539).

Fay, I., ed., 'The Norwich River and Street Accounts, 1557–61 and 1570–80', in *Health and Hygiene in Early Modern Norwich*, ed. E. Phillips and I. Fay, Norfolk Record Society 77 (Norwich, 2013), pp. 105–200.

Fine, Oronce, *Protomathesis* (Paris: Gerard Morrhy and Jean Pierre, 1532).
Fine, Oronce, *De mundi sphaera, sive cosmographia* (Paris: Michel de Vascosan, 1555).
Fortescue, John, *De laudibus legum Anglie*, ed. and trans. S. B. Chrimes (Cambridge, 1949).
Fulke, William, *Antiprognosticon* (London: Henry Sutton, 1560).
Gale, Thomas, *Certaine Workes of Chirurgerie* (London: Rowland Hall, 1563).
Galen, *A Translation of Galen's Hygiene (De sanitate tuenda)*, trans. R. M. Green (Springfield, 1951).
Galen, *Galen: Selected Works*, trans. P. N. Singer (Oxford, 1997).
Galloway, D., ed., *Records of Early English Drama: Norwich 1540–1642* (London, 1984).
Grace, M. ed., *Records of the Gild of St George in Norwich, 1389–1547*, Norfolk Record Society 9 (Norwich, 1937).
Halle, John, ed., *A Most Excellent and Learned Woorke of Chirurgerie, called Chirurgia parua Lanfranci* (London: Thomas Marshe, 1565).
Hippocrates of Cos, *De natura hominis* (Rome: Georg Herolt, *c.* 1481).
Hippocrates of Cos, *Hippocratis octoginta volumina* (Rome: ex aedibus Francisci Minitii Calvi, 1525).
Hippocrates of Cos, *Hippocratis coi medicorum omnium longe principis, opera quae ad nos extant omnia*, trans. Janus Cornarius (Basel: Hieronymus Froben and Nicolaus Episcopius, 1546).
Hippocrates of Cos, *Hippocrates: Volume IV*, trans. W. H. S. Jones (Cambridge, MA, 1931).
Hippocrates of Cos, *Hippocratic Writings*, ed. G. E. R. Lloyd (London, 1978).
Hippocrates of Cos, *Airs, eaux, lieux*, ed. J. Jouanna (Paris, 1996).
Hudson, W., ed., *Leet Jurisdiction in the City of Norwich during the XIIIth and XIVth Centuries*, Selden Society 5 (London, 1892).
Hudson, W., and J. C. Tingey, ed., *The Records of the City of Norwich*, 2 vols. (Norwich, 1906–10).
Hutten, Ulrich von, *De morbo Gallico*, trans. Thomas Paynell (London: Thomas Berthelet, 1533).
Johnson, G., ed., 'Chronological Memoranda Touching the City of Norwich', *Norfolk Archaeology* 1 (1847), 140–66.
Knutsson, Bengt (attrib.), *Here Begynneth a Litill Boke Necessarye and Behovefull Agenst the Pestilence* (London: William de Machlinia, *c.* 1485).
Knutsson, Bengt (attrib.), *A Moche Profitable Treatise against the Pestilence*, trans. Thomas Paynell (London: Thomas Berthelet, 1534).
Luders, A., T. E. Tomlins, J. France, W. E. Taunton and J. Raithby, ed., *Statutes of the Realm, from Original Records and Authentic Manuscripts (1101–1713)*, 11 vols. (London, 1810–28).
Lydgate, John, *The Hystorye, Sege and Dystruccyon of Troye* (London: Richard Pynson, 1513).

Lydgate, John, *The Minor Poems of John Lydgate*, ed. H. N. MacCracken, 2 vols., EETS OS 192 (London, 1911).
Lydgate, John, *Mummings and Entertainments*, ed. C. Sponsler (Kalamazoo, 2010).
Lydgate, John, and John of Burgundy, *In this Tretyse that is Cleped Governayle of Helthe* (Westminster: William Caxton, 1490).
Lydgate, John, and John of Burgundy, *Here Begynneth a Lytell Treatyse called the Governall of Helthe with the Medycyne of the Stomacke* (London: Wynkyn de Worde, *c.* 1506).
Manship, Henry, *The History of Great Yarmouth*, ed. C. J. Palmer (Great Yarmouth, 1854).
Marshall, William, *The Forme and Maner of Subvention or Helpyng for Pore People* (London: Thomas Godfray, 1535).
Mediolano, Joannes de, *Regimen sanitatis Salerni*, trans. Thomas Paynell (London: Thomas Berthelet, 1528).
More, Thomas, *A Fruteful and Pleasaunt Worke of the Beste State of a Publyque Weale and of the newe Yle called Utopia*, trans. Raphe Robynson (London: Abraham Vele, 1551).
Neville, Alexander, *De furoribus Norfolciensium Ketto duce, liber unus; eiusdem Norvicus* (London: Henry Binneman, 1575).
Newton, Thomas, *Approoved Medicines and Cordiall Receiptes with the Natures, Qualities and Operations of Sundry Simples* (London: Thomas Marshe, 1580).
Noble, C. ed., 'Norwich Cathedral Priory Gardeners' Accounts, 1329–1530', *Farming and Gardening in Late Medieval Norfolk*, ed. C. Noble, C. E. Moreton and P. Rutledge, Norfolk Record Society 61 (Norwich, 1997), pp. 1–93.
Owen, D. M., ed., *The Making of King's Lynn: A Documentary Survey*, Records of Social and Economic History, new series 9 (London, 1984).
Phillips, E., ed., 'Account Rolls of The Great Hospital, Norwich, 1549–50 and 1570–71', *Health and Hygiene in Early Modern Norwich*, ed. E. Phillips and I. Fay, Norfolk Record Society 77 (Norwich, 2013), pp. 1–99.
Pound, J., ed., *The Norwich Census of the Poor, 1570*, Norfolk Record Society 40 (Norwich, 1971).
Ptolemy, Claudius, *Ptolemy's Geography: An Annotated Translation of the Theoretical Chapters*, ed. J. L. Berggren and A. Jones (Princeton, 2000).
Recorde, Robert, *The Castle of Knowledge* (London: Reginald Wolfe, 1556).
Reynes, Robert, *The Commonplace Book of Robert Reynes of Acle: An Edition of Tanner MS. 407*, ed. C. Louis (New York, 1980).
Riley, H. T., ed., *Memorials of London and London Life, 1276–1419* (London, 1868).
Rodgers, M., and M. Wallace, ed., *Norwich Landgable Assessment 1568–70*, Norfolk Record Society 63 (Norwich, 1999).
Sharpe, R. R., ed., *Calendar of Letter-Books of the City of London, 1275–1498, Books A-L*, 11 vols. (London, 1899–1912).

Skelton, John, *The Poetical Works of John Skelton*, ed. A. Dyce, 2 vols. (London, 1843).
Smith, William, *The Particular Description of England, 1588*, ed. H. B. Wheatley (London, 1879).
Starkey, Thomas, *A Dialogue Between Pole and Lupset*, ed. T. F. Mayer, Camden Society fourth series 37 (London, 1989).
Strachey, J. et al., ed., *Rotuli Parliamentorum*, 6 vols. (London, 1767–77).
Thomas, A. H., and P. E. Jones, ed., *Calendar of Plea and Memoranda Rolls Preserved Among the Archives of the Corporation of the City of London*, 6 vols. (Cambridge, 1926–61).
Tingey, J. C. ed., 'The Hitherto Unpublished Certificates of Norwich Gilds', *Norfolk Archaeology* 16 (1907), 267–305.
Wakefield, W. L., and A. P. Evans, ed., *Heresies of the High Middle Ages: Selected Sources Translated and Annotated* (New York, 1969).
Williams, C., ed., *The Barber-Surgeons of Norwich* (Norwich, 1896).
Young, S., ed., *The Annals of the Barber-Surgeons of London* (London, 1890).

Secondary sources

Addyman, P. V., 'The Archaeology of Public Health at York, England', *World Archaeology* 21 (1989), 244–63.
Agarwal, S. C., and B. A. Glencross, ed., *Social Bioarchaeology* (Oxford, 2011).
Albala, K., *Eating Right in the Renaissance* (Berkeley, 2002).
Allison, K. J., 'The Norfolk Worsted Industry in the Sixteenth and Seventeenth Centuries [Part] 1', *Bulletin of Economic Research* 12 (1960), 73–83.
Ames, J., W. Herbert and T. F. Dibdin, *Typographical Antiquities: The History of Printing in England, Scotland and Ireland*, 4 vols. (London, 1810–19).
Anderson, T., 'A Medieval Bladder Stone from Norwich, Norfolk', *International Journal of Osteoarchaeology* 13 (2003), 165–7.
Arrizabalaga, J., J. Henderson and R. French, *The Great Pox: The French Disease in Renaissance Europe* (New Haven, 1997).
Arrizabalaga, J., 'Problematizing Retrospective Diagnosis in the History of Disease', *Asclepio* 54 (2002), 51–70.
Atherton, I., E. Fernie, C. Harper-Bill and H. Smith, ed., *Norwich Cathedral: Church, City, Diocese 1096–1996* (London, 1996).
Atkin, M., 'The Chalk Tunnels of Norwich', *Norfolk Archaeology* 38 (1983), 313–20.
Atkin, M., A. Carter and D. H. Evans, ed., *Excavations in Norwich 1971–1978: Part II*, East Anglian Archaeology 26 (Norwich, 1985).
Atkin, M., and D. H. Evans, ed., *Excavations in Norwich 1971–1978: Part III*, East Anglian Archaeology 100 (Norwich, 2002).
Austin, D., 'The "Proper Study" of Medieval Archaeology', in *From the Baltic to the Black Sea: Studies in Medieval Archaeology*, ed. D. Austin and L. Alcock (London, 1990), pp. 9– 42.

Ayers, B., *Excavations at St. Martin-at-Palace Plain, Norwich, 1981*, East Anglian Archaeology 37 (Dereham, 1987).

Ayers, B., 'Building a Fine City: The Provision of Flint, Mortar and Freestone in Medieval Norwich', in *Stone: Quarrying and Building in England, AD 43–1525*, ed. D. Parsons (Chichester, 1990), pp. 217–27.

Ayers, B., 'Norwich: A City and its Image', in *East Anglian Studies: Essays Presented to J. C. Barringer on his Retirement*, ed. A Longcroft and R. Joby (Norwich, 1995), pp. 1–10.

Ayers, B., 'The Infrastructure of Norwich from the 12th to the 17th Centuries', *Lübecker Kolloquium zur Stadtarchäologie im Hanseraum IV: Die Infrastruktur*, ed. M. Gläser (Lübeck, 2004), pp. 31–40.

Ayers, B., 'The Urban Landscape', *Medieval Norwich*, ed. C. Rawcliffe and R. Wilson (London, 2004), pp. 1–28.

Ayers, B., *Norwich: Archaeology of A Fine City* (Stroud, 2009).

Bailey, B. J., J. T. Johnson and S. D. Newlands, *Head and Neck Surgery: Otolaryngology*, 2 vols., 4th edn (Philadelphia, 2006).

Bassett, S., ed., *Death in Towns: Urban Responses to the Dying and the Dead, 100–1600* (Leicester, 1992).

Bates, D., and R. Liddiard, ed., *East Anglia and its North Sea World in the Middle Ages* (Woodbridge, 2013).

Beeching, H. C., and M. Rhodes James, 'The Library of the Cathedral Church of Norwich', *Norfolk Archaeology* 19 (1917), 67–116.

Bensly, W. T., 'St Leonard's Priory, Norwich', *Norfolk Archaeology* 12 (1895), 190–227.

Biller, P., 'Medicine and Heresy', in *Religion and Medicine in the Middle Ages*, ed. P. Biller and J. Ziegler, York Studies in Medieval Theology 3 (York, 2001), pp. 155–74.

Biller, P., 'Proto-Racial Thought in Medieval Science', *The Origins of Racism in the West*, ed. M. Eliav-Feldon, B. Isaac and J. Ziegler (Cambridge, 2009), pp. 157–80.

Bindoff, S. T., ed., *The History of Parliament: The House of Commons 1509–1558*, 3 vols. (London, 1982).

Blomefield, F., *An Essay Towards a Topographical History of the County of Norfolk*, 11 vols. (London, 1805–10).

Boldsen, J. L., and L. Mollerup, 'Outside St Jørgen: Leprosy in the Medieval Danish City of Odense', *American Journal of Physical Anthropology* 130 (2006), 344–351.

Bollingbrook, L. G., 'St John Maddermarket, Norwich: Its Streets, Lanes and Ancient Houses and their Old-Time Associations', *Norfolk Archeaology* 20 (1921), 215–39.

Bühler, C. F., 'A Middle English Medical Manuscript from Norwich', in *Studies in Medieval Literature in Honor of Albert Croll Baugh*, ed. M. Leach (Philadelphia, 1961), pp. 285–98.

Buzon, M. R., 'The Bioarchaeological Approach to Palaeopathology', in *A Companion to Paleopathology*, ed. A. L. Grauer (Chichester, 2012) pp. 58–75.

Campbell, J., 'Norwich', in *The Atlas of Historic Towns: Volume II*, ed. M. Lobel (London, 1975).

Campbell, J., 'Norwich before 1300', in *Medieval Norwich*, ed. C. Rawcliffe and R. Wilson (London, 2004), pp. 29–48.

Capp, B., *Astrology and the Popular Press: English Almanacs 1500–1800* (London, 1979).

Carter, A., 'The Anglo-Saxon Origins of Norwich: The Problems and Approaches', *Anglo-Saxon England* 7 (1978), 175–204.

Cavallo, S., *Charity and Power in Early Modern Italy: Benefactors and their Motives in Turin, 1541–1789* (Cambridge, 1995).

Cavallo, S., and D. Gentilcore, ed. *Spaces, Objects and Identities in Early Modern Italian Medicine, Renaissance Studies* 21 (1998).

Cavallo, S., and T. Storey, *Healthy Living in Late Renaissance Italy* (Oxford, 2013).

Chrimes, S. B., *English Constitutional Ideas in the Fifteenth Century* (Cambridge, 1936).

Cipolla, C. M., *Public Health and the Medical Profession in the Renaissance* (Cambridge, 1976).

Clark, P., 'Improvement, Policy and Tudor Towns', *Authority and Consent in Tudor England: Essays Presented to* C. *S. L. Davies*, ed. G. W. Bernard and S. J. Gunn (Aldershot, 2002), pp. 233–47.

Conheeney, J., 'The Human Bone', in C. Thomas, B. Sloane and C. Phillpotts, *Excavations at the Priory and Hospital of St Mary Spital, London*, Museum of London Archaeology Service Monograp. 1 (London, 1997).

Cooper, C. H., T. Cooper and G. J. Gray, *Athenae Cantabrigienses*, 3 vols. (Cambridge, 1858–1913).

Cozens-Hardy, B., and E. A. Kent, *The Mayors of Norwich, 1403 to 1835, Being Bibliographical Notes on the Mayors of the Old Corporation* (Norwich, 1938).

Creelman, V., '"Ryght Worchepfull Mastres": Letters of Request and Servants' Scripting of Margaret Paston's Social Self', *Parergon* 26 (2009), 91–113.

Cunningham, A., 'Identifying Disease in the Past: Cutting the Gordian Knot', *Asclepio* 54 (2002), 13–34.

Cunningham, A., *The Identity of the History of Science and Medicine* (Farnham, 2012).

Curtis, R., B. Elton, J. Lloyd and R. Atkinson, *Blackadder: The Whole Damn Dynasty* (London, 1998).

Darley, G., 'John Evelyn's Norwich Garden', *Garden History* 34 (2006), 249–53.

Debus, A. G., 'The Paracelsian Compromise in Elizabethan England', *Ambix* 8 (1960), 71–97.

Dixon, T., *From Passions to Emotions: The Creation of a Secular Psychological Category* (Cambridge, 2003).

Dorey, M., 'Controlling Corruption: Regulating Meat Consumption as a Preventative to Plague in Seventeenth-Century London', *Urban History* 36 (2009), 24–41.

Douglas, M., *Purity and Danger: An Analysis of Concepts of Pollution and Taboo* (London, 1966).

Duffy, E., *The Voices of Morebath: Reformation and Rebellion in an English Village* (New Haven, 2001).

Dunn, P., 'Trade', in *Medieval Norwich*, ed. C. Rawlcliffe and R. Wilson (London, 2004), pp. 213–34.

Dutka, J., 'The Lost Dramatic Cycle of Norwich and the Grocers' Play of the Fall of Man', *Review of English Studies* 35 (1984), 1–13.

Dyer, A., *Decline and Growth in English Towns, 1400–1640* (Cambridge, 1995).

Dyer, C., *Standards of Living in the Later Middle Ages: Social Change in England c. 1200–1520*, 2nd edn (Cambridge, 1998).

Dyer, A., 'Appendix: Ranking Lists of English Medieval Towns', in *The Cambridge Urban History of Britain*, ed. D. M. Palliser, 3 vols. (Cambridge, 2000), I, 747–70.

Ekholm, K., 'Anatomy, Bloodletting and Emblems: Interpreting the Title-Page of Nathaniel Highmore's *Disquisitio* (1651)', in *Observing the World Through Images: Diagrams and Figures in the Early-Modern Arts and Sciences*, ed. N. Jardine and I. Fay (Leiden, 2014), pp. 87–123.

Elton, G. R., 'An Early-Tudor Poor Law', *Economic History Review*, 2nd s. 6 (1953), 55–67.

Elton, G. R., *Reform and Renewal: Thomas Cromwell and the Common Weal* (Cambridge, 1973).

Emery, P. A., *Norwich Greyfriars: Pre-Conquest Town and Medieval Friary*, East Anglian Archaeology 120 (Dereham, 2007).

Evenden, E., *Patents, Pictures and Patronage: John Day and the Tudor Book Trade* (Aldershot, 2008).

Fay, I., 'Text, Space and the Evidence of Human Remains in English Late Medieval and Tudor Disease Culture: Some Problems and Possibilities', in *Social Archaeology of Funerary Remains*, ed. R. Gowland and C. Knüsel (Oxford, 2006) pp. 190–208.

Finch, J., 'The Churches', in *Medieval Norwich*, ed. C. Rawcliffe and R. Wilson (London, 2004), pp. 49–72.

Fiorato, V., A. Boylston and C. Knüsel, ed., *Blood Red Roses: The Archaeology of a Mass Grave from the Battle of Towton, AD 1461* (Oxford, 2000).

Fitch, R., 'Norwich Pageants: The Grocers' Play', *Norfolk Archaeology* 5 (1859), 8–31.

Frost, R., 'The Urban Elite', in *Medieval Norwich*, ed. C. Rawcliffe and R. Wilson (London, 2004), pp. 235–53.

Frostick, R., *The Printed Plans of Norwich, 1558–1840: A Carto-Bibliography* (Norwich, 2002).

Furnivall, F. J., 'Forewords', in *The Fyrst Boke of the Introduction of Knowledge*, ed. F. J. Furnivall. EETS ES 10 (London, 1870), pp. 11–110.

Gage, F., 'Exercise for Mind and Body: Giulio Mancini, Collecting, and the Beholding of Landscape Painting in the Seventeenth Century', *Renaissance Quarterly* 61 (2008), 1167–207.

Garibaldi, C., 'The Guildhall of the Norwich Company of Goldsmiths', in *East Anglian Silver 1550–1750*, ed. C. Hartop (Cambridge, 2004) pp. 31–5.

Getz, F. M., 'Medical Practitioners in Medieval England', *Social History of Medicine* 3 (1990), 245–83.

Gilchrist, R., 'Christian Bodies and Souls: The Archaeology of Life and Death in Later Medieval Hospitals', in *Death in Towns: Urban Responses to the Dying and the Dead, 100–1600*, ed. S. Bassett (Leicester, 1992) pp. 101–18.

Gilchrist, R., 'Medieval Bodies in the Material World: Gender, Stigma and the Body', *Framing Medieval Bodies*, ed. S. Kay and M. Rubin (Manchester, 1994) pp. 43–61.

Gilchrist, R., *Norwich Cathedral Close: The Evolution of the English Cathedral Landscape* (Woodbridge, 2005).

Gilchrist, R., *Medieval Life: Archaeology and the Life Course* (Woodbridge, 2012).

Gilchrist, R. and B. Sloane, *Requiem: The Medieval Monastic Cemetery in Britain* (London, 2005).

Giles, K., 'Framing Labour: The Archaeology of York's Medieval Guildhalls', in *The Problem of Labour in Fourteenth-Century England*, ed. J. Bothwell, P. J. P. Goldberg and W. M. Ormrod. (York, 2000), pp. 65–83.

Gittings, C., *Death, Burial and the Individual in Early Modern England* (London, 1984).

Goldberg, P. J. P., 'Pigs and Prostitutes: Streetwalking in Comparative Perspective', in *Young Medieval Women*, ed. K. J. Lewis, N. J. Menuge and K. M. Philips (Stroud, 1999), pp. 172–93.

Goldberg, P. J. P., 'Coventry's "Lollard" Programme of 1492 and the Making of *Utopia*', in *Pragmatic Utopias: Ideals and Communities 1200–1630*, ed. R. Horrox and S. Rees Jones (Cambridge, 2001), pp. 97–116.

Goldberg, P. J. P., 'Migration, Youth and Gender in Later Medieval England', in *Youth in the Middle Ages*, ed. P. J. P Goldberg and F. Riddy (York, 2004), pp. 85–99.

Gordon, B., and Marshall, P., ed., *The Place of the Dead: Death and Remembrance in Late Medieval and Early Modern Europe* (Cambridge, 2000).

Gowland, R., 'The Social Identity of Health in Late Roman Britain', in *TRAC 2003: Proceedings of the Thirteenth Annual Theoretical Archaeology Conference*, ed. B. Croxford, H. Eckhardt, J. Meade and J. Weekes (Oxford, 2004) pp. 135–46.

Grafton, A., *Cardano's Cosmos: The Worlds and Works of a Renaissance Astrologer* (Cambridge MA, 1999).

Grainger, I., D. Hawkins, L. Cowal and R. Mikulski, *The Black Death Cemetery, East Smithfield, London*, Museum of London Archaeology Service Monograph. 43 (London, 2008).

Grauer, A. L., 'Patterns of Life and Death: The Palaeodemography of Medieval York', in *Health in Past Societies. Biocultural Interpretations of Human Skeletal Remains in Archaeological Contexts*, ed. H. Bush and M. Zevelebil. British Archaeological Reports, International Series 567 (Oxford, 1991), pp. 67–80.

Grauer, A. L., and C. Roberts, 'Paleoepidemiology, Healing and Possible Treatment of Trauma in the Medieval Cemetery Population of St. Helen-on-the-Walls, York, England', *American Journal of Physical Anthropology* 100 (1996), 531–44.

Greatrex, J., 'Monk Students from Norwich Cathedral Priory at Oxford and Cambridge, *c*. 1300 to 1530', *English Historical Review* 106 (1991), 555–83.

Greatrex, J., 'The Almonary School of Norwich Cathedral Priory in the Thirteenth and Fourteenth Centuries', in *The Church and Childhood*, ed. D. Wood, Studies in Church History 31 (Oxford, 1994), pp. 169–81.

Greatrex, J., *Biographical Register of the English Cathedral Priories of the Province of Canterbury, c. 1066–1540* (Oxford, 1997).

Greatrex, J., 'Horoscopes and Healing at Norwich Cathedral Priory in the later Middle Ages', in *The Church and Learning in Later Medieval Society: Essays in Honour of R. B. Dobson*, ed. C. M. Barron and J. Stratford, Harlaxton Medieval Studies 11 (Donington, 2002), pp. 170–7.

Green, M., 'Integrative Medicine: Incorporating Medicine and Health into the Canon of Medieval European History', *History Compass* 7 (2009), 1218–45.

Grieg, J., 'The Investigation of a Medieval Barrel-Latrine from Worcester', *Journal of Archaeological Science* 8 (1981), 265–82.

Griffiths, P., 'Masterless Young People in Norwich, 1560–1645', in *The Experience of Authority in Early Modern England*, ed. P. Griffiths, A. Fox and S. Hindle (Basingstoke, 1996), pp. 146–86.

Griffiths, P., 'Inhabitants', in *Norwich Since 1550*, ed. C. Rawcliffe and R. Wilson (London, 2004) pp. 63–88.

Guy, J. R., 'The Episcopal Licensing of Physicians, Surgeons and Midwives', *Bulletin of the History of Medicine* 56 (1982), 528–42.

Harding, V., 'Whose Body? A Study of Attitudes Towards the Dead Body in Early Modern Paris', *The Place of the Dead: Death and Remembrance in Late Medieval and Early Modern Europe*, ed. B. Gordon and P. Marshall (Cambridge, 2000) pp. 170–87.

Harding, V., *The Dead and the Living in Paris and London, 1500–1670* (Cambridge, 2002).

Harley, D., 'Rhetoric and the Social Construction of Sickness and Healing', *Social History of Medicine* 12 (1999), 407–35.

Harley, J. B., 'Meaning and Ambiguity in Tudor Cartography', in *English Map-Making, 1500–1650*, ed. S. Tyacke (London, 1982), pp. 22–45.

Harper, K. N., M. K. Zuckerman, M. L. Harper, J. D. Kingston and G. J. Armelagos, 'The Origin and Antiquity of Syphilis Revisited: An Appraisal of Old World Pre-Columbian Evidence for Treponemal Infection', *Yearbook of Physical Anthropology* 54 (2011), 99–133.

Harper-Bill, C., and C. Rawcliffe, 'The Religious Houses', in *Medieval Norwich*, ed. C. Rawcliffe and R. Wilson (London, 2004), pp. 73–119.

Harris, J. G., *Foreign Bodies and the Body Politic: Discourses of Social Pathology in Early Modern England* (Cambridge, 1998).

Harvey, J., *Medieval Gardens* (London, 1981).

Harvey, P. D. A., *Maps in Tudor England* (London, 1993).

Hawes, T., *An Index to Norwich City Officers, 1453–1835*, Norfolk Record Society 52 (Norwich, 1989).

Hawkins, J., 'Sights for Sore Eyes: Vision and Health in Medieval England', in *On Light*, ed. K. P. Clarke and S. Baccianti (Oxford, 2013) pp. 137–56.

Henderson, J., 'The Black Death in Florence: Medical and Communal Responses', in *Death in Towns: Urban Responses to the Dying and the Dead, 100–1600*, ed. S. Bassett (Leicester, 1992), pp. 136–50.

Henderson, J., 'Public Health, Pollution and the Problem of Waste Disposal in Early Modern Tuscany', in *Economic and Biological Interactions in Pre-industrial Europe from the Thirteenth to the Eighteenth Centuries*, ed. S. Cavaciocchi (Florence, 2010), pp. 373–82.

Henderson, J., 'Coping with Epidemics in Renaissance Italy: Plague and the Great Pox', in *The Fifteenth Century XII: Society in an Age of Plague*, ed. L. Clark and C. Rawcliffe (Woodbridge, 2013), pp. 175–93.

Heninger, S. K., *The Cosmographical Glass: Renaissance Diagrams of the Universe* (San Marino, 1977).

Henrey, B., *British Botanical and Horticultural Literature Before 1800*, 3 vols. (Oxford, 1975).

Hill, C., *Women and Religion in Late Medieval Norwich* (Woodbridge, 2010).

Hoggett, R., *The Archaeology of the East Anglian Conversion* (Woodbridge, 2010).

Holbrook, S. E., 'A Medieval Scientific Encyclopaedia "Renewed by Goodly Printing": Wynkyn de Worde's English "De proprietatibus rerum"', *Early Science and Medicine* 3 (1998), 119–55.

Höltgen, K. J., 'Sir Robert Dallington (1561–1637): Author, Traveler and Pioneer of Taste', *Huntington Library Quarterly* 47 (1984), 147–77.

Horden, P., 'The Millennium Bug: Health and Medicine around the Year 1000', *Social History of Medicine* 13 (2000), 201–19.

Horden, P. , 'Ritual and Public Health in the Early Medieval City', in *Body and City: Histories of Urban Public Health*, ed. S. Sheard and H. Power (Aldershot, 2000), pp. 17–40.

Houlbrooke, R., and McClendon, M., 'The Reformation', in *Medieval Norwich*, ed. C. Rawcliffe and R. Wilson (London, 2004), pp. 255–76.

Hudson, W., 'The "Norwich Taxation" of 1254, so far as Relates to the Diocese of Norwich', *Norfolk Archaeology* 17 (1910), 46–155.

Humphreys, K. W., ed., *The Friars' Libraries*. Corpus of British Medieval Library Catalogues (London, 1990).

Hurst, J. G., and J. Golson, 'Excavations at St Benedict's Gates, Norwich, 1951 and 1953', *Norfolk Archaeology* 31 (1957), 1–112.

James, M., 'Ritual, Drama and Social Body in the Late Medieval English Town', *Past and Present* 98 (1983), 3–29.

Jenner, M., 'The Politics of London Air: John Evelyn's *Fumifugium* and the Restoration', *The Historical Journal* 38 (1995), 535–51.

Jenner, M. S. R., 'The Great Dog Massacre', *Fear in Early Modern Society*, ed. W. G. Naphy and P. Roberts (Manchester, 1997), pp. 44–61.

Jenner, M., 'Underground, Overground: Pollution and Place in Urban History: Review Essay', *Journal of Urban History* 24 (1997), 97–110.

Jenner, M., 'From Conduit Community to Commercial Network? Water in London, 1500–1725', in *Londonopolis: Essays in the Cultural and Social History of Early Modern London*, ed. P. Griffiths (Manchester, 2000), pp. 250–72.

Jenner, M., 'Environment, Health and Population', in *The Healing Arts: Health, Disease and Society in Europ. 1500–1800*, ed. P. Elmer (Manchester, 2004), pp. 284–314.

Johnson, F. R., '*A Newe Herball of Macer* and Banckes's *Herbal*: Notes on Robert Wyer and the Printing of Cheap Handbooks of Science in the Sixteenth Century', *Bulletin of the History of Medicine* 15 (1944), 246–60.

Jørgensen, D., 'Cooperative Sanitation: Managing Streets and Gutters in Late Medieval England and Scandinavia', *Technology and Culture* 49 (2008), 547–67.

Jørgensen, D., ' "All Good Rule of the Citee": Sanitation and Civic Government in England, 1400–1600', *Journal of Urban History* 36 (2010), 300–15.

Jurkowski, M., ed., 'Income Tax Assessments of Norwich, 1472 and 1489', in *Poverty and Wealth: Sheep, Taxation and Charity in Late Medieval Norfolk*, ed. M. Bailey, M. Jurkowski and C. Rawcliffe, Norfolk Record Society 71 (Norwich, 2007), pp. 99–156.

Kassell, L., *Medicine and Magic in Elizabethan London: Simon Forman: Astrologer, Alchemist and Physician* (Oxford, 2005).

Kassell, L., 'Almanacs and Prognostications', in *The Oxford History of Popular Print Culture, Volume One: Cheap Print in Britain and Ireland to 1660*, ed. J. Raymond (Oxford, 2011), pp. 431–42.

Keene, D., 'The Medieval Urban Environment in Documentary Records', *Archives* 16 (1983), 137–44.

Keene, D., 'Issues of Water in Medieval London to *c.* 1300', *Urban History* 28 (2001), 161–79.

Keiser, G. R., *A Manual of the Writings in Middle English 1050–1500: Vol. 10, Works of Science and Information* (New Haven, 1998).

Keiser, G. R., 'Two Medieval Plague Treatises and Their Afterlife in Early Modern England', *Journal of the History of Medicine and Allied Sciences* 58 (2003), 292–324.

Kelly, S., 'The Economic Topography and Structure of Norwich *c.* 1300', in *Men of Property: An Analysis of the Norwich Enrolled Deeds 1285–1311*, ed. U. Priestly (Norwich, 1983), pp. 12–21.

Kent, E. A., 'The Houses of the Dukes of Norfolk in Norwich', *Norfolk Archaeology* 24 (1932), 73–87.

Kibre, P., 'Hippocratic Writings in the Middle Ages', *Bulletin of the History of Medicine* 18 (1945), 371–412.

King, C., 'The Interpretation of Urban Buildings: Power, Memory and Appropriation in Norwich Merchants' Houses, *c.* 1400–1660', *World Archaeology* 41 (2009), 471–88.

Kirkpatrick, John, *The Streets and Lanes of the City of Norwich*, ed. W. Hudson (Norwich, 1889).

Knüsel, C. J., 'Orthopaedic Disability: Some Hard Evidence', in *Disability and Archaeology*, ed. N. Finlay, *Archaeological Review from Cambridge* 15 (1999), 31–53.

Knüsel, C. J., and S. Göggel, 'A Cripple from the Medieval Hospital of Sts James and Mary Magdalen, Chichester', *International Journal of Osteoarchaeology* 3 (1993), 155–65.

Knüsel, C. J., R. L. Kemp and P. Budd, 'Evidence for Remedial Medical Treatment of a Severe Knee Injury from Fishergate Gilbertine Monastery in the City of York', *Journal of Archaeological Science* 22 (1995), 369–84.

Kohnen, T., 'Commonplace-Book Communication: Role Shifts and Text Functions in Robert Reynes's Notes Contained in MS Tanner 407', in *Communicating Early English Manuscripts*, ed. P. Pahta and A. H. Jucker (Cambridge, 2011), pp. 13–24.

Kosak, J. C., '*Polis nosousa*: Greek Ideas about the City and Disease in the fifth century BC', in *Death and Disease in the Ancient City*, ed. V. M. Hope and E. Marshall (London, 2000), pp. 35–54.

Kurath, H., and S. M. Kuhn, ed., *Middle English Dictionary* (Ann Arbor, 1952–2001).

Kusukawa, S., 'Aspectio divinorum operum: Melanchthon and Astrology for Lutheran Medics', in *Medicine and the Reformation*, ed. O. P Grell and A. Cunningham (London, 1993), pp. 33–56.

Kusukawa, S., 'Andreas Nolthius's *Almanach* for 1575', *Journal for the History of Astronomy* 42 (2011), 91–110.

Land, K. van 't, 'Internal Yet Extrinsic: Conceptions of Bodily Space and their Relation to Causality in Late Medieval University Medicine', in *Medicine and Space: Body, Surroundings and Borders in Antiquity and the Middle Ages*, ed. P. A. Baker, H. Nijdam and K. van 't Land (Leiden, 2012), pp. 85–116.

Landsberg, S., *The Medieval Garden* (London, *c.* 1995).

Leader, D. R., V. Morgan and P. Searby, *A History of the University of Cambridge*, 4 vols. (Cambridge, 1988–2004).

Leong, E., 'Collecting Knowledge for the Family: Recipes, Gender and Practical Knowledge in the Early Modern English Household', *Centaurus* 55 (2013), 81–103.

L'Estrange, J., ed., *The Eastern Counties Collectanea* (Norwich, 1872–73).

Lewis, M., *Urbanisation and Child Health in Medieval and Post-Medieval England*, British Archaeological Reports, British Series 339 (Oxford, 2002).

Linnell, C. L. S., 'The Commonplace Book of Robert Reynys of Acle', *Norfolk Archaeology* 32 (1962), 111–27.

Maddern, P. 'Order and Disorder', in *Medieval Norwich*, ed. C. Rawcliffe and R. Wilson (London, 2004), pp. 189–212.

Magilton, J., and F. Lee, 'The Leper Hospital of St James and St Mary Magdalene, Chichester', in *Burial Archaeology: Current Research, Methods and Developments*, ed. C. A. Roberts, F. Lee and J. Bintliff, British Archaeological Reports, British Series 211 (Oxford, 1989), pp. 249–65.

Magilton, J., F. Lee and A. Boylston, *Lepers Outside the Gate: Excavations at the Cemetery of the Hospital of St James and St Mary Magdalene, Chichester, 1986–87 and 1993*, Council for British Archaeology Research Report 158 (York, 2008).

Magnusson, R. J., *Water Technology in the Middle Ages: Cities, Monasteries and Waterworks after the Roman Empire* (London, 2001).

Maloney, G., and R. Savoie, *Cinq cents ans de bibliographie Hippocratique 1473–1982* (Quebec, 1982).

Manchester, K., 'Infective Bone Changes in Leprosy', *The Past and Present of Leprosy: Archaeological, Historical, Palaeopathological and Clinical Approaches*, ed. C. A. Roberts, M. E. Lewis and K. Manchester, British Archaeological Reports, International Series 1054 (Oxford, 2002), pp. 69–72.

Margeson, S., *Norwich Households: The Medieval and Post-Medieval Finds from Norwich Survey Excavations, 1971–1978*, East Anglian Archaeology 58 (Norwich, 1993).

Marr, A. ed., *The Worlds of Oronce Fine: Mathematics, Instruments and Print in Renaissance France* (Donington, 2009).

Maslen, R. W., 'The Healing Dialogues of Doctor Bullein', *The Yearbook of English Studies* 38 (2008), 119–35.

Matheson L. M., and A. Shannon, 'A Treatise on the Election of Times', in *Popular and Practical Science of Medieval England*, ed. L. M. Matheson (East Lansing, 1994), pp. 23–59.

McClendon, M. C., 'Against God's Word: Government, Religion and the Crisis of Authority in Early Reformation Norwich', *Sixteenth Century Journal* 25 (1994), 353–69.

McClendon, M. C., *The Quiet Reformation: Magistrates and the Emergence of Protestantism in Tudor Norwich* (Stanford, 1999).

McLean, A., *The Cosmographia of Sebastian Münster: Describing the World in the Reformation* (Aldershot, 2007).
McRee, B. R., 'Religious Gilds and Civic Order: The Case of Norwich in the Late Middle Ages', *Speculum* 67 (1992), 69–97.
McRee, B., 'Peacemaking and its Limits in Late Medieval Norwich', *English Historical Review* 109 (1994), 831–66.
McVaugh, M. R., *Medicine Before the Plague: Practitioners and their Patients in the Crown of Aragon 1285–1345* (Cambridge, 1993).
Metzler, I., *Disability in Medieval Europe: Thinking About Physical Impairment During the High Middle Ages, c. 1100–1400* (London, 2006).
Meyer, H., *Die Enzyklopädie des Bartholomäus Anglicus: Untersuchungen zur Überlieferungs- und Rezeptionsgeschichte von 'De Proprietatibus Rerum'* (Munich, 2000).
Mikkeli, H., *Hygiene in the Early Modern Medical Tradition* (Helsinki, 1999).
Mitchell, P. D., 'Integrating Historical Sources with Paleopathology', in *A Companion to Paleopathology*, ed. A. L. Grauer (Chichester, 2012), pp. 310–23.
Moens, W. J. C., *The Walloons and their Church at Norwich*, 2 vols. (London, 1887).
Montford, A., *Health, Sickness, Medicine and the Friars in the Thirteenth and Fourteenth Centuries* (Aldershot, 2004).
Mooney, L. R., 'Diet and Bloodletting: A Monthly Regimen', *Popular and Practical Science of Medieval England*, ed. L. M. Matheson (East Lansing, 1994), pp. 245–61.
Mosley, A., 'Early Modern Cosmography: Fine's *Sphaera mundi* in Content and Context', in *The Worlds of Oronce Fine: Mathematics, Instruments and Print in Renaissance France*, ed. A. Marr (Donington, 2009), pp. 114–36.
Murray Jones, P., 'Information and Science', in *Fifteenth-Century Attitudes: Perceptions of Society in Late Medieval England*, ed. R. Horrox (Cambridge, 1994), pp. 97–111.
Murray Jones, P., 'Reading Medicine in Tudor Cambridge', in *The History of Medical Education in Britain*, ed. V. Nutton and R. Porter (Amsterdam GA, 1995), pp. 153–81.
Murray Jones, P., 'Book Ownership and the Lay Culture of Medicine in Tudor Cambridge', in *The Task of Healing: Medicine, Religion and Gender in England and the Netherlands, 1450–1800*, ed. H. Marland and M. Pelling (Rotterdam, 1996), pp. 49–68.
Murray Jones, P., 'Medical Literacies and Medical Culture in Early Modern England', in *Medical Writing in Early Modern English*, ed. I. Taavitsainen and P. Pahta (Cambridge, 2011), pp. 30–43.
Newton, H., *The Sick Child in Early Modern England, 1580–1720* (Oxford, 2012).
Novak, S. A., 'Battle-Related Trauma', in *Blood Red Roses: The Archaeology of a Mass Grave from the Battle of Towton, AD 1461*, ed. V. Fiorato, A. Boylston and C. Knüsel (Oxford, 2000), pp. 90–102.

Novak, S. A., 'Beneath the Façade: A Skeletal Model of Domestic Violence', in *Social Archaeology of Funerary Remains*, ed. R. Gowland and C. Knüsel (Oxford, 2006), pp. 238–52.

Nutton, V., *John Caius and the Manuscripts of Galen* (Cambridge, 1987).

Nutton, V., 'Medical Thoughts on Urban Pollution', in *Death and Disease in the Ancient City*, ed. V. M. Hope and E. Marshall (London, 2000), pp. 65–73.

Nutton, V. , *Ancient Medicine*, 2nd edn (Abingdon, 2013).

O'Boyle, C., *The Art of Medicine: Medical Teaching at the University of Paris, 1250–1400* (Leiden, 1998).

Obrist, B., 'Wind Diagrams and Medieval Cosmology', *Speculum* 72 (1997), 33–84.

Palliser, D. M., 'Civic Mentality and the Environment in Tudor York', *Northern History* 18 (1982), 78–115.

Parker, V., *The Making of King's Lynn: Secular Buildings from the 11th to the 17th Century*, King's Lynn Archaeological Survey 1 (London, 1971).

Pelling, M., 'Appearance and Reality: Barber-Surgeons, the Body and Disease', in *London 1500–1700: The Making of the Metropolis*, ed. A. L. Beier and R. Finlay (London, 1986), pp. 82–112.

Pelling, M., *The Common Lot: Sickness, Medical Occupations and the Urban Poor in Early Modern England* (London, 1998).

Pelling, M., *Medical Conflicts in Early Modern London: Patronage, Physicians and Irregular Practitioners, 1550–1640* (Oxford, 2003).

Pelling, M., 'Health and Sanitation to 1750', in *Norwich Since 1550*, ed. C. Rawcliffe and R. Wilson (London, 2004), pp. 117–37.

Pelling, M., and C. Webster, 'Medical Practitioners', in *Health, Medicine and Mortality in the Sixteenth Century*, ed. C. Webster (Cambridge, 1979), pp. 165–235.

Peyroux, C., 'The Leper's Kiss', in *Monks and Nuns, Saints and Outcasts: Religion in Medieval Society: Essays in Honor of Lester K. Little*, ed. S. Farmer and B. H. Rosenwein (Ithaca, 2000), pp. 172–88.

Pickett, J. P., 'A Translation of the "Canutus" Plague Treatise', in *Popular and Practical Science of Medieval England*, ed. L. M. Matheson (East Lansing, 1994), pp. 263–82.

Pomata, G. and N. G. Siraisi, 'Introduction', in *Historia: Empiricism and Erudition in Early Modern Europe*, ed. G. Pomata and N. G. Siraisi (Cambridge MA, 2005), pp. 1–38.

Pound, J. F., 'The Social and Trade Structure of Norwich 1525–1575', *Past and Present* 34 (1966), 49–69.

Pound, J., *Tudor and Stuart Norwich* (Chichester, 1988).

Pound, J., 'Government to 1660', in *Norwich Since 1550*, ed. C. Rawcliffe and R. Wilson (London, 2004), pp. 35–61.

Prest, J., *The Garden of Eden: The Botanic Garden and the Re-creation of Paradise* (Yale, 1981).

Pugh, R. B., 'The Knights Hospitallers of England as Undertakers', *Speculum* 56 (1981), 566–74.

Rappaport, S., *Worlds Within Worlds: Structures of Life in Sixteenth-Century London* (Cambridge, 1989).

Rawcliffe, C., *Medicine and Society in Later Medieval England* (Stroud, 1995).

Rawcliffe, C., *The Hospitals of Medieval Norwich*, Studies in East Anglian History 2 (Norwich, 1995).

Rawcliffe, C., 'Hospital Nurses and their Work', in *Daily Life in the Late Middle Ages*, ed. R. Britnell (Stroud, 1998), pp. 42–64.

Rawcliffe, C., *Medicine for the Soul: The Life, Death and Resurrection of an English Medieval Hospital: St. Giles's, Norwich, c. 1249–1550* (Stroud, 1999).

Rawcliffe, C., 'On the Threshold of Eternity: Care for the Sick in East Anglian Monasteries', in *East Anglia's History: Essays in Honour of Norman Scarfe*, ed. C. Harper-Bill, C. Rawcliffe and R. G. Wilson (Woodbridge, 2000), pp. 41–72.

Rawcliffe, C., 'Curing Bodies and Healing Souls: Pilgrimage and the Sick in Medieval East Anglia', in *Pilgrimage: The English Experience from Becket to Bunyan*, ed. C. Morris and P. Roberts (Cambridge, 2002), pp. 108–40.

Rawcliffe, C., 'The Eighth Comfortable Work: Education and the Medieval English Hospital', in *The Church and Learning in Later Medieval Society: Essays Presented in Honour of R. B. Dobson*, ed. C. M. Barron and R. Stratford, Harlaxton Medieval Studies 11 (Donington, 2002), pp. 371–98.

Rawcliffe, C., 'The Seventh Comfortable Work: Charity and Mortality in the Medieval Hospital', *Medicina e Storia* 3 (2003), 11–35.

Rawcliffe, C., 'Introduction', in *Medieval Norwich*, ed. C. Rawcliffe and R. Wilson (London, 2004), pp. xix-xxxvii.

Rawcliffe, C., 'Sickness and Health', in *Medieval Norwich*, ed. C. Rawcliffe and R. Wilson (London, 2004), pp. 301–26.

Rawcliffe, C., 'Health and Safety at Work in Late Medieval East Anglia', in *Medieval East Anglia*, ed. C. Harper-Bill (Woodbridge, 2005), pp. 130–51.

Rawcliffe, C., *Leprosy in Medieval England* (Woodbridge, 2006).

Rawcliffe, C., ed., 'The Cartulary of St Mary's Hospital, Great Yarmouth', in *Poverty and Wealth: Sheep, Taxation and Charity in Late Medieval Norfolk*, ed. M. Bailey, M. Jurkowski and C. Rawcliffe, Norfolk Record Society 71 (Norwich, 2007), pp. 157–230.

Rawcliffe, C., 'Delectable Sightes and Fragrant Smelles: Gardens and Health in Late Medieval and Early Modern England', *Garden History* 36 (2008), 3–21.

Rawcliffe, C., *Urban Bodies: Communal Health in Late Medieval English Towns and Cities*, (Woodbridge, 2013).

Rawcliffe, C., and R. Wilson, ed., *Medieval Norwich* (London, 2004).

Rawcliffe, C., and R. Wilson, ed., *Norwich Since 1550* (London, 2004).

Rees Jones, S., 'York's Civic Administration, 1354–1464', in *The Government of*

Medieval York: Essays in Commemoration of the 1396 Royal Charter, ed. S. Rees Jones, Borthwick Studies in History 3 (York, 1997), pp. 108–40.

Rees Jones, S., 'Household, Work and the Problem of Mobile Labour: The Regulation of Labour in Medieval English Towns', in *The Problem of Labour in Fourteenth-Century England*, ed. J. Bothwell, P. J. P. Goldberg and W. M. Ormrod (York, 2000), pp. 133–53.

Rees Jones, S., 'The Household and English Urban Government in the Later Middle Ages', in *The Household in Late Medieval Cities: Italy and North-Western Europe Compared*, ed. M. Carlier and T. Soens (Leuven, 2001), pp. 71–88.

Rees Jones, S., 'Thomas More's *Utopia* and Medieval London', in *Pragmatic Utopias: Ideals and Communities, 1200–1630*, ed. R. Horrox and S. Rees Jones (Cambridge 2001), pp. 117–35.

Resnick, D., *Diagnosis of Bone and Joint Disorders*, 3 vols. (Philadelphia, 1981).

Rexroth, F., *Deviance and Power in Late Medieval London*, trans. P. E. Selwyn (Cambridge, 2007).

Rigby, S. H., 'Urban "Oligarchy" in Late Medieval England', in *Towns and Townspeople in the Fifteenth Century*, ed. J. A. F. Thomson (Gloucester, 1988), pp. 62–86.

Roberts, C., 'The Bioarchaeology of Leprosy and Tuberculosis: A Comparative Study of Perceptions, Stigma, Diagnosis and Treatment', in *Social Bioarchaeology*, ed. S. C. Agarwal and B. A. Glencross (Oxford, 2011), pp. 252–81.

Roberts, C., and M. Cox, *Health and Disease in Britain From Prehistory to the Present Day* (Stroud, 2003).

Rutledge, E., 'Immigration and Population Growth in Early Fourteenth-Century Norwich: Evidence from the Tithing Roll', *Urban History Yearbook* 15 (1988), 15–30.

Rutledge, E., 'Landlords and Tenants: Housing and the Rented Property Market in Early Fourteenth-Century Norwich', *Urban History* 22 (1995), 7–24.

Rutledge, E., 'Introduction', in *Norwich Landgable Assessment 1568–70*, ed. M. Rodgers, and M. Wallace, Norfolk Record Society 63 (Norwich, 1999).

Rutledge, E., 'Economic Life', in *Medieval Norwich*, ed. C. Rawcliffe and R. Wilson (London, 2004), pp. 157–88.

Rutledge, E., 'Documentary Evidence', in *Norwich Greyfriars: Pre-Conquest Town and Medieval Friary*, ed. P. A. Emery, East Anglian Archaeology 120 (Dereham, 2007), pp. 86–92.

Rutledge, E., 'An Urban Environment: Norwich in the Fifteenth Century', in *The Fifteenth Century XII: Society in an Age of Plague*, ed. L. Clark and C. Rawcliffe (Woodbridge, 2013), pp. 79–93.

Ryrie, A., *The Sorcerer's Tale: Faith and Fraud in Tudor England* (Oxford, 2008).

Sabine, E. L., 'City Cleaning in Medieval London', *Speculum* 12 (1937), 19–43.

Sandred, K. I. and B. Lindstrøm, *The Place-Names of Norfolk Part I: The Place-Names of the City of Norwich* (Nottingham, 1989).

Schechner, S. J., *Comets, Popular Culture and the Birth of Modern Cosmology* (Princeton, 1997).
Schweich, M., and C. Knüsel, 'Bio-cultural Effects in Medieval Populations', *Economics and Human Biology* 1 (2003), 367–77.
Seymour, M. C., 'Some Medieval English Owners of *De proprietatibus rerum*', *Bodleian Library Record* 9 (1974), 156–65.
Shepherd Popescu, E., *Norwich Castle: Excavations and Historical Survey 1987–98*, East Anglian Archaeology 132, 2 vols. (Dereham, 2009).
Siraisi, N. G., *The Clock and the Mirror: Girolamo Cardano and Renaissance Medicine* (Princeton, 1997).
Siraisi, N. G., *History, Medicine and the Traditions of Renaissance Learning* (Ann Arbor, 2007).
Slack, P., 'Mirrors of Health and Treasures of Poor Men: The Uses of the Vernacular Medical Literature of Tudor England', in *Health, Medicine and Mortality in the Sixteenth Century*, ed. C. Webster (Cambridge, 1979), pp. 237–73.
Slack, P., *The Impact of Plague in Tudor and Stuart England* (Oxford, 1985).
Slack, P., 'Dearth and Social Policy in Early Modern England', *Social History of Medicine* 5 (1992), 1–17.
Slack, P., *From Reformation to Improvement: Public Welfare in Early Modern England* (Oxford, 1998).
Sloane, B., *The Black Death in London* (Stroud, 2011).
Smith, H., 'Concept and Compromise: Sir Nicholas Bacon and the Building of Stiffkey Hall', in *East Anglia's History: Studies in Honour of Norman Scarfe*, ed. C. Harper-Bill, C. Rawcliffe and R. Wilson (Woodbridge, 2002), pp. 159–88.
Soden, I., *Life and Death on a Norwich Backstreet, AD 900–1600: Excavations in St Faith's Lane*, East Anglian Archaeology 133 (Northampton, 2010).
Sofaer, J. R., *The Body as Material Culture: A Theoretical Osteoarchaeology* (Cambridge, 2006).
Stirland, A., 'Evidence for Pre-Columbian Treponematosis in Medieval Europe', in *L'Origine de la syphilis en Europe: avant ou après 1493?*, ed. O. Dutour, G. Pálfi, J. Bérato and J-P Brun (Paris, 1994), pp. 109–15, 300.
Stirland, A., 'Patterns of Trauma in a Unique Medieval Parish Cemetery', *International Journal of Osteoarchaeology* 6 (1996), 92–100.
Stirland, A., 'Care in the Medieval Community', in *International Journal of Osteoarchaeology* 7 (1997), 587–90.
Stirland, A., with contributions by B. Ayers and J. Bown, *Criminals and Paupers: The Graveyard of St Margaret Fyebriggate in combusto, Norwich*, East Anglian Archaeology 129 (Dereham, 2009).
Stroud, G., 'Human Bone', in R. Price with M. Ponsford, *St Bartholomew's Hospital, Bristol: The Excavation of a Medieval Hospital, 1976–8*, Council for British Archaeology Research Report 110 (York, 1998), pp. 175–81.
Sullivan, A., 'Reconstructing Relationships Among Mortality, Status and

Gender at the Medieval Gilbertine Priory of St Andrew, Fishergate, York', *American Journal of Physical Anthropology* 124 (2004), 330–45.

Taavitsainen, I., 'A Zodiacal Lunary for Medical Professionals', in *Popular and Practical Science of Medieval England*, ed. L. M. Matheson (East Lansing, 1994), pp. 283–300.

Tanner, N. P., *The Church in Late Medieval Norwich, 1370–1532*, Studies and Texts 66 (Toronto, 1984).

Tanner, N., 'The Cathedral and the City', in *Norwich Cathedral: Church, City, Diocese, 1096–1996*, ed. I. Atherton, E. Fernie, C. Harper-Bill, and H. Smith (London, 1996), pp. 255–80.

Tanner, N., 'Religious Practice', in *Medieval Norwich*, ed. C. Rawcliffe and R. Wilson (London, 2004), pp. 137–55.

Taub, L., *Ancient Meteorology* (London, 2003).

Tavormina, M. T., 'The Twenty-Jordan Series: An Illustrated Middle English Uroscopy Text', *ANQ: A Quarterly Journal of Short Articles, Notes and Reviews* 18 (2005), 43–67.

Taylor, E. G. R., *Tudor Geography, 1485–1583* (London, 1930).

Taylor, E. G. R., 'The South-Pointing Needle', *Imago Mundi* 8 (1951), 1–7.

Taylor, E. G. R., *The Mathematical Practitioners of Tudor and Stuart England* (Cambridge, 1967).

Thøfner, M., 'Catholics, Protestants and Strangers', in *The Art of Faith: 3,500 Years of Art and Belief in Norfolk*, ed. A. Moore and M. Thøfner (London, 2010), pp. 34–43.

Thomas, K., *Religion and the Decline of Magic: Studies in Popular Beliefs in Sixteenth- and Seventeenth-Century England* (London, 1991).

Thrupp, S. L., *The Merchant Class of Medieval London, 1300–1500* (Chicago, 1948).

Tillyard, M. with E. Shepherd Popescu and N. Ives, *Norwich Castle: Excavation and Historical Survey Part IV: People and Property in the Documentary Record*, East Anglian Archaeology 23 (Dereham, 2009) [CD ROM].

Tittler, R., *Nicholas Bacon: The Making of a Tudor Statesman* (Ohio, 1976).

Tittler, R., 'For the "Re-edification of Townes": The Rebuilding Statutes of Henry VIII', *Albion* 22 (1990), 591–605.

Tittler, R., *Architecture and Power: The Town Hall and the English Urban Community c. 1500–1640* (Oxford, 1991).

Tittler, R., 'Reformation, Resources and Authority in English Towns: An Overview', in *The Reformation in English Towns 1500–1640*, ed. P. Collinson and J. Craig (Basingstoke, 1998), pp. 190–201.

Tittler, R., *The Reformation and the Towns in England: Politics and Political Culture, c. 1540–1640* (Oxford, 1998).

Tittler, R., 'Henry Manship: Constructing the Civic Memory in Great Yarmouth', in *Townspeople and Nation: English Urban Experiences 1540–1646*, ed. R. Tittler (Stanford, 2001), pp. 121–39.

Tyacke, S., 'Introduction', in *English Map-Making 1500–1650*, ed. S. Tyacke (London, 1983), pp. 13–18.

Updike, D. B., *Printing Types: Their History, Forms and Use*, 2 vols. (Cambridge, 1922).

Valkema Blouw, P., *Dutch Typography in the Sixteenth Century: The Collected Works of Paul Valkema Blouw*, ed. T. Croiset van Uchelen and P. Dijstelberge (Leiden, 2013).

Venn, J., 'Memoir of John Caius', in *The Works of John Caius, M.D*, ed. E. S. Roberts (Cambridge, 1912), pp. 1–78.

Vogel, K. A., 'Cosmography', in *The Cambridge History of Science*, ed. K. Park and L. Daston, 7 vols. (Cambridge, 2003–), III, 469–96.

Voigts, L. E., 'Multitudes of Middle English Medical Manuscripts, or the Englishing of Science and Medicine', in *Manuscript Sources of Medieval Medicine*, ed. M. R. Schleissner (New York, 1995), pp. 183–95.

Waldron, T., *Palaeopathology* (Cambridge, 2009).

Waters, D. W., *The Art of Navigation in England in Elizabethan and Early Stuart Times* (London, 1958).

Wear, A., *Knowledge and Practice in English Medicine, 1550–1680* (Cambridge, 2000).

Wear, A., 'Place, Health, and Disease: The *Airs, Waters, Places* Tradition in Early Modern England and North America', *Journal of Medieval and Early Modern Studies* 38 (2008), 443–65.

Webster, C., 'Thomas Linacre and the Foundation of the College of Physicians', in *Essays on the Life and Work of Thomas Linacre, c. 1460–1524*, ed. F. Maddison, M. Pelling and C. Webster (Oxford, 1977), pp. 198–222.

Wheeler, J., 'Stench in Sixteenth-Century Venice', in *The City and the Senses: Urban Culture Since 1500*, ed. A. Cowan and J. Steward (Aldershot, 2007), pp. 26–38.

Whyte, N., 'The Deviant Dead in the Norfolk Landscape', *Landscapes* 1 (2003), 24–39.

Wieck, R. S., 'The Death Desired: Books of Hours and the Medieval Funeral', in *Death and Dying in the Middle Ages*, ed. E. E. DuBruck and B. J. Gusick (New York, 1999), pp. 431–76.

Wilson, R., 'The Textile Industry', in *Norwich Since 1550*, ed. C. Rawcliffe and R. Wilson (London, 2004), pp. 219–41.

Wood, A., 'Kett's Rebellion', in *Medieval Norwich*, ed. C. Rawcliffe and R. Wilson (London, 2004), pp. 277–99.

Wood, A., *The 1549 Rebellions and the Making of Early Modern England* (Cambridge, 2007).

Wood, J. W., G. R. Milner, H. C. Harpending and K. M. Weiss, 'The Osteological Paradox: Problems of Inferring Prehistoric Health from Skeletal Samples', *Current Anthropology* 33 (1992), 343–70.

Woodward, D., *Men at Work: Labourers and Building Craftsmen in the Towns of Northern England, 1450–1750* (Cambridge, 1995).

Unpublished reports and theses

Bown, J., and A. Stirland, 'Criminals and Paupers: Excavations at the Site of the Church and Graveyard of St Margaret *in combusto*, Norwich, 1987' (unpublished site excavation report, Norfolk Archaeological Unit, Norfolk Museums Service).

Caffell A., and M. Holst, 'Osteological Analysis, Whitefriars, Norwich' (unpublished archaeological report 0806, York Osteoarchaeology Ltd, 2007).

Dunn, P., 'After the Black Death: Society and Economy in late Fourteenth-Century Norwich' (unpublished PhD thesis, University of East Anglia, 2003).

Emery, G., 'A Medieval Mass Grave on the Site of the Chapelfield Shopping Centre, Norwich'. (unpublished archaeological report 1562, NAU Archaeology, 2010).

Fay, I., 'Health and Disease in Medieval and Tudor Norwich' (unpublished PhD thesis, University of East Anglia, 2007).

Jenner, M., 'Early Modern English Conceptions of "Cleanliness" and "Dirt" as Reflected in the Environmental Regulations of London, *c.* 1530–1700' (unpublished DPhil thesis, University of Oxford, 1991).

King, C., 'House and Society in an English Provincial City: The Archaeology of Urban Households in Norwich, 1300–1700' (unpublished PhD thesis, University of Reading, 2006).

Mays, S., 'Part II: Appendix for the Medieval Burials from the Blackfriars Friary, School Street, Ipswich, Suffolk (Excavated 1983–85)' (unpublished Ancient Monuments Laboratory Report 16/91, English Heritage, 1991).

Needham, C. D., 'Drawing on the Past: Reconstructing the Visual Manifestations of Disease and Trauma from Archaeological Human Remains' (unpublished MPhil thesis, University of Manchester, 2002).

Noble, C., 'Aspects of Life at Norwich Cathedral Priory in the Late Medieval Period' (unpublished PhD thesis, University of East Anglia, 2001).

Phillips, E. M., 'Charitable Institutions in Norfolk and Suffolk, *c.* 1350–1600' (unpublished PhD thesis, University of East Anglia, 2001).

INDEX

Page numbers in **bold type** refer to illustrations and their captions.

YORK MEDIEVAL PRESS: PUBLICATIONS

God's Words, Women's Voices: The Discernment of Spirits in the Writing of Late-Medieval Women Visionaries, Rosalynn Voaden (1999)

Pilgrimage Explored, ed. J. Stopford (1999)

Piety, Fraternity and Power: Religious Gilds in Late Medieval Yorkshire 1389–1547, † David J. F. Crouch (2000)

Courts and Regions in Medieval Europe, ed. Sarah Rees Jones, Richard Marks and A. J. Minnis (2000)

Treasure in the Medieval West, ed. Elizabeth M. Tyler (2000)

Nunneries, Learning and Spirituality in Late Medieval English Society: The Dominican Priory of Dartford, Paul Lee (2000)

Prophecy and Public Affairs in Later Medieval England, Lesley A. Coote (2000)

The Problem of Labour in Fourteenth-Century England, ed. James Bothwell, P. J. P. Goldberg and W. M. Ormrod (2000)

New Directions in Later Medieval Manuscript Studies: Essays from the 1998 Harvard Conference, ed. Derek Pearsall (2000)

Cistercians, Heresy and Crusade in Occitania, 1145–1229: Preaching in the Lord's Vineyard, Beverly Mayne Kienzle (2001)

Guilds and the Parish Community in Late Medieval East Anglia, c. 1470–1550, Ken Farnhill (2001)

The Age of Edward III, ed. J. S. Bothwell (2001)

Time in the Medieval World, ed. Chris Humphrey and W. M. Ormrod (2001)

The Cross Goes North: Processes of Conversion in Northern Europe, AD 300–1300, ed. Martin Carver (2002)

Henry IV: The Establishment of the Regime, 1399–1406, ed. Gwilym Dodd and Douglas Biggs (2003)

Youth in the Middle Ages, ed. P. J. P Goldberg and Felicity Riddy (2004)

The Idea of the Castle in Medieval England, Abigail Wheatley (2004)

Rites of Passage: Cultures of Transition in the Fourteenth Century, ed. Nicola F. McDonald and W. M. Ormrod (2004)

Creating the Monastic Past in Medieval Flanders, Karine Ugé (2005)

St William of York, Christopher Norton (2006)

Medieval Obscenities, ed. Nicola F. McDonald (2006)

The Reign of Edward II: New Perspectives, ed. Gwilym Dodd and Anthony Musson (2006)

Old English Poetics: The Aesthetics of the Familiar in Anglo-Saxon England, Elizabeth M. Tyler (2006)

The Late Medieval Interlude: The Drama of Youth and Aristocratic Masculinity, Fiona S. Dunlop (2007)

The Late Medieval English College and its Context, ed. Clive Burgess and Martin Heale (2008)

The Reign of Henry IV: Rebellion and Survival, 1403–1413, ed. Gwilym Dodd and Douglas Biggs (2008)

Medieval Petitions: Grace and Grievance, ed. W. Mark Ormrod, Gwilym Dodd and Anthony Musson (2009)

St Edmund, King and Martyr: Changing Images of a Medieval Saint, ed. Anthony Bale (2009)

Language and Culture in Medieval Britain: The French of England c.1100–c.1500, ed. Jocelyn Wogan-Browne et al. (2009)

The Royal Pardon: Access to Mercy in Fourteenth-Century England, Helen Lacey (2009)

Texts and Traditions of Medieval Pastoral Care: Essays in Honour of Bella Millett, ed. Cate Gunn and Catherine Innes-Parker (2009)

The Anglo-Norman Language and its Contexts, ed. Richard Ingham (2010)

Parliament and Political Pamphleteering in Fourteenth-Century England, Clementine Oliver (2010)

The Saints' Lives of Jocelin of Furness: Hagiography, Patronage and Ecclesiastical Politics, Helen Birkett (2010)

The York Mystery Plays: Performance in the City, ed. Margaret Rogerson (2011)

Wills and Will-Making in Anglo-Saxon England, Linda Tollerton (2011)

The Songs and Travels of a Tudor Minstrel: Richard Sheale of Tamworth, Andrew Taylor (2012)

Sin in Medieval and Early Modern Culture: The Tradition of the Seven Deadly Sins, ed. Richard G. Newhauser and Susan J. Ridyard (2012)

Socialising the Child in Late Medieval England, c. 1400–1600, Merridee L. Bailey (2012)

Barking Abbey and Medieval Literary Culture: Authorship and Authority in a Female Community, ed. Jennifer N. Brown and Donna Alfano Bussell (2012)

Christians and Jews in Angevin England: The York Massacre of 1190, Narratives and Contexts, ed. Sarah Rees Jones and Sethina Watson (2013)

Reimagining History in Anglo-Norman Prose Chronicles, John Spence (2013)

Henry V: New Interpretations, ed. Gwilym Dodd (2013)

Rethinking Chaucer's Legend of Good Women, Carolyn P. Collette (2014)

The Prelate in England and Europe, 1300–1560, ed. Martin Heale (2014)

The Revolt of Owain Glyndŵr in Medieval English Chronicles, Alicia Marchant (2014)

York Studies in Medieval Theology

I *Medieval Theology and the Natural Body*, ed. Peter Biller and A. J. Minnis (1997)

II *Handling Sin: Confession in the Middle Ages*, ed. Peter Biller and A. J. Minnis (1998)

III *Religion and Medicine in the Middle Ages*, ed. Peter Biller and Joseph Ziegler (2001)

IV *Texts and the Repression of Medieval Heresy*, ed. Caterina Bruschi and Peter Biller (2002)

York Manuscripts Conference

Manuscripts and Readers in Fifteenth-Century England: The Literary Implications of Manuscript Study, ed. Derek Pearsall (1983) [Proceedings of the 1981 York Manuscripts Conference]

Manuscripts and Texts: Editorial Problems in Later Middle English Literature, ed. Derek Pearsall (1987) [Proceedings of the 1985 York Manuscripts Conference]

Latin and Vernacular: Studies in Late-Medieval Texts and Manuscripts, ed. A. J. Minnis (1989) [Proceedings of the 1987 York Manuscripts Conference]

Regionalism in Late-Medieval Manuscripts and Texts: Essays celebrating the publication of 'A Linguistic Atlas of Late Mediaeval English', ed. Felicity Riddy (1991) [Proceedings of the 1989 York Manuscripts Conference]

Late-Medieval Religious Texts and their Transmission: Essays in Honour of A. I. Doyle, ed. A. J. Minnis (1994) [Proceedings of the 1991 York Manuscripts Conference]

Prestige, Authority and Power in Late Medieval Manuscripts and Texts, ed. Felicity Riddy (2000) [Proceedings of the 1994 York Manuscripts Conference]

Middle English Poetry: Texts and Traditions. Essays in Honour of Derek Pearsall, ed. A. J. Minnis (2001) [Proceedings of the 1996 York Manuscripts Conference]

Manuscript Culture in the British Isles

I *Design and Distribution of Late Medieval Manuscripts in England*, ed. Margaret Connolly and Linne R. Mooney (2008)

II *Women and Writing, c.1340–c.1650: The Domestication of Print Culture*, ed. Anne Lawrence-Mathers and Phillipa Hardman (2010)

III *The Wollaton Medieval Manuscripts: Texts, Owners and Readers*, ed. Ralph Hanna and Thorlac Turville-Petre (2010)

IV *Scribes and the City: London Guildhall Clerks and the Dissemination of Middle English Literature, 1375–1425*, Linne R. Mooney and Estelle Stubbs (2013)

V *Robert Thornton and his Books: Essays on the Lincoln and London Thornton Manuscripts*, ed. Susanna Fein and Michael Johnston (2014)

VI *Middle English Texts in Transition: A Festschrift dedicated to Toshiyuki Takamiya on his 70th birthday*, ed. Simon Horobin and Linne R. Mooney (2014)

Heresy and Inquisition in the Middle Ages

Heresy and Heretics in the Thirteenth Century: The Textual Representations, L. J. Sackville (2011)

Heresy, Crusade and Inquisition in Medieval Quercy, Claire Taylor (2011)

Heresy, Inquisition and Life-Cycle in Medieval Languedoc, Chris Sparks (2014)